Comprehensive Review of Headache Medicine

The Headache Cooperative of New England

Comprehensive Review of Headache Medicine

Edited by

MORRIS LEVIN, MD

Authors

Steven M. Baskin, PhD
Marcelo E. Bigal, MD, PhD
Richard B. Lipton, MD, FAAN
Herbert G. Markley, MD, FAAN, FAHS
Brian E. McGeeney, MD, MPH
Lawrence C. Newman, MD
Alan M. Rapoport, MD
Mark J. Rapoport, MD
Robert E. Shapiro, MD, PhD
Fred D. Sheftell, MD
Stewart J. Tepper,MD
Thomas N. Ward, MD
Randall E. Weeks, PhD

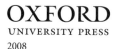
UNIVERSITY PRESS
2008

OXFORD

UNIVERSITY PRESS

Oxford University Press, Inc., publishes works that further
Oxford University's objective of excellence
in research, scholarship, and education.

Oxford   New York
Auckland   Cape Town   Dar es Salaam   Hong Kong   Karachi
Kuala Lumpur   Madrid   Melbourne   Mexico City   Nairobi
New Delhi   Shanghai   Taipei   Toronto

With offices in
Argentina   Austria   Brazil   Chile   Czech Republic   France   Greece
Guatemala   Hungary   Italy   Japan   Poland   Portugal   Singapore
South Korea   Switzerland   Thailand   Turkey   Ukraine   Vietnam

Copyright © 2008 by Oxford University Press, Inc.

Published by Oxford University Press, Inc.
198 Madison Avenue, New York, New York 10016
www.oup.com

Oxford is a registered trademark of Oxford University Press

Library of Congress Cataloging-in-Publication Data
Comprehensive review of headache medicine / edited by Morris Levin.
p.; cm.
Includes bibliographical references and index.
ISBN 978-0-19-536673-0
1. Headache—Examinations, questions, etc. I. Levin, Morris, 1955-
[DNLM: 1. Headache Disorders—diagnosis—Problems and Exercises. 2. Headache Disorders—therapy—
Problems and Exercises. WL 18.2 C737 2008]
RB128.C67 2008
616.8'4910076—dc22
                          2007036891

9 8 7 6 5 4 3 2 1

Printed in the United States of America
on acid-free paper

To my wife, Karen, for her support and love, and to my patients, students, and colleagues in the field of headache medicine

Preface

Headache medicine has lately become a focus of interest for many neurologists, pain medicine physicians, physiatrists, psychiatrists, primary care physicians and other practitioners. For those of us who have been in the field for many years this is not surprising. HM is not only intellectually challenging, with a varied and intriguing population of patients, but is also extremely gratifying most of the time. Clinical practice or research oriented around headache disorders is rewarding on many levels, and this is of course evidenced by the increase in training programs and trainees in HM.

The recent decision by the United Council for Neurologic Subspecialties (UCNS) to accredit HM fellowship programs and to offer certification in HM is a crucial step in the process of validating HM as a serious subspecialty. The American Headache Society (AHS) has taken a number of steps to make HM academic resources available to residents and fellows, as well as interested clinicians in practice. The American Academy of Neurology and American Pain Society emphasize teaching of headache medicine in their conferences. A number of other headache related conferences and symposia are available around the world, and headache research is growing dramatically.

There are several noted texts in the field of HM, including those by Silberstein *et al*, Olesen *et al* and Lance and Goadsby. There are also several patient and family oriented books about headache and its treatment. However, there is no one concise synopsis of HM at the time of writing, hence the impetus for this work.

The Headache Cooperative of New England first conceived this project as a key resource for those planning on sitting for the HM certification examination. Soon however other purposes seemed appropriate. There seemed to be a need for a concise but authoritative resource for clinicians who practice headache medicine. In addition, with the increasing interest in HM, it seemed important that there be a readable comprehensive text which could serve as an introduction to the field.

This book is divided into sections similar to those outlined by the UCNS in their excellent curriculum for HM training and follows the summary of topics covered in the UCNS HM examinations. Part I deals with the anatomy, physiology, pathophysiology and epidemiology of the headache disorders. Part II covers classification and diagnosis in the primary headaches. Part III discusses diagnosis of non-primary headache. Part IV deals with treatment of primary headache types, and Part V includes chapters concerning treatment of special populations and treatments that are advanced or specialized.

This ordering of topics was not chosen only for its appropriateness in preparing headache specialists for the certification examination. I and my fellow authors decided that it also mirrored the decision-making processes we all go through in the practice of HM on a day-to-day basis. First, we think about diagnosis. Is it a primary headache (Part II)? If so, which category does it fall into? —migraine, tension type, trigeminal autonomic cephalalgia, indomethacin responsive headaches, etc. If primary headache diagnosis is not certain, what are the possibilities for secondary causes (Part III)? Once we have firmed up a diagnosis, treatment decision-making begins (Part IV). This will be based on diagnosis again but the twin treatment decisions in headache management — acute relief and prevention, are really different processes. When treatment fails or when it is particularly challenging, decision making follows some different paths (Part V).

We hope that this book fills a need for this type of information and presentation. We think that reading it in order will be very helpful and we hope enjoyable. But the authors and editors have strive to make each chapter independent and thus the reader can skip from one chapter or section to another. Please let us know if you have any comments or suggestions. Thanks for reading!

Morris Levin, MD
Dartmouth Medical School
Hanover, New Hampshire

Acknowledgments

This book is a true team effort. The Headache Cooperative of New England is a professional organization to which I have been privileged to belong for a number of years. It is composed of many of the foremost headache clinicians, researchers, teachers and writers in the United States and this book represents their vast experience in the field of headache medicine. In order to compose a coherent review of headache medicine, I coerced the authors to constrain themselves to specific topics, many of which overlapped. I also tended to impose my own vision for this project, and invariably my co-authors were kind enough to go along. They will always have my gratitude for their generosity.

We have all been the recipients of mentoring by our teachers, many of whom were true pioneers in the field. I would like to extend our esteem and thanks to our role models in the field. And speaking of teaching, our best teachers have actually been our patients. We benefit daily from their partnership in the quest to understand and manage their headaches and are most appreciative of their perseverance.

Finally, I would like to warmly thank our editor at Oxford University Press, Craig Panner. First, for taking on this project and, more importantly, for maintaining his unfailing patience and support throughout the process of producing this book.

Morris Levin, MD
Hanover, New Hampshire

Contents

Part I Headache Medicine Basic Science: Anatomy, Physiology, and Epidemiology

1. Head Pain Anatomy and Physiology – Morris Levin *3*
2. Pathophysiology and Genetics of Migraine and Cluster Headache – Robert E. Shapiro *21*
3. The Epidemiology and Burden of Headache – Marcelo E. Bigal, and Richard B. Lipton *39*

Part II Diagnosis of Primary Headache Disorders

4. The International Classification of Headache Disorders and Classification and Diagnosis of Migraine – Morris Levin *59*
5. Classification and Diagnosis of Chronic Daily Headache and Tension-Type Headache – Herbert G. Markley *73*
6. Classification and Diagnosis of Trigeminal Autonomic Cephalalgias and Other Primary Headaches – Lawrence C. Newman *91*

Part III Diagnosis of Secondary Headache Disorders

7. Classification and Diagnosis of Secondary Headaches: Traumatic and Vascular Causes – Alan M. Rapoport and Mark J. Rapoport *115*
8. Classification and Diagnosis of Secondary Headaches: Altered Intracranial Pressure, Neoplasm, and Infection – Brian E. McGeeney *149*
9. Classification and Diagnosis of Secondary Headaches: Substances, Metabolic Disorders, EENT Causes, and Neuralgias – Lawrence C. Newman *177*
10. Psychiatric Comorbidity and Causes of Headache – Steven M. Baskin *193*

Part IV Headache Treatment

11. Pharmacologic Treatment of Acute Migraine – Alan M. Rapoport *209*

12. Preventive Pharmacologic Treatment of Migraine and Tension-Type
     Headache – Stewart J. Tepper *231*
13. Pharmacologic Treatment of Trigeminal Autonomic
     Cephalalgias and Other Primary Headaches – Brian E.
     McGeeney *255*
14. Treatment of Chronic Daily Headache – Fred D. Sheftell *265*

Part V   Treatment of Intractable Headache and Special Populations

15. Headache Treatment in Children, Pregnancy and Lactation,
     the Elderly, and Renal Disease – Thomas N. Ward *277*
16. Inpatient Headache Treatment – Thomas N. Ward *285*
17. Non-Pharmacologic Headache Treatment – Randall E.
     Weeks *293*
18. Procedures for Headache – Thomas N. Ward *303*

Index *311*

Contributors

STEVEN M. BASKIN, PhD
Co-Director
New England Institute for Behavioral
    Medicine
Stamford, CT

MARCELO E. BIGAL, MD, PhD
Assistant Professor
Department of Neurology
Albert Einstein College of Medicine
Director of Research
The New England Center for Headache
Stamford, CT

MORRIS LEVIN, MD
Co-Director, Headache Clinic
Associate Professor of Neurology
Department of Neurology
Dartmouth-Hitchcock Medical Center
Lebanon, NH

RICHARD B. LIPTON, MD, FAAN
Professor of Neurology, Epidemiology
    and Social Medicine
The Saul R. Korey Department of Neurology
Albert Einstein College of Medicine
Bronx, NY

HERBERT G. MARKLEY, MD, FAAN
Director
New England Regional Headache Center
Worcester, MA

BRIAN E. MCGEENEY, MD, MPH
Assistant Professor of Neurology
Boston University School of Medicine
Department of Neurology
Boston University School of Medicine
Boston, MA

LAWRENCE C. NEWMAN, MD
Associate Clinical Professor of Neurology
Albert Einstein College of Medicine
Director, The Headache Institute
St. Luke's – Roosevelt Hospital Center
New York, NY

ALAN M. RAPOPORT, MD
Clinical Professor of Neurology
David Geffen School of Medicine at UCLA
Los Angeles, CA
Founder and Director-Emeritus
The New England Center for Headache, P.C.
Stamford, CT

MARK J. RAPOPORT, MD
Department of Radiology
Northwestern University
Feinberg School of Medicine
Chicago, IL

ROBERT E. SHAPIRO, MD, PhD
Associate Professor of Neurology
Medical Director, UVM Office of Clinical
    Trials Research
Department of Neurology
University of Vermont
College of Medicine
Burlington, VT

FRED D. SHEFTELL, MD
Assistant Clinical Professor of Neurology
    and Psychiatry
Albert Einstien College of Medicine
Bronx, NY
Founding Director
New England Center for Headache
Stamford, CT

Stewart J. Tepper, MD
Center for Headache and Pain
Cleveland Clinic
Cleveland, OH

Thomas N. Ward, MD
Co-Director, Headache Clinic
Professor of Neurology
Department of Neurology
Dartmouth-Hitchcock Medical Center
Lebanon, NH

Randall E. Weeks, PhD
Co-Director
New England Institute for Behavioral
    Medicine
Stamford, CT

I
Headache Medicine Basic Science: Anatomy, Physiology, and Epidemiology

1
Head Pain Anatomy and Physiology

Morris Levin, MD

Virtually all tissues of the head, face, and neck are pain-sensitive, with only a few exceptions (Table 1–1). Pain sensation from the front of the head and face, as well as the anterior skull contents, is mostly carried by the trigeminal nerve. Pain from the posterior scalp and more posterior and inferior intracranial structures is carried by the upper cervical roots C2 and C3 (see Table 1–2 for innervation of specific regions and Fig. 1–1 for dermatomes of the head). In this chapter, pain-sensitive structures and their innervation will be described, followed by a discussion of pain physiology as it relates to headache pain.

SOURCES OF HEAD PAIN AND THEIR NOCICEPTIVE INNERVATION

Scalp and skull inflammation can produce head pain, generally of obvious cause. Bone is relatively insensate, but periostea are quite painful. Scalp muscles, vessels, and skin are highly sensitive as well. Muscular causes of pain are often considered in patients with head pain but are generally not significant. Scalp muscles are basically all connected by aponeurosis, with the frontalis and occipitalis forming the anterior and posterior portions (Fig. 1–2). A number of upper cervical region muscles can be pain sources as well. Suboccipital muscles connect the atlas and the posterior base of the skull. The long capitis muscles (longissimus and longus) run along the spine and connect to the skull base, and the splenius muscles also connect the spine to the skull (mastoid). The sterno-cleidomastoid and scalene muscles connect clavicle and rib cage elements to the skull and upper spine. The muscles attached to the hyoid bone include the stylohyoid, mylohyoid, and geniohyoid and can also be sources of facial pain, generally around the jaw and pharynx. The temporalis muscle, interestingly a very common site of perceived pain in headache, is one of the most prominent of the scalp region muscles. The temporalis as well as the other muscles of mastication (masseter and lateral and medial pterygoids) can also be painful. Facial expression muscles are complex, but all are innervated by the facial nerve, which serves both motor and sensory functions of these muscles (see Fig. 1–2).

Dural pain is particularly intense and is probably the cause of most pain related to increased intracranial pressure and intracranial mass effect. The arachnoid is also very pain-sensitive, which explains the intense headache of meningitis and subarachnoid hemorrhage. Above the tentorium, meningeal

Table 1–1 Pain-Sensitive Structures of the Head

Dura
Dural veins and arteries
Intracranial arteries
Cranial nerves V, VII, IX, X
Cervical root C1–3
Periosteum of the skull
Scalp
Scalp muscles
Scalp vessels
Sinuses
Eyes
Ears
Teeth and gums
Carotid and vertebral arteries
Cervical spine
Cervical muscles and tendons
Pain-Insensitive Structures:
Parenchyma
Pia, ventricles
Skull, cervical spine

sensation is subserved by the first division of the trigeminal nerve, but below the tentorium there is more complex innervation, with contributions from the facial, glossopharyngeal, and vagal nerves as well as C2 and C3.

The cerebral arteries are particularly sensitive, which explains the presence of significant headache in virtually all cases of cerebral vasculitis (either primary or secondary). Arteries of the circle of Willis are innervated by the first division of the trigeminal nerve. Dural veins and cortical arteries are served by meningeal nerves (either ophthalmic nerve or C2–3-derived).

Table 1–2 Nociceptive Innervation of Specific Head Regions

Face and frontal head regions	V1-3
Eyes	V1
Sinuses	
Frontal and anterior ethmoid	V1
Maxillary, sphenoid, post-ethmoid	V2
Muscles of facial expression	VII
Throat	IX, X
Arteries of circle of Wills	V1
Cortical and meningeal arteries	V1, C2-3
Dura above tentorium	V1
Dura in posterior fossa	C2-3, VII, IX, X

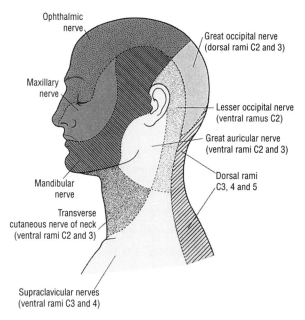

Ophthalmic nerve

Great occipital nerve (dorsal rami C2 and 3)

Maxillary nerve

Lesser occipital nerve (ventral ramus C2)

Great auricular nerve (ventral rami C2 and 3)

Dorsal rami C3, 4 and 5

Mandibular nerve

Transverse cutaneous nerve of neck (ventral rami C2 and 3)

Supraclavicular nerves (ventral rami C3 and 4)

Figure 1–1 Dermatomes of the head and neck. (Used with permission from Standring, S. *Gray's anatomy: The anatomical basis of clinical practice*. Elsevier, 2004)

Meningeal arteries can be branches of the internal carotid, external carotid, or vertebral artery and can be pain sources; they are also innervated by the first division of the trigeminal nerve and upper cervical roots. Referral patterns of these intracranial arteries can be complex (Fig. 1–3). Blood vessels of the scalp include the occipital artery, the auriculotemporal artery, and the temporal artery. All are derived from the external carotid artery and are pain-sensitive. (There are some anterior branches derived from the ophthalmic artery, an internal carotid artery branch.) The most important of the scalp arteries is the temporal artery, which, when inflamed, can be intensely painful (Fig. 1–4). Typical of other cervical and cranial arteries, the cervical portion of the carotid artery is pain-sensitive (innervated by C2, C3, and C4), but interestingly, as shown by Raskin in 1978, processes affecting it can produce surprising pain referral patterns, including areas of the scalp, teeth, gums, eye, nose, cheek, and jaw.

Involvement of any of several cranial nerves can lead to significant headache. The trigeminal nerve is most important. Its dermatomal distribution covers most of the face and frontal scalp (see Fig. 1–1). The ophthalmic nerve carries sensation from the frontal scalp, forehead, upper eyelid, the conjunctiva and cornea of the eye, the nose, nasal mucosa, the frontal sinuses, and parts of the meninges as above. The maxillary nerve carries sensation from the lower eyelid; nares; nasal mucosa; the maxillary, ethmoid, and sphenoid sinuses; cheek;

6

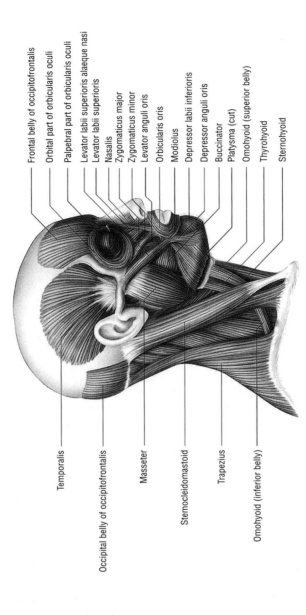

Frontal belly of occipitofrontalis
Orbital part of orbicularis oculi
Palpebral part of orbicularis oculi
Levator labii superioris alaeque nasi
Levator labii superioris
Nasalis
Zygomaticus major
Zygomaticus minor
Levator anguli oris
Orbicularis oris
Modiolus
Depressor labii inferioris
Depressor anguli oris
Buccinator
Platysma (cut)
Omohyoid (superior belly)
Thyrohyoid
Sternohyoid

Temporalis
Occipital belly of occipitofrontalis
Masseter
Sternocleidomastoid
Trapezius
Omohyoid (inferior belly)

Figure 1–2 Muscles of the head and face. (Used with permission from Standring, S. *Gray's anatomy: The anatomical basis of clinical practice.* Elsevier, 2004)

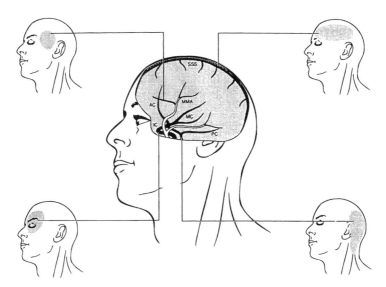

Figure 1–3 Cortical and meningeal arteries and their pain referral patterns. (Used with permission from Lance, J.W., & Goadsby, P.J. *Mechanisms and management of headache*. Elsevier, 2004)

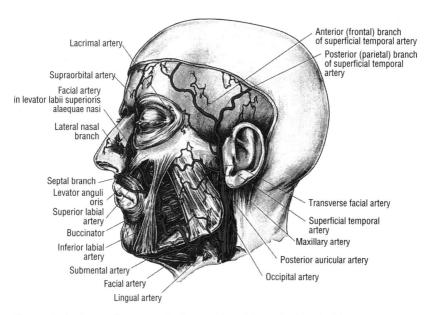

Figure 1–4 Temporal artery and other arteries of the scalp. (Used with permission from Standring, S. *Gray's anatomy: The anatomical basis of clinical practice*. Elsevier, 2004)

8

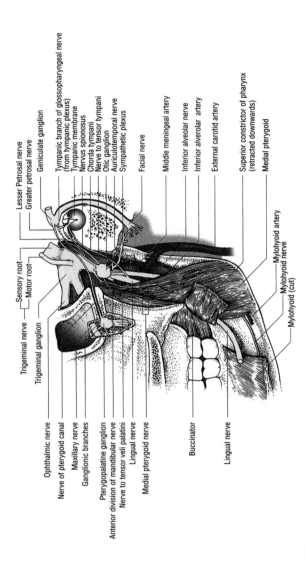

Figure 1–5 Trigeminal (Gasserian) ganglion, sphenopalatine (pterygopalatine) ganglion, and associated structures. (Used with permission from Standring, S. *Gray's anatomy: The anatomical basis of clinical practice*. Elsevier, 2004)

upper lip; upper teeth and gums; the palate; and parts of the meninges. The mandibular nerve carries sensory information from the lower lip, the lower teeth and gums, the floor of the mouth, the anterior two thirds of the tongue, the chin and jaw (except the angle of the jaw, which is innervated by C2 and C3), anterior parts of the external ear, and parts of the meninges. Innervation of the tympanic membrane has been controversial but is probably almost entirely trigeminal.

The ophthalmic branch passes through the superior orbital fissure and the cavernous sinus. The maxillary branch passes through the foramen rotundum and also the cavernous sinus. The mandibular division passes through the foramen ovale, bypassing the cavernous sinus. The three branches of the trigeminal nerve converge within Meckel's cave (located at the tip of the petrous part of the temporal bone) to form the trigeminal ganglion (also known as the Gasserian or semilunar ganglion) (Fig. 1–5). The proximal processes of the nociceptive neurons of the trigeminal nerve enter the brain stem at the level of the pons. They descend in the spinal trigeminal tract to synapse in the spinal trigeminal nucleus (STN), located in the upper cervical spinal cord and lower medulla. Processes affecting any of the branches of the trigeminal nerve anywhere along their course can result in pain in the distribution of that branch as well as referred pain to other parts of the head. These include disease processes of the facial bones, eye, cavernous sinus, meninges, skull base, and brain stem.

Some nociceptive sensation from the anterior head is carried by cranial nerves VII, IX, and X, which synapse in the STN as well. Lesions or dysfunction of the sensory portions of these nerves can thus also lead to head pain. Sensory branches of VII innervate facial muscles of expression and parts of the external auditory canal and pharynx. Their bodies are located in the geniculate ganglion in the facial canal. Glossopharyngeal and vagal afferents carry some pharyngeal and palatal sensation and posterior tongue sensation is carried by IX. The glossopharyngeal nerve also innervates the middle ear. Cranial nerves IX and X also innervate the dura of the posterior fossa. Both pass through the jugular foramen on their way to the brain stem.

Upper cervical roots, primarily C2 and C3, carry pain sensation from posterior portions of the head as well as the dura in the posterior fossa (see Fig. 1–1). C2 passes between the atlas and axis, and C3 in the foramen between C2 and C3 bodies, on their way to the spinal cord. C1 emerges between the base of the skull and the atlas and is essentially a motor nerve innervating several suboccipital muscles.

Certain branches of the trigeminal nerve and cervical roots in the scalp are prone to trauma and other dysfunction. Particularly vulnerable are the occipital nerve (derived from C2) and the supratrochlear and supraorbital nerves (derived from V1) since their path is minimally protected (Fig. 1–6).

Paranasal sinuses are liberally innervated with nociceptive afferents, generally derived from the first two divisions of the trigeminal nerve (frontal and

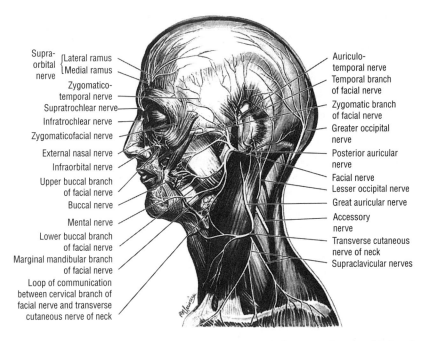

Supra-orbital nerve {Lateral ramus, Medial ramus}
Zygomatico-temporal nerve
Supratrochlear nerve
Infratrochlear nerve
Zygomaticofacial nerve
External nasal nerve
Infraorbital nerve
Upper buccal branch of facial nerve
Buccal nerve
Mental nerve
Lower buccal branch of facial nerve
Marginal mandibular branch of facial nerve
Loop of communication between cervical branch of facial nerve and transverse cutaneous nerve of neck

Auriculo-temporal nerve
Temporal branch of facial nerve
Zygomatic branch of facial nerve
Greater occipital nerve
Posterior auricular nerve
Facial nerve
Lesser occipital nerve
Great auricular nerve
Accessory nerve
Transverse cutaneous nerve of neck
Supraclavicular nerves

Figure 1–6 Nerves of the scalp, including greater occipital nerve and supraorbital and supratrochlear nerves. (Used with permission from Standring, S. *Gray's anatomy: The anatomical basis of clinical practice.* Elsevier, 2004)

anterior ethmoid sinuses—V1; maxillary, sphenoid, and posterior ethmoid—V2). The nose and nasal mucosa are generally innervated by V1 and V2. The sphenopalatine ganglion (also known as the pterygopalatine ganglion) is a complex group of nerves with parasympathetic, sympathetic, sensory, and motor roots. It lies in the pterygopalatine fossa (which the maxillary nerve passes through) (see Fig. 1–5). The sensory roots are maxillary branches. Its anatomy is worth knowing as anesthesia of this ganglion is easily accomplished with sometimes beneficial results for anterior head pain.

The bony and ligamentous anatomy of the upper cervical spine and its articulation with the base of the skull is complex (Fig. 1–7). Deformity or dysfunction in these areas is often blamed for head pain. Certainly bony elements, synovial joints, intervertebral discs, nerve roots, tendons, and muscular structures can all be the source of pain. Atlantoaxial deformity and dislocation can affect the roots C2 and/or C3 with resulting posterior head pain (and possibly anteriorly referred pain). However, the articulating atlanto-occipital, atlantoaxial, and intervertebral joints are highly innervated with nociceptive afferents and can be painful when inflamed, even without any root involvement.

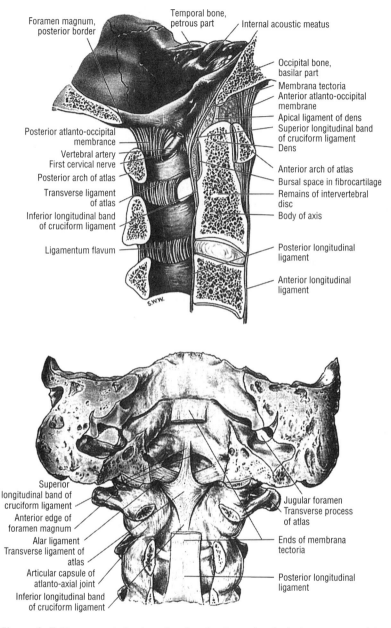

Figure 1–7 Upper cervical spine, showing C2, C3, and articulating processes. (a) Lateral view. (b) Coronal view. (Used with permission from Standring, S. *Gray's anatomy: The anatomical basis of clinical practice*. Elsevier, 2004)

The eyes are another pain source and can radiate pain sensation to other sites. For unclear reasons, they are also a site of referred pain from a number of other structures, including the posterior fossa, carotid arteries, and other trigeminal sources. Nociceptive receptors are numerous in the conjunctivae, cornea, and retina as well as surrounding tissues in the orbit, including extraocular muscles and tissues surrounding the optic nerve. The pain of optic neuritis is probably mediated by dural inflammation.

Pharyngeal sensation is generally carried by the glossopharyngeal nerve and of course can radiate to other regions. Dental pain is common and may also be the source of referred head pain. Maxillary and mandibular nerves mediate dental pain and when these nerves are involved by non-dental process, referral of pain to the teeth may ensue. Structures in the submandibular region such as the parotid gland, other salivary glands, and the stylohyoid ligament can be significant pain sources.

PHYSIOLOGY OF HEAD PAIN

Both the trigeminal and upper cervical spinal root systems contain bipolar nociceptive nerves whose distal axons are undifferentiated nerve endings and whose proximal axons synapse in the dorsal horn region of the upper cervical

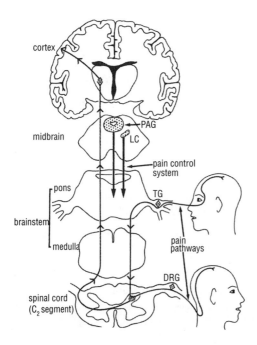

Figure 1–8 Nociceptive anatomy of the face and head, illustrating the convergence of upper cervical and trigeminal components. *Note:* DRG, Dorsal root ganglion; TG, Trigeminal ganglion; PAG, Periaqueductal gray; LC, Locus ceruleus. (Used with permission from Lance, J. W., & Goadsby, P.J. *Mechanisms and management of headache.* Elsevier, 2004)

spinal cord, a portion of which contains the spinal trigeminal nucleus. The bodies of the bipolar primary afferents of the trigeminal nerve lie in the trigeminal ganglion, and those of the cervical roots are in the analogous dorsal root ganglia. The first synapse in the nociceptive system of the face, head, and upper cervical areas takes place in the dorsal horn region of the upper cervical spinal cord, both for trigeminally based neurons as well as for those in the C2 and C3 roots. In fact, the populations of second-order neurons for the two systems are virtually indistinguishable. As a result, these systems are functionally intermixed to some extent, which explains the often complex pain referral patterns seen in pain conditions of the head, face, and upper neck (Fig. 1–8).

For the trigeminal afferents to reach the STN they must descend to the upper cervical dorsal horn region via the spinal trigeminal tract. Interestingly, afferents of cranial nerves IX and X and the sensory roots of VII also all run in the spinal tract of the trigeminal nerve and synapse in the STN (leading again to potential complex referral patterns for pain in the regions served by these various afferent systems). The projections of the second-order pain neurons of the upper cervical and trigeminal systems ascend in several tracts, the best understood being the spinothalamic tract and trigeminothalamic tracts respectively, which terminate in the ventral posterolateral (for cervical-derived tracts) and ventral posteromedial (for trigeminal-derived tracts) nuclei. These paths cross in the spinal cord (C2- and C3-derived neurons in the anterior commissure) or brain stem (trigeminal-derived neurons) before terminating in the thalamus.

However, there are other tracts that are bilateral and terminate in midline portions of the thalamus. Projections from more lateral thalamic nuclei tend to carry more specific localizing information of a more somatic nature, and terminate in parietal and other cortical areas. Projections from the more medial thalamic nuclei carry less specific but more "emotional" painful information and terminate in a number of other cerebral areas, including limbic structures such as the cingulate gyrus, prefrontal cortex, and insula.

So, in summary, nociception from the anterior and posterior head is transmitted via a three-neuron pathway—the bipolar afferent neuron, the dorsal horn/STN neuron, and the thalamic neuron—but unlike most other sensation, pain does not have a specific map or "homunculus" represented in the cortex. And the intermixing of these two systems leads to the clinical observation that pain in the head, face, and neck is poorly localizing.

It is useful to define *nociceptive pain* as pain due to actual activation of the peripheral nociceptive afferents, leading to nociception and pain, and *neuropathic pain* as pain arising from aberrant sensory processing in the peripheral or central nervous system (peripheral versus central nociceptive pain). Nociceptive pain examples include pain due to skeletal fractures, tendinitis, dermatitis, and osteoarthritis. Peripheral neuropathic pain examples would be painful polyneuropathy, entrapment neuropathy pain, and neuralgia. Central neuropathic pain examples include thalamic pain syndrome and the pain of syringomyelia.

Table 1–3 Pain Pathways

Medial/Affective	Lateral/Discriminative
Polymodal receptors	Mechano-, thermoreceptors
C axons (unmyelinated)	A delta (small, myelinated)
"Second pain"	"First pain"
Burning, nonlocalized pain	Sharp, localized pain
Dorsal horn neuron wide dynamic range	Dorsal horn neuron nociceptive only
Dorsal horn neuron—large field	Small field
Spinoreticular tracts	Spinothalamic tract
Medial thalamic nuclei	Lateral thalamic nuclei
Multiple cortical projections	Postcentral gyrus projection

Referred pain is thought to be due to convergence of multiple first-order afferents on a population of second-order neurons, leading to false or mixed localization. Referred pain is often a visceral–somatic convergence that is then typically perceived as somatic (e.g., cardiac pain perceived as arm pain in the same root distribution). As noted above, referral patterns in the head, face, and neck can include any site innervated by cranial nerves V, VII, IX, and X and C2 and C3.

Broadly, there are actually two afferent pain systems. One is served by primary afferents which can be activated by a range of stimuli (wide dynamic range) and second-order neurons with a responsive to large receptive field, and the other by primary afferents responsive to more specific stimuli (such as pressure) and second-order neurons with a small field. The first pathway is termed the "discriminative" pain pathway because of its better localizing ability and the second, "affective" pain because it leads to a more emotional "suffering" pain perception. The affective pathway is generally subserved by C fibers, thus slow, and the discriminative pathway by A delta fibers, leading to a faster perception. Since the discriminative pathway involves lateral thalamic nuclei and the "affective" pathway more medial thalamic nuclei they are also called lateral and medial pathways respectively (Table 1–3).

What stimulates the afferent nociceptive nerve endings? A number of agents are released by damaged or irritated tissue (and mast cells), including potassium ions, prostaglandins, bradykinin, serotonin, leukotrienes, substance P, and histamine, all of which can stimulate or sensitize the nociceptive afferents. Pressure, even from local dilation of vessels, can also contribute and so can other changes in the local milieu, particularly when the nociceptors are sensitized. At the first synapse in the nociceptive system, the key neurotransmitter is glutamate. Stimulation of the first-order neuron leads to release of glutamate as well as neuropeptides like substance P (SP) and calcitonin gene-related peptide (CGRP), at the synaptic cleft in the dorsal horn/trigeminal nucleus caudalis region. The release of these leads to depolarization of the second-order neuron.

There are two main types of glutamate receptors: *ionotropic* (directly linked to sodium and calcium channels, which when stimulated lead to rapid influx of calcium, and excitation of the neuron) and *metabotropic* (which when stimulated lead to protein kinase second-messenger activity that ultimately leads to displacement of magnesium at calcium channels and then sodium and calcium influx, and excitation of the neuron). The ionotropic glutamate receptors are subdivided into three categories: *NMDA* (N-methyl-D-aspartate), *kainate*, and *AMPA* (alpha-amino-3-hydroxy-5-methyl-4-isoxazolepropionic acid).

MODULATION AND SENSITIZATION OF PAIN

The activity of the second-order nociceptive cells (dorsal horn/STN cells) can be heightened by a number of factors. With repeated stimulation, they become more active in certain situations (this is referred to as "wind-up" and also appears to occur at the level of the third-order thalamic neuron). When this is prolonged it can become relatively fixed and is known as central sensitization. This process is thought to be mediated by the NMDA receptor complex. When receptors are damaged and dorsal horn/STN neurons become "deafferented," they become hyperactive. This denervation hypersensitivity is a widespread phenomenon in the nervous system.

Presynaptic inhibition from incoming non-nociceptive afferents occurs at the level of the first synapse too. This is the result of primarily A beta fibers and is termed the *gating* mechanism (i.e., non-nociceptive afferent activity can "close the gate" on nociceptive activity) (Fig. 1–9). Clinical examples of pain treatments that employ the gating mechanism are massage, transcutaneous nerve stimulation, and heat/cold therapy.

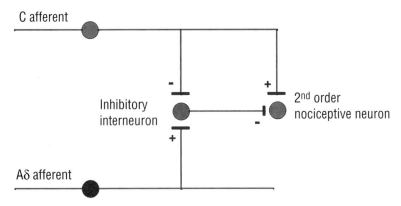

Figure 1–9 The gating mechanism of pain modulation. Incoming nociceptive signals (carried by C fibers) are modulated by afferent non-nociceptive sensory input (carried by A delta fibers) via inhibitory interneurons, which are *excited* by non-nociceptive axons and *inhibited* by nociceptive axons.

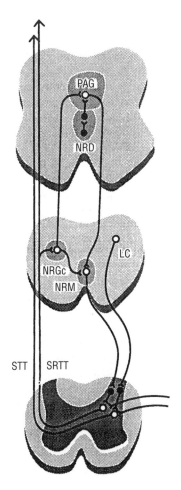

Figure 1–10 The descending antinociceptive system, originating in the brain stem and higher centers, descending to modulate the first synapse in the nociceptive pathway in the dorsal horn/spinal trigeminal nucleus complex. *Note:* NRM, Nucleus raphe magnus; LC, Locus ceruleus; SRTT, Spinoreticulothalamic tract; STT, Spinothalamic tract; NRGc, Nucleus reticularis gigantocellularis; NRD, Nucleus raphe dorsalis. (Used with permission from Lance, J.W., & Goadsby, P.J. *Mechanisms and management of headache.* Elsevier, 2004)

Inhibition of pain transmission also results from descending inhibition of the second-order neuron. Inhibitory presynaptic opiate receptors are found on the first-order axon. Other opiate receptors are found throughout the neuroaxis, including the brain stem. These respond to the descending "antinociceptive system," which originates in a number of higher centers, including the cortex, thalamus, and brain stem (Fig. 1–10). The midbrain periaqueductal gray region (PAG) is crucial in this system; it includes the serotonergic nucleus raphe magnus of the medulla and an area referred to as the rostral ventromedial medulla (RVM). The RVM contains so-called on cells that fire during nociception and off-cells that seem to ameliorate nociceptive transmission. Opioids inhibit on-cells and activate off-cells. Opioid antagonists impair the antinociceptive system.

It is well accepted now that pain is a "biopsychosocial" experience. In other words, psychological and social factors can modulate or intensify the perception of pain. Certainly there may be cortical reinterpretation of pain sensations depending upon an individual's psychological state. However, cortical activity may be exerting a more proximal effect at the level of the first synapse. A key example is the placebo effect, which seems to be related to the descending antinociceptive system. Evidence for this is the ability of naloxone, the opioid antagonist, to block placebo-related pain reduction.

SUMMARY

Pain sources in the head, face, and neck are numerous. Both nociceptive and neuropathic pain processes can occur, and may coexist. The pain sensory innervation in these areas is complex and there is a significant degree of convergence between the trigeminal and upper cervical nociceptive systems. As a result, pain referral patterns can be misleading. Modulation and sensitization are active forces that alter pain processing. These are best understood at the level of the second-order nociceptive neuron, but clearly the story is just beginning to unfold. Knowledge of the anatomy of pain-sensitive structures of the head, face, and neck is important to bring to the diagnostic side of clinical headache medicine, and understanding of the concepts of pain control in the nervous system should inform treatment decisions.

Review Questions

1. Which of the following cranial nerves does not contain afferent nociceptive nerves?
   a. II
   b. VII
   c. IX
   d. X
2. Which of the following contains nociceptors?
   a. Skull
   b. Brain parenchyma
   c. Circle of Willis
   d. Pia
3. Cortical centers that are known to be active in nociception include all but:
   a. Cingulate gyrus
   b. Posterior parietal lobe
   c. Insula
   d. Prefrontal cortex
4. Nociceptive off-cells are known to exist in the:
   a. Tectal nuclei

  b. Locus ceruleus
  c. Nucleus raphe magnus
  d. Rostral ventromedial medulla
5. The "affective" pain system contains:
  a. A delta fibers
  b. Wide dynamic range nociceptors
  c. Second-order neurons with small receptive fields
  d. Lateral thalamic nuclei
6. Which of the following is not a glutamate receptor type?
  a. AMPA
  b. Kainate
  c. Kappa
  d. NMDA
7. Central sensitization is generally a phenomenon that occurs at the level of the:
  a. First-order nociceptive neuron
  b. Second-order nociceptive neuron
  c. Thalamus
  d. Cortex
8. The maxillary nerve:
  a. Passes through the pterygopalatine fossa
  b. Enters the skull at the foramen ovale
  c. Passes through the superior orbital fissure
  d. Innervates the orbicularis oculi
9. A 42-year-old man with lung cancer begins to have pain in his distal right upper extremity. Exam and radiological workup reveals no neoplastic involvement of the arm. He is most likely to be suffering from:
  a. Referred pain
  b. Central neuropathic pain
  c. Peripheral neuropathic pain
  d. Nociceptive pain
10. A 73-year-old woman has chronic posterior head pain due to severe upper cervical involvement by rheumatoid arthritis. She is able to reduce the pain by having a massage, using heat, visualizing pain reduction, and meditating. She is employing all of the following mechanisms except:
  a. Placebo effect
  b. Descending antinociceptive system
  c. Gating mechanism
  d. Behavioral medicine

10. a
9. c

8. a
7. b
6. c
5. b
4. d
3. b
2. c
1. a

SUGGESTED READING

Burstein, R., Levy, D., Jakubowski, M., & Woolf, C.J. "Peripheral and central sensitization related to headaches." In *The Headaches*, eds. J. Olesen, P.J. Goadsby, N.M. Ramadan et al. Philadelphia: Lippincott Williams & Wilkins, 2006.

Fausett, H. "Anatomy and physiology of pain." In *Principles and Practice of Pain Medicine*, eds. C.A. Warfield & Z.H. Bajwa. 2nd ed., pp. 28–34. New York: McGraw Hill, 2004.

Lance, J.W., & Goadsby, P.J. "Mechanisms and management of headache." Chapter 8 in *Migraine: Pathophysiology*, pp. 87–121. Philadelphia: Elsevier, Butterworth Heinemann, 2005.

Levine, J.D., Gordon, N.C., & Fields, H.L. The mechanism of placebo analgesia. *Lancet* 2 (1978): 654–657.

Levin, M. The many causes of headache. *Postgraduate Medicine* 112, no. 6 (2002): 67–82.

Raskin, N.H., & Prusiner, S. Carotidynia. *Neurology* 27 (1977): 43–46.

Saunders, R.L., & Weider, D. Tympanic membrane sensation. *Brain* 108 (1985): 387–404.

Woolf, C.J. Pain: Moving from symptom control toward mechanism-specific pharmacologic management *Annals of Internal Medicine* 140, no. 6 (2004): 441–451.

2

Pathophysiology and Genetics of Migraine and Cluster Headache

Robert E. Shapiro, MD, PhD

Migraine and cluster headache are episodic states of the nervous system. Each state is dominated by head pain but also associated with multiple other neurologic and systemic features, including behavioral, cognitive, perceptual, and autonomic signs and symptoms. The expression of these brain states is governed by both heritable and environmental factors.

MIGRAINE

Migraine is an episodic neurologic state with widespread effects on other body systems. The experience of migraine episodes or attacks is often recurrent and stereotypical for an individual sufferer, or migraineur. However, it is also true that migraine symptom patterns are clinically heterogeneous and highly idiosyncratic to each migraineur. Consequently, there is no single obligate clinical feature that defines the common form of migraine state by the diagnostic criteria now codified in the *International Classification of Headache Disorders*, 2nd edition (ICHD-2). Migraine is diagnostically categorized based upon the presence (MA) or absence (MO) of aura symptoms (see below) with attacks, though overlap between these entities is common since patients who experience aura rarely do so with every attack. In addition to MO and MA, there are multiple rarer varieties such as hemiplegic migraine, a disorder where aura symptoms may include temporary but prolonged hemiparesis.

Many symptoms and signs of migraine occur with sufficient frequency across migraineurs that for any theory of migraine pathogenesis to be truly comprehensive, it will need to account for them. These features include the following: (1) migraine attacks often occur as a sequence of phases (e.g., premonitory, aura, headache, and postdrome or resolution), (2) premonitory symptoms often include alterations in affect, cravings, yawning, and so forth, (3) aura typically comprises positive sensory symptoms (usually visual or somesthetic) that migrate dynamically across a sensory field over minutes, (4) headache, when present, is often throbbing, unilateral, severe, and/or worsened with exertion or physical activity, (5) attacks are often generally associated with distorted cognition and mood, as well as heightened perception that usually renders sensations aversive across modalities, and (6) autonomic control may be dys-functionally manifest as nausea, vomiting, gastric dysmotility, or sinusitis. In addition, migraine may be provoked in many migraineurs by any of a host of external stimuli (e.g., weather changes, food and odor triggers, stressors, ambi-ent diurnal cues) and endogenous stimuli (e.g., hormonal fluctuations, level of arousal, circadian rhythms), thereby lending some predictability to the timing of attacks.

Currently our knowledge of the pathophysiology of migraine is very incom-plete and our ability to explain many, if not most, of these clinical phenomena is rudimentary at best. However, a number of recent advances in genetics, imag-ing, and physiology allow a picture of migraine pathophysiology to begin to emerge.

Genetics

Migraine is considered to be a genetically complex disorder—that is, the clinical expression of common forms of migraine is a consequence of multiple factors acting in concert. These factors may include the summated and integrated small contributions of multiple genetic mutations and variations (i.e., polygenic inheritance) as well as influences of environment.

Studies of migraine in families have sought to determine whether it is more frequently seen among first-degree relatives of migraineurs than would be expected by chance. Many of these studies have had methodologic limitations such as varying diagnostic criteria or ascertainment questionnaires. However, a large Danish study from the mid-1990s addressed many of these concerns and found that first-degree relatives of individuals with MO had a 1.9-fold higher risk of MO and a 1.4-fold higher risk of MA, whereas first-degree relatives of individuals with MA had a nearly 4-fold higher risk of MA but no greater risk of MO. These authors concluded that for MO, both genetic and environmental factors are important determinants, whereas MA is largely determined by genetic factors.

Twin studies have compared the likelihood of migraine co-occurring (con-cordance rates) between pairs who were either related monozygotically (genet-ically identical) or dizygotically (genetically as similar as non-twin siblings). Across multiple studies, monozygotic pairs have consistently been reported to show higher concordance rates than dizygotic pairs, regardless of whether the pairs were raised separately or together. Together, these studies have indicated that the contribution of genetic factors to this variance of migraine expression (heritability estimate) may range from 28% to 65%; however, a figure of 50% heritability is a generally accepted overall estimate.

Linkage analysis genome-wide screening studies have sought to identify genetic markers (polymorphisms) that segregate with the trait of migraine with the goal of narrowing chromosomal regions where migraine susceptibility genes must lie. A number of such studies have identified chromosomal loci for genes for MO (4q21, 14q21–22), MA (4q24, 11q24), and mixed MO/MA

(1q31, 6p12–21, 18p11, Xq24–28). Case–control association studies have also been performed to determine whether mutations in candidate genes (based on hypotheses of migraine pathogenesis) segregate with migraine traits within a family or cohort at a frequency higher than expected by chance. Many genes have been reported to have association with migraine in such studies, including those for the dopamine type 2 receptor, dopamine type 4 receptor, tumor necrosis factor-β/lymphotoxin α, serotonin transporter, methylenetetrahydrofolate reductase, low-density lipoprotein, dopamine-β hydroxylase, angiotensin-converting enzyme, insulin receptor, progesterone receptor, and glutathione-S-transferase. However, caution must taken when interpreting the results of such genome-wide screening and association studies of common forms of migraine, since many of these findings have been difficult to replicate. This variability is likely a consequence of multiple factors, including differing genetic backgrounds, ages, and environments across studied populations.

"Monogenic" Forms

The identification of susceptibility genes for common forms of migraine has proven to be very challenging because of the likely contributions of many interacting genetic loci and environmental factors to the expression of the clinical phenotypes. Fortunately for our understanding of migraine, and by contrast to the circumstances with a number of other common complex polygenic disorders (e.g., depression, anxiety, diabetes), variant migraine syndromes exist that segregate in families in an autosomal dominant pattern with a high degree of penetrance according to classic Mendelian inheritance. In other words, susceptibility genes exist for some migraine variant disorders where a genetic mutation of only one allele of the two possible copies on somatic (i.e., non-sex) chromosomes is sufficient to confer a high likelihood of the clinical expression of the disorder. Study of these variant syndromes and identification of such susceptibility genes have allowed significant insights to be made into the pathogenesis of these disorders. These insights are being extended to our understanding of more common migraine forms.

The most fruitful genetic studies of migraine have been those of rare families where hemiparesis is a migraine aura trait—that is, familial hemiplegic migraine (FHM). Since the initial report by Ophoff and colleagues of the gene for FHM1 in 1996, two further genes (FHM2, FHM3) have been identified that contain mutations resulting in essentially the identical FHM phenotype. All three of these genes code for ion transporters or ion channels and these disorders are collectively regarded as "channelopathies." Considering the anatomic and functional consequences of these ion channels together, Moskowitz and colleagues have proposed an attractive hypothesis for the molecular pathogenesis of migraine susceptibility: potentiation of excitatory neurotransmission at glutamatergic synapses in the cerebral cortex. All of the identified FHM mutations either increase (gain of function) or decrease (loss of function) molecular processes, which then result in enhanced glutamatergic transmission and elevated concentrations of extracellular potassium.

As an introduction to this area, it is helpful to briefly review the biophysics of these cortical structures (Fig. 2–1). Depolarization of cortical neurons and the initiation and propagation of their axonal action potentials is dependent upon the opening of neuronal voltage-gated sodium channels, which facilitate the influx of sodium into the cytosol and depolarization of the membrane and markedly increase extracellular concentrations of potassium. The firing rate of neurons is dependent upon the repolarization time for the membrane potential, which is in part secondary to the recovery time of these sodium channels. As an action potential reaches a glutamatergic axon terminal, it encounters and opens voltage-gated calcium channels in the presynaptic membrane, thereby leading to an influx of calcium into the presynaptic cytosol. This calcium influx triggers fusion of glutamate-containing vesicles with the synaptic membrane and release of glutamate into the synaptic cleft. Released glutamate then acts as an excitatory transmitter at postsynaptic (e.g., NMDA) receptors, leading to depolarization of the postsynaptic neuron. Glutamate remaining in the synaptic cleft is cleared by glutamate transporters in the plasma membranes of

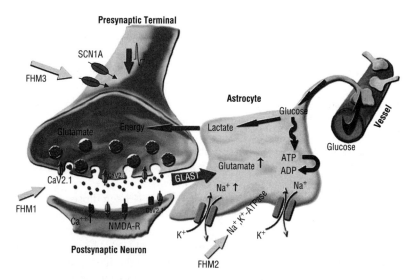

Figure 2–1 Putative mechanisms for generation of cortical hyperexcitability in familial hemiplegic migraine. Mutations in three genes—SCNIA, CACNA1A, and ATP1A2—result in similar FHM phenotypes. All three gene products are localized to serve functions that can result in increased extracellular potassium concentrations and increased neurotransmission at glutamatergic synapses in cerebral cortex. See text for details. (Reprinted and modified from *Ann Neurol* Vol. 55, No. 2, 2004, pp. 276–280. Copyright 2004 American Neurological Association; with permission of John Wiley & Sons, Inc.)

adjacent astrocytes, where the glutamate is then recycled. The glutamate transporters passively carry glutamate and sodium into astrocytes in exchange for the release of intracellular potassium ions. The transporters are driven by an ion gradient of relatively high intracellular potassium and high extracellular sodium established by Na$^+$/K$^+$-ATPase pumps, which are also located on astrocytic membranes. These Na$^+$/K$^+$-ATPases pump three sodium ions out of the astrocyte for every two ions of potassium pumped into the astrocyte.

As hypothesized, each FHM mutation can influence a crucial event in this synaptic sequence and each can lead to the same result: increased glutamatergic neurotransmission (see Fig. 2–1). Mutations in the SCN1A gene (FHM3; chromosome locus 2q24) coding for the α1 subunit of Na$_v$1.1 voltage-gated sodium channels lead to faster recovery (gain of function) of these sodium channels after depolarization, thus allowing more action potentials to be propagated per unit time. Mutations in the CACNA1A gene (FHM1; chromosome locus 19p13) coding for the α1A subunit of the Ca$_v$2.1 P/Q calcium channel lead to increased calcium transport into presynaptic elements (gain of function) of glutamatergic synapses, resulting in more glutamate release per action potential. Mutations in the ATP1A2 gene (FHM2; chromosomal locus 1q21) coding for the astrocytic Na$^+$/K$^+$-ATPase pump lead to pump failure (loss of function), loss of the astrocyte membrane ionic gradient, and then failure of the glutamate transporter (GLAST/EAAT1) to be able to clear excess glutamate from the synapse. The consequence is prolonged elevations in synaptic glutamate concentrations and enhanced excitatory neurotransmission. The significance of enhanced excitatory transmission and elevated extracellular potassium concentrations in the cerebral cortex in migraine is relevant to current models of the pathogenesis of migraine aura, particularly the phenomenon of cortical spreading depression (see below).

Of note, Baloh and colleagues have identified a patient with a clinical triad phenotype of hemiplegic migraine, episodic ataxia, and seizures (EA-6). This patient has a point mutation in the gene coding for the glutamate transporter (GLAST/EAAT1) that also leads to loss of transporter function consistent with the loss hypothesized for FHM2. Furthermore, some other mutations in CACNA1A lead to ataxic phenotypes (EA-2, SCA6), whereas other mutations in SCN1A and in ATP1A2 lead to epilepsy phenotypes. Collectively, these results indicate that the molecular pathogenesis of FHM is closely linked to the pathogeneses of other paroxysmal neurologic disorders such as epilepsy and episodic ataxia. While mutations in the FHM genes have not been found to confer increased susceptibility to common forms of migraine, the high degree of comorbidity of epilepsy with migraine would suggest that these paroxysmal disorders may also share pathogenetic mechanisms involving channelopathies.

A number of other heritable disorders include migraine attacks as syndromic symptoms. Two of these disorders are cerebral autosomal dominant arteriopathy with subcortical infarcts and leukoencephalopathy (CADASIL), due to mutations in the Notch3 gene located at chromosome locus 19p13.2, and mitochondrial encephalopathy lactic acid and stroke (MELAS), due to mutations in the ND4 gene within the mitochondrial genome.

Migraine Aura and Cortical Spreading Depression

In 1941, Karl Lashley took careful note of the visual disturbance of his own migraine aura as it spread slowly across his visual field. He hypothesized that if this disturbance was due to events originating in his primary visual cortex, then it would reflect a process that was propagating across the cortex at a rate of approximately 3 mm/min. In 1944, Leão, studying rabbits, observed a self-propagating wave of profound depolarization that continued at a rate of approximately 3 mm/min across the cerebral cortex and that was followed within seconds by suppression of neuronal activity lasting minutes. He termed this phenomenon cortical spreading depression (CSD). For over 60 years, CSD has been hypothesized to be the physiologic phenomenon underlying migraine aura.

CSD in animal models can be elicited by focal irritation of the cortex directly by mechanical or electrical stimuli or by high potassium concentrations. Experimentally induced CSD also produces marked changes in the chemical composition of the cortex: extracellular concentrations of potassium ions, nitric oxide, arachidonic acid, and prostaglandins are increased and intracellular concentrations of calcium are increased. CSD also results in activation of genes for pro-inflammatory agents such as tumor necrosis factor-α and interleukin-1β and leads to the focal disruption of the blood–brain barrier through activation of matrix metalloprotease 9. Whether due to these chemical changes or other processes, such as the actions of astrocytes through their vascular foot processes, CSD is associated with dramatic and complex blood flow shifts in the cerebral and meningeal vasculature as well as changes in vascular permeability leading to localized meningeal edema and plasma protein extravasation.

While differences exist in some details between the CSD phenomenon observed in animals and that inferred from human observations, the current weight of evidence supports CSD as the physiologic correlate of migraine aura symptoms. This evidence comes from several independent sources. First, human brain noninvasive functional imaging studies across multiple modalities, including positron emission tomography (PET), blood oxygen-level dependent (BOLD) fMRI, and magnetoencephalography, all consistently show a migraine-associated slowly propagating wave of hyperactivity followed by suppressed activity that begins near the occipital pole and extends anteriorly at a rate of approximately 2 to 3 mm/min. Secondly, knock-in mice bearing an FHM1 (R192Q CACNA1A) mutation also have lower thresholds for stimulation of CSD and faster propagation speeds of CSD across the cortex. Finally, diverse medications that have shown clinical benefit as migraine prophylactic agents (e.g., amitriptyline, divalproex sodium, DL-propranolol, topiramate, methysergide) also demonstrate an ability to suppress spontaneous CSD events in rats. Moreover, D-propranolol, which is a clinically ineffective substance for migraine prophylaxis, was also ineffective in suppressing CSD in the rat model.

It is unclear whether CSD in humans is triggered by excessive glutamatergic excitatory neurotransmission in the cerebral cortex, by enhanced extracellular concentrations of potassium, or by a combination of these and other factors (e.g., mechanical head trauma, plasma-borne factors). However, many but not all studies employing transcranial magnetic stimulation techniques have reported that the cerebral cortex in migraineurs has increased excitability between migraine attacks. Other studies using evoked potential methodologies have suggested that the brains of migraineurs do not habituate (i.e., decrease amplitude and increase latency of potentials) appropriately to repetitive stimulation and that this may predispose them to synchronized cortical activity. Collectively, these studies suggest that the brains of migraineurs are predisposed or "primed" to develop synchronized cortical events such as CSD. Whether CSD plays a role in migraine attacks in the absence of the clinical symptoms of aura is unresolved; however, blood flow shifts in the occipital cortex consistent with CSD have been recorded by PET imaging during at least one attack of migraine *without* aura.

Migraine Pain Phase

Sixty years ago, Harold Wolff observed that the pain-sensitive structures within the cranium were restricted to the cranial nerves, dura mater, meningeal vessels, and venous sinuses. These observations led him to hypothesize that migraine symptoms were a consequence of changes in cerebrovascular tone. In other words, the aura of migraine might be caused by transient vasoconstriction of extracerebral vessels and oligemia, followed by headache caused by vasodilation of these vessels and hyperemia. Olesen's 1990 angiographic studies of cerebrovascular tone during migraine attacks clarified that headache onset is not strictly associated with the onset of hyperemia, and that a vascular hypothesis for migraine pathogenesis is insufficient.

It is clear, however, that prominent changes in meningeal vascular tone occur during migraine headache. Attention has been focused on the nociceptive innervation of these vessels by the ophthalmic division of the trigeminal nerve (anterior and middle cranial fossa) and upper cervical roots (posterior cranial fossa), as well as by cranial parasympathetic postganglionic fibers (Fig. 2–2). Moskowitz has coined the term *trigeminovascular system* (TGVS) to describe this anatomic entity. Considerable evidence points to this system as integral to the pain phase of migraine.

Stimulation of the trigeminal ganglion in rat results in release of vasoactive neuropeptides (calcitonin gene-related peptide [CGRP], substance P, neurokinin A) by trigeminal fibers in the vicinity of these dural vessels, leading to extravasation of plasma proteins and localized edema or so-called sterile inflammation. These vascular changes can be blocked by application of agonists for serotonin $5HT_{1b/1d/1f}$ receptors (triptans), ergot alkaloids, and

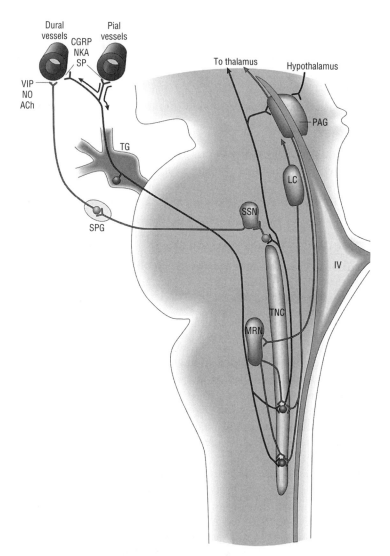

Figure 2–2 Intracerebral and extracerebral neural connectivity in migraine. See text
for details. IV, fourth ventricle; ACh, acetylcholine; CGRP, calcitonin gene-related
peptide; LC, locus ceruleus; PAG, periaqueductal gray region; MRN, magnus raphe
nucleus; NKA, neurokinin A; NO, nitric oxide; SP, substance P; SPG, superior
sphenopalatine ganglion; SSN, superior salivatory nucleus; TG, trigeminal ganglion;
TNC, trigeminal nucleus pars caudalis; VIP, vasoactive intestinal peptide. (Reprinted
with permission from Macmillan Publishers Ltd: *Nat Rev Neurosci* 4:386–398,
Copyright 2003)

anti-inflammatory agents (e.g., acetylsalicylic acid, indomethacin), all of which have demonstrated efficacy as acute antimigraine agents in humans. Triptans can also inhibit the release of CGRP into plasma following trigeminal ganglion or sagittal sinus stimulation in animal models. Notably, antagonists of substance P, but not CGRP, can block plasma protein extravasation in rodent models. However, during the headache phase of human migraine attacks, whether these attacks arise spontaneously or have been induced by nitroglycerine (nitric oxide-donor), significant elevations in CGRP, but not substance P, neuropeptide Y, or vasoactive intestinal polypeptide (VIP), are detected in jugular plasma. Furthermore, exogenous CGRP delivered intravenously can provoke migraine attacks. Finally, CGRP antagonists, but not substance P antagonists, have shown efficacy as acute antimigraine agents in humans. Taken together, these data support a role for CGRP in migraine pathogenesis but raise questions about a role for sterile inflammation.

As mentioned previously, CSD induced in rat can result in increased permeability and vasodilatation of dural vessels. Moskowitz and colleagues have shown that these processes are neurogenic and mediated by the cranial innervation of these vessels. More specifically, CSD triggered in rat induces vasodilatation of pial vessels, leading to activation of trigeminal fibers with collaterals branching to innervate dural vessels, which then extravasate plasma protein. Trigeminal activation also leads to stimulation of second-order trigeminal neurons in the nucleus caudalis of the trigeminal nucleus of the spinal tract in the medulla oblongata. This then leads, via brain stem circuits, to activation of cranial parasympathetic fibers arising in the superior salivatory nucleus and projecting to the dural vasculature via the cranial nerve VII and a relay in the sphenopalatine (pterygopalatine) ganglion. These parasympathetic fibers release VIP, nitric oxide, and/or acetylcholine, producing prompt vasodilatation of dural vessels. This circuitry is sometimes referred to as the *trigeminoparasympathetic reflex.*

The role of serotonin in migraine is complex, and consideration of this role led to the development of the triptans. Reduced concentrations of serotonin are measurable in plasma during migraine attacks and serotonin metabolites are increased in urine following attacks. Drugs that deplete serotonin such as reserpine can provoke headache events that are migrainous in quality, and intravenous serotonin can relieve symptoms of migraine headache. Conditions that are comorbid with migraine such as depression and anxiety have presumptive serotoninergic mechanisms, and a number of antidepressant drugs with actions on serotoninergic systems are effective migraine prophylactic agents (e.g., tricyclics and monoamine oxidase [MAO] inhibitors). Whereas triptans are useful abortive agents for migraine and are agonists at $5HT_{1b/1d/1f}$ receptors, other drugs (e.g., methysergide) are effective migraine prophylactic agents and are antagonists at $5HT_2$ receptor subtypes, and some antiemetic agents (e.g. ondansetron) therapeutically useful in migraine are antagonists at the $5HT_3$ receptor subtype.

Sensitization in Migraine

Burstein and colleagues have studied the process of sensitization of the trigeminovascular system that occurs in migraine. They have shown that early in the activation of peripheral trigeminovascular fibers, headache typically adopts a throbbing quality, reflecting the sensitization of these peripheral trigeminal fibers to the mechanical stimulation of the rhythmically pulsing dural vessels. This peripheral sensitization is presumably the result of inflammatory mediators, perhaps released from brain by CSD, or by histamine or other mediators following degranulation of dural mast cells. When migraine attacks are prolonged beyond 1 hour, approximately two thirds of migraineurs will describe the onset of marked scalp or periorbital skin sensitivity to otherwise innocuous tactile stimuli. This cutaneous allodynia is a reflection of central sensitization of second-order trigeminal afferent neurons in the nucleus caudalis whose activity is now independent of trigeminal input. These activated nucleus caudalis neurons receive convergent input from trigeminal fibers innervating the scalp and facial skin to which they are now hyperresponsive. With further prolongation of a migraine attack, some patients describe development of allodynia on extracranial cutaneous locations such as the arm. These expansions of allodynic sensory fields likely reflect the convergence of sensory afferent systems from both the arm and dura on centrally sensitized third-order nociceptive neurons within the ventroposterolateral and ventroposteromedial nuclei of the thalamus.

The molecular site(s) of action of triptans in the acute relief from migraine symptoms has been a matter of controversy. $5HT_{1b}$ receptors are located on smooth muscle cells of dural vessels, where their activation by triptan agonists leads to vasoconstriction. $5HT_{1d}$ and $5HT_{1f}$ are located on trigeminal fibers (generally presynaptically in the brain stem), where their activation by triptan agonists leads to reduced trigeminal activity and blockade of plasma protein extravasation, but not vasoconstriction of dural vessels. A $5HT_{1f}$-selective triptan with no vasoconstrictive activity has been found to have antimigraine efficacy in phase II trials, implying that vasoconstriction of dural vessels is not an obligate action of triptans in relieving migraine symptoms. $5HT_{1d}$ and $5HT_{1f}$ are also found at several sites within the brain stem, where they could be activated by triptans that are brain-permeable. Burstein and colleagues have shown that triptans, whether they are brain-permeable or not, are essentially ineffective when administered after allodynia and central sensitization have developed during migraine attacks. They concluded that the crucial site of action of triptans for therapy of migraine symptoms is on peripheral trigeminal afferents.

Brain Stem Mechanisms of Migraine

The second-order nociceptive neurons of the nucleus caudalis receive both direct and indirect modulatory input from multiple structures in the brain stem, including the ventrolateral periaqueductal gray matter of the midbrain (PAG), noradrenergic neurons of the locus ceruleus of the pons (LC), the rostral ventromedial nucleus of the medulla (RVM), and the serotoninergic neurons of the nucleus raphe magnus (RM), among others. Some of these inputs likely inhibit and some likely potentiate activity in the nucleus caudalis. For example, the RVM contains both "on-cells" and "off-cells" in terms of their influence on promoting or inhibiting ascending nociceptive afferent inputs. The probable role of the brain stem centers in migraine has been reinforced by PET studies from Diener and colleagues. These studies demonstrate the activation of dorsal midbrain (including PAG) and dorsal pons (likely including LC) structures ipsilateral to migraine headache that persisted after treatment with sumatriptan but were not active between attacks. These same midbrain regions were found to have increased concentrations of non-heme iron (a marker of neurodegeneration) on magnetic resonance studies of individuals with long histories of migraine attacks. Electrical stimulation of this region in some patients has also resulted in the provocation of headache. Collectively, these studies have prompted speculation that the dorsal midbrain and pons contains a migraine "generator." While this interpretation is attractive, another possible interpretation would be that these structures are permissive for migraine because of dysfunction in their ability to modulate or dampen ascending nociceptive sensory systems. Either interpretation supports a view that migraine is fundamentally a disorder of sensory processing.

Summary

Available data indicate that both abnormal cortical activity (e.g., CSD) and abnormal brain stem activity (e.g., midbrain/pons modulation of ascending nociceptive input) likely play key roles in the pathophysiology of migraine (Fig. 2–3). Whether or how dysmodulation of sensory systems might influence thresholds for the induction of CSD is unknown. Other endogenous processes may influence or modulate either ascending sensory processing or CSD thresholds as well. For example, the female predominance of migraine and the strong temporal relationship of migraine attacks to fluctuations in hormonal levels (i.e., estrogen and to some extent progesterone) could reflect modulation of either brain stem or cortical processes, or both. Recent data from Brennan and Charles indicate that female rats have lower thresholds to induce CSD, and Moskowitz has shown that ovariectomized female rats have CSD thresholds comparable to male rats. Other endogenous, perhaps bloodborne, substances may influence thresholds for migraine induction as well. Patients with migraine with aura have a significantly higher likelihood of having large potential cardiac right-to-left shunts due to patent foramen ovale or other atrial septal defects. Whether this relationship is causal is not known but may be clarified with ongoing studies of the effect of patent foramen ovale closure on migraine attack frequency. If the relationship is indeed causal, it might well reflect the presence of substances in venous blood capable of provoking CSD.

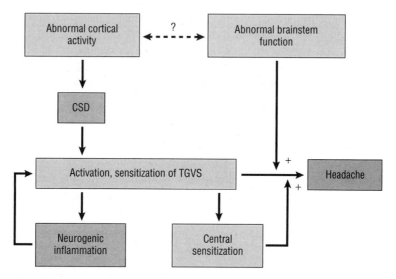

Figure 2–3 Hypothetical schema for integration of cortical, brain stem, and trigeminovascular mechanisms in the generation of migraine. See text for details. (Reprinted by permission from Macmillan Publishers Ltd: *Nat Rev Neurosci* 4:386–398, Copyright 2003)

The genesis of migraine remains an enigma. At its root, migraine is a condition marked by spontaneous pain and associated symptoms that prompt profound behavioral consequences, including prolonged withdrawal from social interactions. Elizabeth Loder has pointed out that the exceptionally high prevalence of this syndrome among women of childbearing age begs the question of whether migraine has been retained due to adaptive evolutionary benefit. The potential evolutionary advantages of a number of other pain conditions are readily apparent: for example, nociceptive pain protects us from injury. What might migraine protect us from? One possibility is that early human fecundity was enhanced by the withdrawal of women from social interactions at the time of menses, thereby reducing the probability of nonprocreative sexual intercourse and/or detection by predators.

CLUSTER HEADACHE

Cluster headache is an episodic primary headache disorder characterized by four cardinal features:

1. It is widely appreciated to be perhaps the most severe pain condition known to humans. The pain is typically boring, periorbital or otherwise localized to the dermatome of the ophthalmic division of the trigeminal nerve, and without variation in location from attack to attack.

2. It occurs in relatively brief episodes (mean less than 1 hour, but between 15 and 180 minutes) often with highly predictable timing. In particular individuals, attacks will occur daily or nearly daily, for up to eight attacks per day, often occurring at the same times each day and typically during sleep. These daily attacks will also occur during periods lasting from weeks to a few months, and these periods will often recur on an annual or biannual basis during the same seasons, which are often perisolsticial.

3. Cluster attacks are associated with dramatic autonomic features ipsilateral to the pain, including increased conjunctival injection, rhinorrhea, facial sweating, lacrimation, partial Horner's syndrome, and periorbital edema.

4. Attacks are associated with restlessness or agitation.

As with the clinical features of migraine, any comprehensive theory of cluster headache pathogenesis will need to account for these cardinal features.

Genetics

Cluster headache has a population prevalence of 0.5%, with a male:female predominance of approximately 3:1. First-degree relatives of patients with cluster headache have approximately a 17-fold higher risk of also having the disorder. Five monozygotic twin pairs have been described with 100% concordance. Association studies from Italy and Germany have found increased odds ratios of 6.79 and 1.97 respectively for cluster headache and the G1246A polymorphism in the HCRTR2 gene that codes for the orexin-2 receptor. This association was not observed in a third large cohort from northern Europe. The potential further significance of orexinergic systems in cluster headache will be reviewed below.

Brain Mechanisms

The understanding of the pathophysiology of cluster headache was dramatically advanced over the past decade by the imaging studies of Goadsby and colleagues. PET imaging studies demonstrated focal activation during cluster attacks of a small region ipsilateral to the headache pain within the posteromedial inferior diencephalon that has been typically interpreted as being a hypothalamic structure but may actually lie within the thalamus. Voxel-weighted T1 magnetic resonance imaging studies have identified this same region as having a higher tissue density. On the basis of this anatomic localization, Leone and colleagues have applied deep brain stimulation to this region in patients with intractable chronic cluster headache, often resulting in dramatic amelioration of symptoms.

The nature of this diencephalic structure has been the focus of much speculation. The level of resolution of these imaging studies makes precise identification of the involved nuclei impossible for such small structures.

Hypothalamic mechanisms have long been hypothesized for cluster headache. Levels of a number of hormones under hypothalamic influence have been reported to be abnormal in cluster headache patients, including melatonin, testosterone, beta-endorphin, prolactin, beta-lipotropin, growth hormone, and cortisol. Moreover, the suprachiasmatic nucleus located in the anterior hypothalamus is the site of the brain's master pacemaker neurons that regulate human circadian rhythms.

One very attractive candidate for this diencephalic structure in cluster headache is the group of neurons in the perifornical region of the hypothalamus that contain orexins as neurotransmitters. Orexins are two peptides derived from a common preprohormone, hypocretin. Orexin A is 34 amino acids and orexin B is 28 amino acids. Two g protein-coupled receptors bind the orexins: orexin-1 receptor binds orexin A, and orexin-2 receptor binds orexin A and orexin B. Orexinergic neurons project to a wide variety of neural structures previously implicated in mechanisms of migraine, including locus ceruleus, raphe nuclei, cerebral cortex, and autonomic structures such as the nucleus tractus solitarius and the intermediolateral cell column of the spinal cord. Moreover, orexinergic neurons are lost in narcolepsy, a disorder characterized by symptoms of loss of coordinated circadian brain state boundaries, including sleep and waking. They are also markedly diminished in multiple system atrophy, a condition of autonomic failure. Orexin A concentrations are increased in the cerebrospinal fluid (CSF) of patients with restless leg syndrome. Orexin B applied to rat hypothalamus potentiates trigeminal responses to dural stimulation or noxious facial stimulation, whereas orexin A has the opposite effect. Activation of the orexin-1 receptor produces analgesic effects in the rat formalin test. Could cluster headache, a condition characterized by extreme pain, autonomic hyperactivity, and motor restlessness and governed by strict timing, be a condition of transient orexinergic hyperactivity? Measurements of CSF orexins during cluster headache attacks and pathologic examination of the brains of cluster headache patients should answer this question.

An alternative diencephalic structure has been proposed by Clifford Saper as the region of increased metabolic activity and hypertrophy in cluster headache: the subparafascicular nucleus of the thalamus. This small structure notably contains CGRP neurons with widespread projections to other regions, including the amygdala, which might relate to mechanisms of the affective nature of pain.

The autonomic manifestations of cluster headache are likely a consequence of an imbalance in autonomic tone, with parasympathetic hyperactivity (e.g., increased lacrimation, rhinorrhea, conjunctival injection, periorbital edema) combined with sympathetic hypoactivity (e.g., miosis, ptosis) and possibly sympathetic hyperactivity (e.g., sweating). Activation of cranial parasympathetic fibers is implicated as in migraine, and the possibility of compromise of postganglionic sympathetic fibers due to marked vasodilation of the ipsilateral carotid artery has been proposed as well, though the latter mechanism carries little empiric support. Moskowitz has proposed that the anatomic convergence of sympathetic, parasympathetic, and ophthalmic division trigeminal nerve fibers within the cavernous sinus implicates this region as a focal site of cluster headache pathophysiology. However, conventional magnetic resonance imaging of this region during cluster periods has been normal, and the basis for the excruciating pain of cluster headache remains unexplained. The mobilization of both trigeminal and cranial parasympathetic nerves in cluster headache is also supported by the detection of elevated levels of CGRP and VIP in plasma following cluster attacks.

SUMMARY

Cluster headache is a relatively uncommon disorder with prominent nociceptive, autonomic, biorhythmic, and motor manifestations. Diencephalic mechanisms are certainly involved, as evidenced by imaging studies. Further progress in understanding the pathophysiology of this disorder can be expected over the next few years with the likely identification of the functions of these diencephalic structures.

Study Questions

1. Genes for familial hemiplegic migraine have been identified at all of the following chromosomal loci except:
   a. 1q21
   b. 8p11
   c. 2q24
   d. 19p13
2. Identified FHM mutations have been found in genes for membrane channels or pumps regulating all of the following ions except:
   a. Magnesium
   b. Potassium
   c. Calcium
   d. Sodium
3. All of the following have been proposed to increase susceptibility to hemiplegic migraine except:
   a. Mutations in the CACNA1A gene produce a pathologic gain of function.
   b. Mutations in the SCN1A gene produce a pathologic gain of function.
   c. Mutations in the ATP1A2 gene produce a pathologic gain of function.
   d. Mutations in the GLAST gene produce a pathologic loss of function.
4. All of the following statements are true regarding serotonin and migraine except:
   a. Urine metabolites of serotonin rise during migraine attacks.
   b. Intravenous serotonin can relieve migraine attacks.

    c. Some drugs that deplete serotonin can trigger migraine-like attacks.

    d. Drugs that antagonize $5HT_{1b/1d/1f}$ receptors can relieve migraine attacks.

5. Data from all of the following provide evidence in favor of CSD constituting the physiologic event underlying migraine aura except:

    a. fMRI BOLD imaging during human migraine aura

    b. R192Q CACNA1A knock-in mutant mice with lower thresholds for inducing CSD

    c. Surface electroencephalograms recorded during human migraine aura

    d. Migraine prophylactic pharmaceuticals suppressing spontaneous CSD in mice

6. All of the following statements provide evidence in favor of a midbrain role in the pathophysiology of migraine except:

    a. PET studies show activation in the dorsal PAG during migraine.

    b. MR studies have found non-heme iron deposition in the midbrain of patients with long histories of migraine.

    c. Electrical stimulation of the midbrain can provoke headache.

    d. Mutant mice lacking a midbrain have lower thresholds for CSD.

7. All of the following are true regarding the genetics of cluster headache except:

    a. First-degree relatives of cluster headache patients have an ~50-fold increased risk of developing cluster headache compared to the general population risk.

    b. Among monozygotic twin pairs reported to date, there is a 100% concordance for expression of cluster headache.

    c. Mutations in the orexin-2 receptor have been associated with increased risk for cluster headache.

    d. The ratio of men to women cluster headache patients is approximately 3:1.

8. All of the following statements regarding the hypothalamus and cluster headache are true except:

    a. The suprachiasmatic nucleus of the hypothalamus contains master pacemaker neurons that regulate human circadian rhythms.

    b. PET studies of cluster headache patients demonstrate suprachiasmatic nucleus activation ipsilateral to the painful side of the head.

    c. Voxel-weighted morphometry magnetic resonance images of cluster headache patients demonstrate hypertrophy of diencephalic structures ipsilateral to the painful side of the head.

    d. Some cluster headache patients have circadian alterations in melatonin, testosterone, prolactin, and cortisol levels.

9. The following statements about autonomic function and cluster headache attacks are all true except:
   a. Postganglionic cranial parasympathetic nerves release vasoactive intestinal polypeptide.
   b. Activation of cranial parasympathetic nerves can result in increased lacrimation, conjunctival injection, and rhinorrhea.
   c. Cranial parasympathetic preganglionic nerves for lacrimation arise in the superior salivatory nucleus.
   d. Activity of cranial preganglionic sympathetic nerves may be compromised by carotid dilatation to result in miosis and ptosis.

10. Functional brain imaging studies have demonstrated activation in all of the following conditions except:
    a. Dorsal pons ipsilateral to head pain in cluster headache
    b. Dorsal pons ipsilateral to head pain in migraine
    c. Diencephalon ipsilateral to head pain in cluster headache
    d. Occipital cortex during cortical spreading depression

10. a
9. d
8. b
7. a
6. c
5. c
4. d
3. c
2. a
1. b

SUGGESTED READING

Burstein, R., Collins, B., & Jakubowski, M. Defeating migraine pain with triptans: A race against the development of cutaneous allodynia. *Annals of Neurology* 55 (2004): 19–26.

Colson, N.J., Fernandez, F., Lea, R.A., & Griffiths, L.R. The search for migraine genes: An overview of current knowledge. *Cellular Molecular Life Sciences* 64 (2007): 331–344.

Dalkara, T., Zervas, N.T., & Moskowitz, M.A. From spreading depression to the trigeminovascular system. *Neurologic Sciences* 27 (2006): S86–S90.

Edvinsson, L. Aspects on the pathophysiology of migraine and cluster headache. *Pharmacology Toxicology* 89 (2001): 65–73.

Goadsby, P.J. Pathophysiology of cluster headache: a trigeminal autonomic cephalgia. *Lancet Neurology* 1 (2002): 251–257.

Goadsby, P.J. Can we develop neurally acting drugs for the treatment of migraine? *Nature Reviews Drug Discovery* 4 (2005):741–750.

Goadsby, P.J. Recent advances in understanding migraine mechanisms, molecules and therapeutics. *Trends in Molecular Medicine* 13 (2006): 39–44.

Moskowitz, M.A., Bolay, H., & Dalkara, T. Deciphering migraine mechanisms: Clues from familial hemiplegic migraine genotypes. *Annals of Neurology* 55 (2004):276–280.

Pietrobon, D., & Striessnig, J. Neurobiology of migraine. *Nature Reviews Neuroscience* 4 (2003): 386–398.

Russell, M.B. Genetics in primary headaches. *Journal of Headache Pain* 8 (2007): 190–195.

3

The Epidemiology and Burden of Headaches

Marcelo E. Bigal, MD, PhD, and Richard B. Lipton, MD

Although almost everyone gets occasional headaches, particular headache disorders vary in incidence, prevalence, duration, and consequent impact (Table 3–1). Headache disorders are divided into primary and secondary disorders. Secondary disorders have an identifiable underlying cause, such as an infection, a brain tumor, or stroke. In primary headache disorders, there is no apparent underlying cause.

Recurrent headache disorders impose a substantial burden on headache sufferers and on society. Epidemiologic studies are used to estimate the frequency, distribution, and burden of disease in the population. Widely used measures of disease frequency include incidence and prevalence. Incidence quantifies the number of new events or cases of disease that develop in a population over a defined period of time. Prevalence refers to the proportion of a population that has the disease over a given period of time. Prevalence is an important measure of the burden of disease.

In this chapter, we will review the epidemiology and burden of headaches, with an emphasis on migraine. We focus on migraine because this is probably the most important primary headache disorder from the perspective of societal burden. We follow by briefly discussing the epidemiology and impact of tension-type headache and of cluster headache.

EPIDEMIOLOGY OF MIGRAINE

Epidemiologic studies focus on the incidence and prevalence of disease in defined populations. Incidence refers to the rate of onset of new cases of a disease in a given population over a defined period. Prevalence is defined as the proportion of a given population that has a disease over a defined period. Prevalence is determined by the average incidence and average duration of disease.

Incidence of Migraine

The incidence of migraine has been investigated in a limited number of studies. Using the reported age of migraine onset from a prevalence study, Stewart and colleagues found that in females the incidence of migraine with aura peaked

Table 3–1 Lifetime Prevalence of Primary and Secondary Headaches

Type (%)	Prevalence
Primary	
Tension-type headache	78
Migraine	16
Secondary	
Fasting	19
Nose/sinus disease	15
Head trauma	4
Nonvascular intracranial disease	0.5
(brain tumor and other disorders)	

between ages 12 and 13 (14.1/1,000 person-years); migraine without aura peaked between ages 14 and 17 (18.9/1,000 person-years). In males migraine with aura peaked in incidence several years earlier, around 5 years of age at 6.6/1,000 person-years; the peak for migraine without aura was 10/1,000 person-years between 10 and 11 years. New cases of migraine were uncommon in men in their 20s (Fig. 3–1). From these data, we can conclude that migraine begins earlier in males than in females and that migraine with aura begins earlier than migraine without aura.

A study performed in a random sample of young adults (21–30 years) found that the incidence of migraine was 5.0 per 1,000 person-years in males and 22.0 in females, supporting the findings reported above.

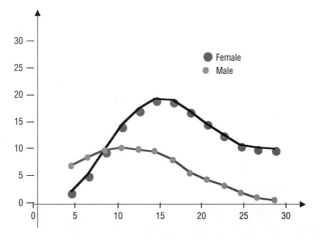

Figure 3–1 Incidence of migraine, by age and sex. (From Stewart et al, 1993)

In the Danish population, the annual incidence of migraine in those aged 25 to 64 years old was 8/1,000 (15/1,000 in males and 3/1,000 in females). Prevalence peaked in younger women (20/1,000). As we are going to discuss below, the gap between peak incidence in adolescence and peak prevalence in middle life indicates that migraine is a condition of long duration.

More recently, Stewart and colleagues used age of onset of migraine, derived from the American Migraine Prevalence and Prevention Study (AMPP, $n = 193,477$) to estimate migraine incidence. Regression-based methods were used to account for systematic errors in underreporting. Two methods were used to estimate age-specific incidence. First, the "naïve method" is based on the assumption that there is no systematic bias in reporting age of onset or errors in underreporting among inactive cases. The second method assumes that these errors occur and uses a statistical model to adjust for their effect on estimates. This method assumes that the probability of error depends on how long ago the event occurred and makes use of patterns in the data by current age and reported duration of time with migraine. The median age of onset using the naïve method was 19 for males and 20 for females (Fig. 3–2a). The cumulative lifetime incidence was 7.4% for males and 21% for females. In contrast, the median age of onset for migraine in the model-based estimates is 23.0 for males and 25.3 for females. The cumulative incidence of migraine by age 85 is 18.5% in males and 44.3% in females (see Fig. 3–2b). Based on these findings, it was suggested that migraine is a dynamic state with high rates of both onset and remission.

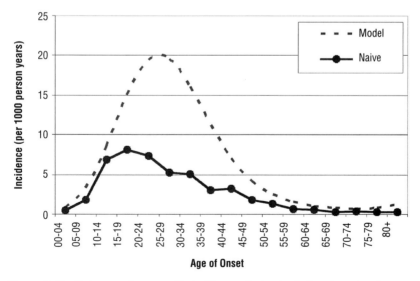

Figure 3–2a Estimates of age-specific incidence of migraine in females using the naïve and model-based estimating procedures.

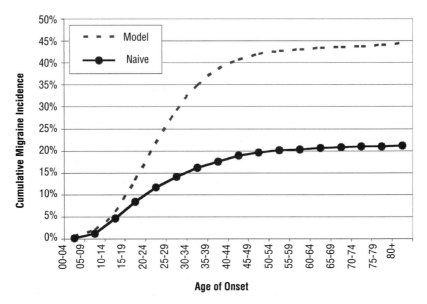

Figure 3–2b Estimates of cumulative incidence of migraine in females using the naïve and model-based estimating procedures.

Prevalence of Migraine

Published estimates of migraine prevalence have varied broadly, probably because of differences in the methodology used.

Before puberty, migraine prevalence is higher in boys than in girls. As adolescence approaches, incidence and prevalence increase more rapidly in girls than in boys. The prevalence increases throughout childhood and early adult life until approximately age 40, after which it declines (Fig. 3–3). Overall, prevalence is highest from 25 to 55, the peak years in terms of economic productivity.

In the United States, three studies assessed the epidemiology of migraine in adults. The American Migraine Study-1 (AMS-1) collected information from 15,000 households representative of the U.S. population in 1989. AMS-II used virtually identical methodology 10 years later. Finally, the American Migraine Prevention and Prevalence study (AMPP) replicated, in its first research phase, the methods of AMS-I and AMS-II. In these three very large studies, the prevalence of migraine was about 18% in women and 6% in men (Fig. 3–4).

Prevalence of Migraine in Children

The prevalence of headache in children has been investigated in a number of school- and population-based studies. By age 3, headache occurs in 3% to 8% of children. At age 5, 19.5% have headaches; by age 7, 37% to 51.5% have headaches. In 7- to 15-year-olds, headache prevalence ranges from 57% to 82%. The prevalence increases from ages 3 to 11 in both boys and girls, with higher headache

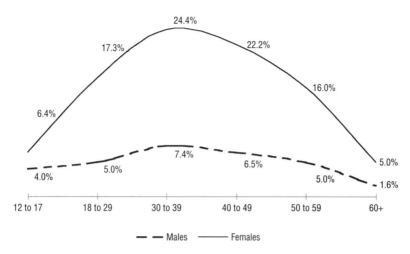

Figure 3–3 One-year period prevalence of migraine by age and gender adjusted for demographics.

prevalence in 3- to 5-year-old boys than in 3- to 5-year-old girls. Thus, the overall prevalence of headache increases from preschool children to mid-adolescence when examined using various cross-sectional studies.

In a recent very large population study (AMPP), a total of 30,215 individuals aged 12 to 19 were identified. The 1-year prevalence for migraine in this age range was 6.3% (5.0% in boys and 7.7% in girls). Table 3–2 displays the crude and adjusted prevalence ratios for several demographic features, stratified by gender. The adjusted prevalence in boys was remarkably stable, ranging from 2.9% to 4.1%; it did not significantly differ in any age. In girls, compared to the age of 12, the prevalence was significantly higher in those at older ages.

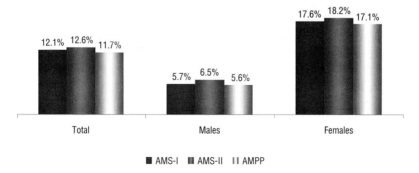

Figure 3–4 Prevalence of migraine in the American Migraine Study (AMS)-1, AMS-2, and American Migraine Prevalence and Prevention Study (AMPP) for total sample and by gender.

Table 3–2 Sex Specific Migraine Prevalence and Prevalence Ratios
in Adolescents: Results from the AMPP study.

	Adjusted Prevalence		Adjusted Prevalence Ratio*	
	Male	Female	Male	Female
Race				
White†	5.1	7.5	1	1
Black	2.6	4.4	0.51 (0.34–0.76)	0.59 (0.44–0.78)
Age				
12†	3.4	3.2	1	1
13	3.6	4.4	1.07 (0.73–1.55)	1.39 (0.95–2.02)
14	4.0	4.6	1.17 (0.82–1.69)	1.45 (1.00–2.09)
15	3.9	6.0	1.16 (0.81–1.67)	1.88 (1.32–2.68)
16	2.9	6.2	0.85 (0.55–1.26)	1.94 (1.37–2.78)
17	4.1	9.8	1.20 (0.83–1.73)	3.09 (2.23–4.26)
18	3.9	7.8	1.16 (0.81–1.67)	2.45 (1.75–3.42)
19	3.2	6.3	0.93 (0.63–1.36)	1.99 (1.40–2.81)
Household Income				
Under $22,500†	5.8	8.1	1	1
$22,500–$39,999	3.5	5.9	0.60 (0.45–0.79)	0.72 (0.57–0.91)
$40,000–$59,999	3.1	6.2	0.53 (0.40–0.72)	0.76 (0.61–0.95)
$60,000–$89,999	3.4	4.8	0.59 (0.45–0.77)	0.59 (0.47–0.75)
$90,000 and Over	2.8	4.4	0.49 (0.36–0.65)	0.54 (0.43–0.67)

† Reference group for Odds Ratio. * Adjusted by age, gender, and sociodemographic features.

For both genders, the prevalence was significantly higher in Caucasians than African Americans.

Prevalence by Race and Geographic Region

Several studies indicate that migraine prevalence varies by race and geographic region. Stewart and colleagues conducted a population-based study in the United States and reported that the lowest prevalence was observed among Asian Americans, intermediate estimates were reported in African Americans, and the highest prevalence estimates were observed among Caucasians, before and after adjusting for demographic covariates. A more recent meta-analysis confirmed these findings: prevalence was lowest in Africa and Asia and higher in Europe and Central/South America. The highest estimates were found in North America.

Since migraine prevalence is low in Africa and Asia and remains low among African Americans and Asians in the United States, it has been hypothesized that there are race-related differences in genetic susceptibility to migraine. However, since the prevalence in Asia is even lower than in the United States, other variables such as environmental risk factors or culturally determined differences in symptom reporting may further explain the international variations.

Prevalence by Socioeconomic Status

In the United States, three very large population-based studies have demonstrated that in the community, migraine prevalence is inversely related to household income: as income or education increased, migraine prevalence declined. This inverse relationship may be explained by two alternative hypotheses. According to the social causation hypothesis, factors associated with low socioeconomic status act to increase disease prevalence. The opposing social selection hypothesis suggests that disease-related dysfunction interferes with educational and occupational functioning, which in turn would lead to low income. Since adolescents make at most a modest contribution to household income, we conducted a population study in this group to address the influence of family income on migraine prevalence. We found that in adolescents with a family history of migraine, household income does not have a significant effect, probably because of the higher biologic predisposition or due to a common stressor event. In those without a strong predisposition, household income is associated with prevalence. This suggests the social causation hypothesis rather than the social selection hypothesis, highlighting the need to explore environmental risk factors related to low income and migraine and to search for specific comorbidities and stressors in this group.

BURDEN OF MIGRAINE

Burden of Migraine to the Individual

Migraine is a public health problem of enormous scope that has an impact on both the individual sufferer and on society. The AMPP, conducted in 2005, estimated that 35 million U.S. residents had migraine headaches, meaning that nearly one in four U.S. households had someone with migraine. Twenty-five percent of women in the United States who had migraine experienced four or more severe attacks a month; 35% experienced one to four severe attacks a month; 38% experienced one, or less than one, severe attack a month. Similar frequency patterns were observed for men.

In the American Migraine Study II, conducted in 2001, 92% of women and 89% of men with severe migraine had some headache-related disability. About half were severely disabled or needed bed rest. In addition to the attack-related disability, many migraineurs live in fear, knowing that at any time an attack could disrupt their ability to work, care for their families, or meet social obligations. Abundant evidence indicates that migraine reduces health-related quality of life.

The results of the American Migraine Study II were confirmed by the AMPP study, the largest epidemiologic study conducted to assess the epidemiology of migraine to date. As a part of the AMPP, more than 160,000 individuals were interviewed. Around 37% of the migraineurs had five or more headache days per month. During migraine attacks, most migraineurs reported severe impairment or the need for bed rest (53.7%); just 7.2% reported no attack-related impairment. Over a 3-month period, 35.1% of the migraineurs had at least 1 day of activity restriction related to headache.

Burden of Migraine to the Family

Because migraine affects women more often than men and is most prevalent between the ages of 25 and 55, the years of childrearing, a substantial impact on family life might be expected. However, of the many studies focusing on the burdens of migraine, relatively few have examined its impact on the families of those directly affected. A Canadian study reported that 90% of people with migraine reported postponing their household work because of headaches, 30% had canceled family and social activities during their last migraine attack, and two thirds feared letting others down because of their headaches. Other studies found that migraine attacks brought significant disruption to family life, with impact on spouses, children, and friends.

In an epidemiologic study conducted in the United Kingdom and the United States, the impact of migraine on family life was assessed from the perspective of those with migraine and from the perspective of their partners. A validated computer-assisted telephone interview (CATI) identified 574 people with migraine from a population sample of 4,007 in mainland England and 568 from 4,376 in Philadelphia in the United States. In a follow-up interview, questions were asked of the proband about the impact of migraine. Similar questions were also asked of the proband's partners regarding the impact of the proband's migraine on participation in social, family, and leisure activities and on family relationships. Of 389 people with migraine living with a household partner, 85% reported substantial reductions in their ability to do household work and chores, 45% missed family social and leisure activities, and 32% avoided making plans for fear of cancellation due to headaches. One half believed that because of their migraine they were more likely to argue with their partners (50%) and children (52%), while majorities (52%–73%) reported other adverse consequences for their relationships with their partner and children, and at work. A third (36%) believed they would be better partners but for their headaches. Participating partners ($n = 100$) partly confirmed these findings: 29% felt that arguments were more common because of headaches and 20% to 60% reported other negative effects on relationships at home. Compared with subjects who did not have migraine regarding their work performance, a statistically significantly higher proportion of migraine partners were unsatisfied with work demands placed on them ($P = 0.02$), with their level of responsibilities and duties ($P = 0.02$), and with their ability to perform ($P = 0.001$). These results suggest that the impact of migraine extends to household partners and other family members.

Societal Impact of Migraine

Migraine has an enormous impact on society. Recent U.S. studies have evaluated both the indirect costs of migraine as well as the direct costs. Indirect costs include the aggregate effects of migraine on productivity at work (paid employment), for household work, and in other roles. The largest component of indirect costs is the productivity losses, which take the form of absenteeism and reduced productivity while at work. Hu and associates estimated that productivity losses due to migraine cost American employers $13 billion per year. These issues have been recently reviewed in more detail elsewhere.

Migraine's impact on healthcare utilization is marked as well. The National Ambulatory Medical Care Survey, conducted from 1976 to 1977, found that 4% of all visits to physicians' offices (over 10 million visits a year) were for headache. Migraine also results in major utilization of emergency rooms and urgent care centers. Vast amounts of prescription and over-the-counter medications are taken for headache disorders. Over-the-counter sales of pain medication (for all conditions) were estimated to be $3.2 billion in 1999 (U.S.), and headaches account for about one third of over-the-counter analgesic use, according to the Consumer Healthcare Products Association (OTC Sales Statistics, 1995–1999, ACNeilsen, April 2000). Gross sales for the triptans are about $1 billion per year in the United States.

Migraine is a lifelong disorder. Bille followed a cohort of children with severe migraine for up to 37 years. As young adults, 62% were migraine-free for more than 2 years, but only 40% continued to be migraine-free after 30 years, suggesting that migraine is often a lifelong disorder. For 15 years, Fry collected information on migraine patients in his general practice in Kent. His data showed a tendency for the severity and frequency of attacks to decrease as the patients got older. After 15 years, 32% of the men and 42% of the women no longer had migraine attacks. Waters noted a similar decrease in migraine prevalence.

EPIDEMIOLOGY OF TENSION-TYPE HEADACHE

Tension-type headache (TTH) is the most prevalent of the primary headaches. It is much more common than migraine, although less disabling and far less frequent in the clinical setting. According to the first studies of Rasmussen, in Denmark the lifetime prevalence of TTH was 69% in men and 88% in women. The 1-year prevalence was respectively 63% and 83%. The male/female ratio was 4:5. The prevalence of episodic TTH decreased with increasing age, and the opposite was seen with chronic TTH.

In the United States, Schwartz and colleagues found that the 1-year prevalence of episodic TTH was 38.3% (33). Women had a higher 1-year episodic TTH prevalence than men in all age, race, and education groups, with an overall prevalence ratio of 1.16. Prevalence peaked in the 30- to 39-year-old age group in both men (42.3%) and women (46.9%). Whites had a higher 1-year prevalence than African Americans in men (40.1% versus 22.8%) and women (46.8% versus 30.9%). Prevalence increased with increasing educational levels in both sexes, peaking in subjects with graduate school educations (48.5% for men and 48.9% for women). The 1-year period prevalence of chronic TTH was 2.2%; the prevalence was higher in women and declined with increasing education. Of subjects with episodic TTH, 8.3% reported lost workdays because of their headaches, while 43.6% reported decreased effectiveness at work, home, or school. Subjects with chronic TTH reported more lost workdays (mean of 27.4 days versus 8.9 days for those reporting lost workdays) and reduced-effectiveness days (mean of 20.4 versus 5.0 days for those reporting reduced effectiveness) compared with subjects with episodic TTH.

The economic impact of TTH is less studied than the impact of migraine. The first population-based study to examine work loss data in episodic TTH was reported by Rasmussen and colleagues in Denmark. Twelve percent of employed participants had been absent from work at least once during the previous year because of episodic TTH. The majority of those who missed work (68%) had been absent for 1 to 7 days during the previous year. Twenty-five percent had been absent between 8 and 14 days during the year, and 16% had been absent more than 14 days during the previous year.

Schwartz and associates also measured the impact of headache in the workplace in a study conducted in Baltimore County, Maryland. Inability to function (actual missed work) and reduced ability to function were measured separately. Of the lost work time associated with headache, 19% of the missed workdays and 22% of the reduced-effectiveness days were specifically due to episodic TTH. Among subjects with episodic TTH, 8.3% reported missed workdays (absenteeism), while 43.6% reported reduced-effectiveness days at work due to headache. Among those with missed workdays, an average of 8.9 missed workdays was reported; subjects with reduced-effectiveness days reported approximately 5.0 reduced-effectiveness days per person. Lavados and Tenhaman found higher levels of missed work among their sample of TTH sufferers: 25% of men and 38.9% of women reported missed work due to their headaches.

The proportions of subjects with chronic TTH and episodic TTH who reported lost and reduced effectiveness days were similar: 11.8% of chronic TTH sufferers reported lost workdays and 46.5% reported reduced-effectiveness days. Chronic TTH sufferers reported more frequent lost workdays and reduced-effectiveness days than episodic TTH sufferers. Subjects with lost workdays reported an average of 27.4 lost workdays per person; subjects with reduced-effectiveness days reported approximately 20.4 reduced-effectiveness days per person.

EPIDEMIOLOGY OF CLUSTER HEADACHE

Cluster headache is the most severe primary headache disorder, although far less common than migraine and TTH. Recent epidemiologic studies indicate that the prevalence of cluster headache is about 0.2%. Genetic epidemiologic surveys indicate that first-degree relatives are 5 to 18 times and second-degree relatives 1 to 3 times more likely to have cluster headache than the general population.

The male/female ratio of cluster headache has been investigated over the years. While the first studies indicated a ratio of 6.2:1 for patients with cluster headache onset before 1960, the ratio fell to 5.6:1, 4.3:1, 3.0:1, and 2.1:1 for patients with cluster headache onset in the 1960s, 1970s, 1980s, and 1990s, respectively.

The impact of cluster headache is enormous. Studies consistently show that it has a higher disability and a higher impact on health-related quality of life than any other primary headache, including migraine and chronic migraine.

Finally, a recent population-based questionnaire study was performed among 224 female cluster headache patients, and the possible effect of hormonal influences on cluster headache attacks was studied. For control data, a similar but adjusted questionnaire was sent to healthy volunteers and migraine patients. It was found that menstruation, use of oral contraceptives, pregnancy, and menopause had a much smaller influence on cluster headache attacks than in migraine. Cluster headache can, however, have a large impact on individual women, for example causing them to refrain from having children.

EPIDEMIOLOGY OF CHRONIC DAILY HEADACHE

Discussing the epidemiology of chronic daily headache in detail is beyond the scope of this chapter. We will focus on chronic daily headache as a syndrome and briefly discuss its subtypes. We use the term "transformed migraine" to refer to the result of migraine progression, in a way analogous to chronic migraine.

The prevalence of chronic daily headache has been surprisingly consistent at about 4% of the adult and elderly population. In children, epidemiologic data are limited and case definitions are variable, but the prevalence of very frequent headache in late childhood and adolescence may approach levels seen in adults. In adulthood, chronic daily headache is about twice as common in women as men, even in elderly populations.

Most people with chronic daily headache have either chronic TTH or transformed migraine headaches, but this also includes rare headache syndromes such as hemicrania continua as well as new daily persistent headache and chronic disorders of short duration. In population studies, chronic TTH and chronic daily headache with migrainous features are equally common. In contrast, the vast majority of chronic daily headache patients in subspecialty care begin with a history of migraine or continue to have migraine features; this has led to the perception that chronic daily headache is a complication of (e.g., mediated through medication overuse) or reflects the natural progression of episodic migraine.

In the population, several risk factors for chronic daily headache have been identified.

Chronic daily headache appears to be more common in individuals with low socioeconomic status. In a U.S. case–control study, the risk was elevated in those with less than a high school education relative to those with a graduate-level education (odds ratio = 3.35 [2.1–5.3]).

Sleep apnea has long been viewed as a headache aggravating factor. This is supported by a case–control study showing that chronic daily headache cases were more likely to be habitual (daily) snorers than episodic headache controls. This association between chronic daily headache and habitual snoring was not explained by cardiovascular factors associated with sleep-disordered breathing (e.g., increasing age, male gender, hypertension, body mass index); nor was it explained by potential confounders such as caffeine consumption, hypertension, or depression.

Stressful life events were associated with chronic daily headache onset in a case–control study. Overall, cases reported more pre-onset events than the controls (2.7 versus 2.0, $P < 0.001$, rank-sum test). No difference was found for post-onset events, strengthening a causal interpretation.

Head and neck injury and high headache frequency have been associated with progression to chronic daily headache.

Obesity, defined as a body mass-index of 30 or more, was predictive of 1-year chronic daily headache incidence in this population. The reason why obesity would predispose individuals to headache progression is uncertain. Subsequent studies have shown that obesity is associated with an increased frequency of attacks among migraineurs, that the prevalence of transformed migraine increases with body mass index, and that the link is between obesity and migraine progression, not with headaches overall.

Scher and colleagues, in a study in the population, showed that in comparison with episodic headache controls, chronic daily headache cases were more likely overall to have been high caffeine consumers before headache onset (odds ratio = 1.50, $P = 0.05$).

SUMMARY

In this chapter, we reviewed the prevalence and burden of primary headaches. For migraine, we emphasized that it is a remarkably common cause of temporary disability. Nonetheless, many migraineurs, even those with disabling headache, have never consulted a physician for the problem. Prevalence is highest in women, in persons between the ages of 25 and 55 years, and, at least in the United States, in individuals from low-income households. Probable migraine is a prevalent form of migraine, and like migraine with and without aura it produces decrements in health-related quality of life and increments in disability relative to control subjects. The emerging evidence that migraine is progressive in a subgroup (evolving to chronic daily headaches) mandates the development of strategies to reduce the risk of progression by addressing modifiable risk factors and by assessing the effects of treatment on headache progression.

Episodic TTH is the most common of the primary headaches, but it is associated with less disability than migraine. Cluster headache is the most disabling of the primary headaches, but it is rare.

Review Questions

1. Regarding the prevalence of migraine, which of the following statements is correct?
    a. After adjustments, the age influence on migraine prevalence is small.
    b. Overall, migraine is twice as common in women than in men.
    c. The prevalence of migraine has been remarkably stable over the past 15 years; there is no evidence of a recent increase in migraine prevalence.
    d. Obesity is a risk factor for migraine. Prevalence is higher in obese than normal-weight migraineurs.
2. Which of the following statements is true?
    a. The incidence of migraine is higher in the female gender at all ages.
    b. The incidence of migraine peaks earlier in boys than in girls.
    c. The incidence of migraine with aura is higher than the incidence of migraine without aura.
    d. None of the above
3. Which of the following statements is false?
    a. Migraine is the most common of the primary headaches.
    b. The burden of migraine affects the individual sufferer, his/her family, and society.
    c. Migraine is a chronic-recurrent disease that sometimes progresses to a state where individuals have headaches on more days than not.
    d. Migraineurs who are obese have a greater chance of developing chronic migraine.
4. Which of the following statements is false?
    a. In the population, most of the chronic daily headaches are associated with medication overuse.
    b. Chronic migraine and chronic tension-type headache are equally prevalent in the population.
    c. The prevalence of chronic migraine is around 2% in the population.
    d. None of the above
5. Which of the following has not been proposed as a risk factor for chronic migraine?
    a. Obesity
    b. Analgesic medication overuse
    c. Caffeine overuse
    d. Male gender

6. Which of the following statements is false?
   a. Episodic tension-type headache is the most prevalent of the primary headaches.
   b. The burden of episodic tension-type headache is almost as important as the burden of migraine.
   c. Tension-type headache is slightly more common in women than in men.
   d. None of the above
7. Which of the following statements is true?
   a. Chronic tension-type headache is less common than chronic migraine in the population.
   b. In the population, chronic tension-type headache is frequently associated with medication overuse.
   c. Chronic tension-type headache usually does not have an impact on the sufferer.
   d. None of the above
8. Which of the following statements is false?
   a. Cluster headache is a rare disease that is associated with extremely severe pain.
   b. Cluster headache is considered to be the most severe of the primary headache disorders.
   c. Cluster headache affects more women than men.
   d. None of the above
9. Which of the following statements is false?
   a. Migraine affects 12% of the adults in the United States.
   b. Chronic daily headaches happen in 2% of the adults in the United States.
   c. Episodic tension-type headache happens in around 40% of the adults in the United States.
   d. None of the above
10. Which of the following statements is true?
    a. The 1-year prevalence of cluster headache is lower than 1%.
    b. Episodic cluster headache is more common than chronic cluster headache.
    c. Cluster headache is more common in men than women.
    d. All of the above

10. d
9. c
8. c
7. d
6. b
5. d
4. a

3. a
2. b
1. c

SUGGESTED READING

Abu-Arefeh, I., & Russell, G. Prevalence of headache and migraine in schoolchildren. *British Medical Journal* 309 (1994): 765–769.

Bigal, M.E., Liberman, J.N., & Lipton, R.B. Obesity and migraine: A population study. *Neurology* Feb 28; 66, no. 4 (2006): 545–550.

Bigal, M.E., & Lipton, R.B. Obesity is a risk factor for transformed migraine but not for chronic tension-type headache. *Neurology* 67 (2006): 252–257.

Bigal, M.E., Lipton, R.B., & Stewart, W.F. The epidemiology and impact of migraine. *Current Neurology Neuroscience Reports* Mar; 4, no. 2 (2004): 98–104.

Bigal, M.E., Lipton, R.B., Winner, P., et al. Epidemiology, burden, and patterns of treatment for adolescents in the United States. *Neurology* 2007 (in press).

Bigal, M.E., Tsang, A., Loder, E., et al. Body mass index and primary headaches. The AMPP study. *Archives of Internal Medicine* 2007 (in press).

Bille B. Migraine in school children. *Acta Paediatrica Scandinavica* 51, Suppl. 136 (1962): 1–151.

Bille B. "Migraine in children: Prevalence, clinical features, and a 30-year follow-up." In: *Migraine and other headaches*, eds. Ferrari, M, & Lataste, X. New Jersey: Parthenon, 1989:29–38.

Bussone, G., Usai, S., Grazzi, L., Rigamonti, A., Solari, A., & D'Amico, D. Disability and quality of life in different primary headaches: results from Italian studies. *Neurologic Science* Oct; 25, Suppl. 3 (2004): S105–107.

Castillo, J., Muñoz, P., Guitera, V., & Pascual, J. Epidemiology of chronic daily headache in the general population. *Headache* 39 (1999): 190–196.

Couch, J., Lipton, R.B., Stewart, W.F., & Lipton, R.B. Head and neck injury as a risk factor for the development of chronic daily headache: A population-based study. *Neurology* 68 (2007): 89.

Ekbom, K., Svensson, D.A., Traff, H., & Waldenlind, E. Age at onset and sex ratio in cluster headache: Observations over three decades. *Cephalalgia* March; 22, no. 2 (2002): 94–100.

Evans, R.W., Lipton, R.B., & Ritz, K.A. A survey of neurologists on self-treatment and treatment of their families. *Headache* Jan; 47, no. 1 (2007): 58–64.

Fry, J. 1996. *Profiles of disease.* Edinburgh: Livingstone.

Goadsby, P.J. Trigeminal autonomic cephalalgias. Pathophysiology and classification. *Review of Neurology (Paris)* July; 161, no. 6–7, (2005): 692–695.

Hazard, E., Serrano, D., Reed, M., Bigal, M.E., Stewart, W.F., & Lipton, R.B. The burden of migraine in the United States. Current and emerging perspectives on disease management and economic analyses (in preparation).

Headache Classification Committee of the International Headache Society. Classification and diagnostic criteria for headache disorders, cranial neuralgias, and facial pain, 2nd ed. *Cephalalgia* 2004 (suppl 1): 1–160.

Hu, X., Markson, L., Lipton, R., Stewart, W., & Berger, M. Burden of migraine in the United States: Disability and economic costs. *Archives of Internal Medicine* 159 (1999): 813–818.

Incidence of migraine headache: a population-based study in Olmstead County, Minnesota. *Neurology* 42 (1992): 1657–1662.

Jensen, R., Lyngberg, A., & Jensen, R. Burden of cluster headache. *Cephalalgia* April 25, 2007 [Epub ahead of print].

Lavados, P.M., & Tenhamm, E. Epidemiology of tension-type headache in Santiago, Chile: A prevalence study. *Cephalalgia* October; 18, no. 8 (1998): 552–558.

Lipton, R., Stewart, W., Diamond, S., Diamond, M., & Reed, M. Prevalence and burden of migraine in the United States: Data from the American Migraine Study II. *Headache* 41 (2001): 646–657.

Lipton, R., Stewart, W., & Simon, D. Medical consultation for migraine: Results of the American Migraine Study. *Headache* 38 (1998): 87–90.

Lipton, R.B., Bigal, M.E., Diamond, M., Freitag, F., Reed, M.L., Stewart, W.F.; AMPP Advisory Group. Migraine prevalence, disease burden, and the need for preventive therapy. *Neurology* Jan. 30; 68, no. 5 (2007): 343–349.

Lipton, R.B., Bigal, M.E., Kolodner, K., Stewart, W.F., Liberman, J.N., & Steiner, T.J. The family impact of migraine: Population-based studies in the USA and UK. *Cephalalgia* July; 23, no. 6 (2003): 429–440.

Lipton, R.B., Bigal, M.E., Steiner, T.J., Silberstein, S.D., & Olesen, J. The classification of the headaches. *Neurology* Aug 10; 63, no. 3 (2004): 427–435.

Lyngberg, A., Jensen, R., Rasmussen, B., & Jorgensen, T. Incidence of migraine in a Danish population-based follow-up study [abstract]. *Cephalalgia* 23 (2003): 596.

MacGregor, E.A., Brandes, J., Eikermann, A., & Giammarco, R. Impact of migraine on patients and their families: the Migraine and Zolmitriptan Evaluation (MAZE) survey—Phase III. *Current Medical Research Opinion* July; 20, no. 7 (2004): 1143–1150.

Mathew, N.T. Drug-induced headache. *Neurology Clinics* 8 (1990):903–912.

Meskunas, C.A., Tepper, S.J., Rapoport, A.M., Sheftell, F.D., & Bigal, M.E. Medications associated with probable medication overuse headache reported in a tertiary care headache center over a 15-year period. *Headache* May;46, no. 5 (2006): 766–772.

Michel, P., Dartigues, J., Duru, G., Moreau, J., Salamon, R., & Henry, P. Incremental absenteeism due to headache in migraine: Results from the Mig Access French national cohort. *Cephalalgia* 19 (1999): 503–510.

Mortimer, J., Kay, J., & Jaron, A. Epidemiology of headache and childhood migraine in an urban general practice using ad hoc, Valquist and IHS criteria. *Developmental Medicine & Child Neurology* 34 (1992): 1095–1101.

Osterhaus, J., Gutterman, D., & Plachetka, J. Healthcare resource and lost labour costs of migraine headache in the U.S. *Pharmacoeconomics* 1 (1992): 67–76.

Raieli, V., Raimondo, D., Cammalleri, R., & Camarda, R. Migraine headaches in adolescents: A student population-based study in Montreal. *Cephalalgia* 15 (1995): 5–12.

Rasmussen, B.K. Epidemiology of headache. *Cephalalgia* 15 (1995): 45–68.

Rasmussen, B.K., & Olesen, J. Epidemiology of migraine and tension-type headache. *Current Opinion in Neurology* June; 7, no. 3 (1994): 264–271.

Scher, A.I., Stewart, W.F., & Lipton, R.B. Prevalence of frequent headache in a population sample. *Headache* 38, no. 7 (1998): 497–506.

Scher, A.I., Stewart, W.F., & Lipton, R.B. "Migraine and headache: A meta-analytic approach." In: *Epidemiology of pain*, ed. Crombie. I.K. Seattle, WA: IASP Press, 1999:159–170.

Scher, A.I., Stewart, W.F., & Lipton, R.B. Caffeine as a risk factor for chronic daily headache: A population-based study. *Neurology* 4; 63, no. 11 (2004): 2022–2027.

Scher, A.I., Stewart, W.F., Ricci, J.A., & Lipton, R.B. Factors associated with the onset remission of chronic daily headache in a population-based study. *Pain* 6 (2003): 81–88.

Schwartz, B.S., Stewart, W.F., Simon, D., & Lipton, R.B. Epidemiology of tension-type headache. *JAMA* Feb 4; 279, no. 5 (1998): 381–383.

Silanpaa, M. Prevalence of migraine and other headache in Finnish children starting school. *Headache* 15 (1976): 288–290.

Silberstein, S.D., Lipton, R.B., & Sliwinski, M. Classification of daily and near-daily headaches: Field trial of revised IHS criteria. *Neurology* 47 (1996): 871–875.

Stang, P.E., Crown, W.H., Bizier, R., Chatterton, M.L., & White, R. The family impact and costs of migraine. *American Journal of Managed Care* May; 10, no. 5 (2004): 313–320.

Stewart, W., Linet, M., Celentano, D., Van Natta, M., & Ziegler, D. Age- and sex-specific incidence rates of migraine with and without visual aura. *American Journal of Epidemiology* 134 (1991): 1111–1120.

Stewart, W., Lipton, R., Celentano, D., & Reed, M. Prevalence of migraine headache in the United States: Relation to age, income, race, and other sociodemographic factors. *JAMA* 267 (1992): 64–69.

Stewart, W.F., Reed, M., Bigal, M.E., & Lipton, R.B. Lifetime migraine incidence. Results from the American Migraine Prevalence and Prevention study. *Headache* 46 (2006): 52.

Stewart, W.F., Scher, A.I., & Lipton, R.B. The Frequent Headache Epidemiology study (FrHE): Stressful life events and risk of chronic daily headache. *Neurology* 56, no. 8 (2001): A138–A139.

Stillman, M. Steroid hormones in cluster headaches. *Current Pain Headache Reports* April; 10, no. 2 (2006): 147–152.

Torelli, P., Beghi, E., & Manzoni, G.C. Cluster headache prevalence in the Italian general population. *Neurology* Feb. 8; 64, no. 3 (2005):469–474.

Von Korff, M., Stewart, W., & Lipton, R. Assessing headache severity: New directions. *Neurology* 44, suppl. 4 (1994): 40–46.

Von Korff, M., Stewart, W., Simon, D., & Lipton, R. Migraine and reduced work performance: A population-based diary study. *Neurology* 50 (1998): 1741–1745.

Waters, W.E. *Headache* (Series in Clinical Epidemiology). Littleton, MA: PSG Co. Inc., 1986.

II

Diagnosis of Primary Headache Disorders

4

International Classification of Headache Disorders and Classification and Diagnosis of Migraine

Morris Levin, MD

In designing a comprehensive and useful headache classification, the largest obstacle is the lack of reliable diagnostic markers for even such thoroughly studied illnesses as migraine. Thus, any diagnostic system must rely on subjective data, which leads to the essentially descriptive approach of all headache classifications to date, including the most recent and best system, the *International Classification of Headache Disorders*, 2nd edition (ICHD-II). This is a limitation of the classification system, but it has become clear that to further our understanding of the headache disorders, we need to divide them into types using some system of classification. To improve upon this system of defining the various headache types, it is important to subject the ICHD-II itself to systematic study. In other words, to learn more about headaches, they must first be separated into more or less discrete categories, then examined with the best tools available; next rearranged into more accurate categories based on evidence accumulated in this way; and then re-examined, in a reiterative process.

Pitfalls easily encountered include the tendency toward "lumping" (making categories too broad) or "splitting" (defining very narrow categories). When categories are too broad, the results of analysis can be all but unusable, since conclusions may be so general as to apply to few individuals or even groups. Tiny categories separated by minute differences would lead to a system far too cumbersome to use. Establishing demarcations between diagnostic categories in the absence of evidence is another challenge. Here, consensus opinions of experts are used, but consensus can be hard to reach. Bearing these obstacles in mind, the ICHD-II has proven reasonably reliable and is dynamic enough to reflect changes in our understanding of the various headache disorders. As a result, an enormous amount of research has been driven by the existence of this useful tool for defining subpopulations in the headache disorders.

This chapter will focus on the format and use of the ICHD in general, and on key areas of the ICHD classification of the spectrum of migraine headaches, both in adults and children. Tables for reference will be highlighted and clinical examples of important diagnostic entities will be presented.

THE HISTORY OF CLASSIFICATION SYSTEMS IN HEADACHE

Thomas Willis, a founder of modern neurologic thought, described headaches, in *De Cephalalgia* in 1672, as "within or without the skull; universal or particular; short, continuous or intermittent; wandering or uncertain; before, behind or the side; and occasional or habitual." Christian Baur in 1787 divided headaches, in a very contemporary-sounding way, into primary headaches ("idiopathic") and secondary headaches ("symptomatic"), with a total of 84 categories.

The first significant modern attempt at classifying headache disorders was done by an ad hoc committee formed by the NIH in 1962. This classification (Table 4–1) consisted of brief, glossary-type definitions of a limited number of headache types. With its relatively vague diagnostic definitions, it required subjective interpretation and relied primarily on accepted ideas of headache diagnostic classes without much in the way of evidence to support them. This classification system, notable for strict differentiation between migraine headaches (pulsatile unilateral headaches with a vascular pathology) and tension headaches (with muscular pathophysiology), became accepted worldwide but by the 1970s began to be seen as more of an impediment to advancing headache understanding than a help.

The International Headache Society (IHS) formed the Classification Committee in 1985, with Dr. Jes Olesen as its chairman. The IHS classification

Table 4–1 Ad Hoc Committee on Classification of Headache of the National Institute of Health. Classification of Headache

1. Vascular Headache
    A. Classic Migraine
    B. Common Migraine
    C. Cluster
    D. Hemiplegic, Ophthalmoplegic Migraine
    E. Lower-Half Headache
2. Muscle Contraction Headache
3. Combined Headache: Vascular and Muscle Contraction Headache
4. Headache of Nasal Vasomotor Reaction
5. Headache of Delusional, Conversion, or Hypochondriacal States
6. Nonmigrainous Vascular Headaches
7. Traction Headache
8. Headache due to Overt Cranial Inflammation
9–13. Headache due to Diseases of Ear, Nose, Sinus, Teeth
14. Cranial Neuritides
15. Cranial Neuralgias

Adapted from Ad Hoc Committee on Classification of Headache of the National Institute of Health. Classification of headache. *JAMA* 179(1962): 717–718.

was published in 1988. It was 96 pages long and consisted of 165 diagnoses. The ICHD-1 unified headache clinicians and researchers around the world, led to a great deal of clinical and basic scientific research, and provided credibility and scientific rigor for the field of headache. In addition, a correspondence to the International Classification of Diseases-10 (ICD-10) of the World Health Organization (WHO) further enabled uniformity and accuracy in diagnosis. (This has not been as helpful in the United States, where ICD-10 is not used to any extent.)

The revision of the IHS's classification was begun in 1999, and the ICHD-II was published in *Cephalalgia* in 2004. The ICHD-II is 160 pages long and contains approximately 200 diagnoses (depending upon what one chooses to call independent illnesses). It can be viewed and downloaded from www.i-h-s.org under "Guidelines."

ICHD-II—Basic Organization

Format

The ICHD-II (now available following several changes as a revision of ICHD—ICHD-2R), like its predecessor, consists of several parts (Table 4–2). In this edition, these comprise the following:

Part 1: Primary headaches
Part 2: Secondary headaches
Part 3: Cranial neuralgias, central and primary facial pain and other
         headache
Appendix.

Part 1, primary headaches, consists of 45 diagnostic categories in Chapters 1 through 4 and includes migraine, tension-type headache, cluster headache and its relatives, and a group of "other primary headaches." These first four groups are considered to have "no other causative disorder."

Part 2, secondary headaches, consists of 120 diagnostic categories in Chapters 5 through 12 and includes headaches "caused by another disorder" such as head trauma, vascular disease, abnormal intracranial pressure, mass lesions, hydrocephalus, and so on. In these chapters we also see headaches due to processes involving a number of structures in and around the head, including the eyes, nose, sinuses, teeth, and neck. In addition there is a brief chapter on headaches presumably caused by psychiatric disorders. As evidence is lacking in this area, postulated psychogenic headaches of other types are contained in the appendix.

Part 3 consists of 29 causes of facial pain or neuralgic illnesses as well as Chapter 14, "empty for now," existing merely as a placeholder for any unclassifiable headache types.

The appendix (Table 4–3) is an interesting collection of diagnoses that are not fully supported by evidence at the time of its writing. These include

Table 4–2 International Classification of Headache Disorders, Second Edition (ICHD-II)

Part 1: Primary headaches, Chapters 1–4 (no other causative disorder)

1. Migraine
2. Tension-type headache
3. Cluster and its relatives (TACs)
4. Other primary headaches — exertional, hemicrania continua, hypnic headache, et al.

Part 2: Secondary headaches, Chapters 5–12 (caused by another disorder)

5. Posttraumatic
6. Vascular disease
7. Other intracranial pathology — including abnormal intracranial pressure, neoplasm, etc.
8. Substances
9. CNS infection
10. Homeostatic disorders — including hypoxia, hypertension, and endocrine dysfunction
11. Cervicogenic, eyes, ENT, sinuses, mouth, teeth, TMJ
12. Psychiatric

Part 3: Cranial neuralgias, central and primary facial pain, other headaches

13. Neuralgias and neuropathy
14. Other headaches (empty for now)

Appendix

Used with permission from the Headache Classification Committee of the International Headache Society. *The International Classification of Headache Disorders*, 2nd edition. *Cephalalgia* 24, Suppl. 1(2004):9–160.

suggested criteria for possible new entities, alternative diagnostic criteria for certain existing categories, and previously accepted disorders with questionable support. The appendix therefore provides fertile ground for research activity aimed at acquiring evidence to firm up, discard, or revise previous definitions for the next ICHD revision.

Decisions about diagnoses and diagnostic criteria of the ICHD were made by the IHS classification subcommittees based on evidence when possible and expert opinion (consensus) when no evidence was available. Definitions for headache disorders are necessarily symptom-based for primary headaches but

Table 4–3 ICHD-II Appendix Contents

1. Suggested criteria for possible new entities
     (e.g., A1.1 Menstrual migraine; A3.3 SUNA)
2. Alternative diagnostic criteria for certain categories (pending evidence)
     (e.g., A2 — two alternative tension - type headache diagnostic criteria)
3. Some previously accepted disorders that have not been supported by evidence
     (e.g., A1.3.4 — Alternating hemiplegia of childhood)

etiology-based for secondary headaches. This will presumably change as etiologies and diagnostic tests for primary headaches become clearer.

In the ICHD, specificity in diagnosis is weighted over sensitivity. Precise inclusion and exclusion criteria for each diagnosis are provided. The classification is hierarchical, with large categories subdivided into smaller categories. A decimal numerical system is used, with finer distinctions to the right of the decimal point. Hence, in the case of ICHD 2.3.1, "Chronic tension-type headache associated with pericranial tenderness," "2" denotes *tension-type headache,* "2.3" denotes *chronic* tension-type headache, and "2.3.1" denotes that this chronic tension-type headache is associated with *pericranial tenderness.* The hierarchical format allows the user to decide how detailed to make the diagnosis, depending on the situation. The Classification Committee felt that in primary care settings, one or two digits of specificity would be useful (e.g., migraine without aura, 1.1), and that for a researcher or specialist, a three-digit diagnosis would be more appropriate (e.g., typical aura with non-migraine, 1.2.2).

In each chapter there is a standard order of information, with an initial general introduction, then discussion of previously used terms and related disorders, followed by a table of explicit diagnostic criteria and finally notes and comments about the particular headache type as necessary (often the most thought-provoking and important part of the section). For a particular diagnosis, all criteria must be fulfilled. At the conclusion of each chapter of the ICHD-II, there is a bibliography for the chapter's topic, with subdivisions by subcategory.

In patients with more than one distinct type of headache, each is coded separately. For example a patient may be coded with 1.1, migraine without aura; 2.1, infrequent episodic tension-type headache; and 3.1, chronic post-traumatic headache. But if a *single* headache type fulfills two different sets of explicit criteria, using other data to decide is recommended, such as the history of the headache onset, family history, menstrual relationship, and so forth. The classification of a patient's headache is based upon his or her current phenomenology, or at least the past 1 year. (This is a bit problematic, since, for example, if there were different headaches in the past [e.g., migraine with aura several years ago], there may be the implication that the patient may have the "trait" for migraine with aura, which could be important both in clinical as well as research settings.)

Secondary headaches (Part 2) should begin to occur close in time to the causative disorder and should go away when the cause is removed. A common problem here is that the cause may not be removable, or that the cause led to permanent changes, such that its removal will not lead to resolution of headaches. For some of these, the ICHD encourages the use of "probable" while this is being sorted out (see below). In clinical practice, of course, the problem is reversed: secondary headaches must always be considered and all possibilities ruled out before migraine or other primary headache treatment can be started.

Nomenclature in the ICHD-II

The ICHD has carefully defined a number of terms. *Chronic* refers to frequency for some of the primary headache disorders; for instance, "chronic migraine" and "chronic tension-type headache" occur on more than 50% of days. But in cluster headache and paroxysmal hemicrania, "chronic" denotes the pattern of continuous vulnerability to individual attacks (e.g., "chronic cluster," which does not remit) as opposed to the more typical recurring cluster or hemicrania cycles (*episodic*). And finally, as is typical in other pain terminology, "chronic" denotes the duration of the problem for some secondary headaches (e.g., greater than 3 months for chronic posttraumatic headache).

Aura is used for the well-described brief pre-headache symptoms of migraine with aura and *premonitory symptoms* for the 2- to 48-hour-long symptoms of forewarning before a migraine. "Prodrome" and "warning symptoms" are not used in the ICHD.

Probable is the term used in the ICHD to indicate that all but one criterion has been met for a particular diagnosis. For example, if a patient has recurrent headaches that meet all but one of the four basic criteria (A through D) for migraine, the diagnosis 1.6, "probable migraine," is used.

Attributed to replaces the *associated with* phrase used for secondary headaches in ICHD-I to imply there is a causal link between the underlying disorder and the headache. As stated above, the difficulty in proving causality will lead to frequent *probable* secondary headache diagnoses. All of the primary headache criteria include the requirement that the headache not be attributed to another disorder. Thus, in patients where there is doubt, two diagnoses may be best—a probable primary headache disorder as well as a probable secondary headache.

DIAGNOSIS OF MIGRAINE AND ITS RELATIVES

Migraine diagnosis depends on a relatively complex set of criteria (Table 4–4). In practice the diagnosis is not difficult, but a number of migraine patients will probably receive the "probable migraine" diagnosis if the ICHD criteria are applied strictly. Commonly reported migraine accompaniments such as nausea and light and sound sensitivity are expected criteria, but other ICHD requirements like exercise intolerance, pulsation, and unilaterality are thought by many to be much less significant clues. Moderate or severe pain intensity is rather broad and the requirement for both photo- and phono-sensitivity seems rather stringent to some. An interesting contrast to the strict use of the ICHD migraine classification is a clever shortcut to migraine diagnosis arrived at by Lipton and his colleagues after analyzing migraine patients' reporting of various historical features. This tool, ID Migraine™, is a three-question survey concerning the presence of nausea, photophobia, and disability. If a patient admits to at least two of these three features, there is a very high likelihood of an ICHD diagnosis of migraine (93%).

Table 4–4 ICHD-II 1.1, Migraine Without Aura

A. At least 5 attacks fulfilling criteria B–D
B. Headache attacks lasting 4–72 hours (untreated or unsuccessfully treated)
C. Headache has at least two of the following characteristics:
   1. Unilateral location
   2. Pulsating quality
   3. Moderate or severe pain intensity
   4. Aggravation by or causing avoidance of routine physical activity (*e.g.,* walking or climbing stairs)
D. During headache at least one of the following:
   1. Nausea and/or vomiting
   2. Photophobia and phonophobia
E. Not attributed to another disorder

Used with permission from the Headache Classification Committee of the International Headache Society. *The International Classification of Headache Disorders,* 2nd edition. *Cephalalgia* 24, Suppl 1(2004):9–160.

The "migraine with aura" category 1.2 includes the odd-sounding "aura with migraine," "aura with non-migraine," and "aura without headache" (Tables 4–5 and 4–6). The goal was to allow for a patient with typical aura but whose headache type otherwise did not meet migraine criteria. Thus, it is possible to assign 2.1, "tension-type headache," and 1.2.2, "aura with non-migraine" to the same patient. Some would consider the aura proof of migraine pathophysiology, and hence this begs the question of whether the migraine criteria are too strict. However, a number of clinical reports document auras in patients with non-migraine headaches, including cluster, hemicrania continua, chronic paroxysmal hemicrania, and hypnic headache. Only approximately 20% of patients with migraine experience clear aura symptoms, but this may be an underestimate due to lack of reporting of some subtle or less typical aura symptoms.

Migraine auras can take many forms, including positive (scintillations, fortification spectra) and negative (scotomata) visual symptoms, sensory symptoms (paresthesias and/or numbness), and dysphasic speech disturbances. Positive symptoms are more common than negative, and sensory symptoms are much more common than motor symptoms. Aura symptoms should last between 5 and 60 minutes. Auras involving any motor weakness are placed in

Table 4–5 ICHD-II 1.2 Migraine with Aura — Subtypes

1.2.1 Typical aura with migraine headache
1.2.2 Typical aura with non-migraine headache
1.2.3 Typical aura without headache
1.2.4 Familial hemiplegic migraine (FHM)
1.2.5 Sporadic hemiplegic migraine
1.2.6 Basilar-type migraine

Table 4–6 ICHD-II 1.2.1 Typical Aura with Migraine Headache

A. At least 2 attacks fulfilling criteria B–D
B. Aura consisting of at least one of the following, but no motor weakness:
    1. Fully reversible visual symptoms including positive features (*e.g.*, flickering lights, spots, or lines) and/or negative features (*i.e.*, loss of vision)
    2. Fully reversible sensory symptoms including positive features (*i.e.*, pins and needles) and/or negative features (*i.e.*, numbness)
    3. Fully reversible dysphasic speech disturbance
C. At least two of the following:
    1. Homonymous visual symptoms and/or unilateral sensory symptoms
    2. At least one aura symptom develops gradually over ≥5 minutes and/or different aura symptoms occur in succession over ≥5 minutes
    3. Each symptom lasts ≥5 and ≤60 minutes
D. Headache fulfilling criteria B–D for 1.1 Migraine without aura begins during the aura or follows aura within 60 minutes
E. Not attributed to another disorder

Used with permission from the Headache Classification Committee of the International Headache Society. *The International Classification of Headache Disorders*, 2nd edition. *Cephalalgia* 24 Suppl 1(2004):9–160.

the separate "hemiplegic migraine" categories ("familial hemiplegic migraine," 1.2.4, and "sporadic hemiplegic migraine," 1.2.5), with the implication that motor auras are different from other auras, a concept that is certainly not proven.

"Persistent aura without infarction" requires an aura to persist longer than a week. "Migrainous infarction" occurs when an aura symptom lasts longer than 60 minutes *and* imaging (MRI or CT) reveals an infarction in the appropriate territory. Persistent aura symptoms without visible stroke are puzzling and should probably lead to further workup for occult vascular, inflammatory, or other pathology. Migraine-triggered seizure is supposed to occur within 1 hour after a migraine aura (Table 4–7).

As stated above, migraine-like headaches that meet all criteria save one are best termed "probable migraine." Ophthalmoplegic migraine, once thought to be a primary headache, is now relegated to the neuralgia section (13.17) based on suggestive clinical and radiologic evidence that the entity is more closely related to neuralgic syndromes. Basilar "type" migraine and retinal migraine are listed in the migraine chapter, however. Basilar migraine should have symptoms and/or signs suggestive of the posterior cerebral circulation, such as bilateral visual symptoms, dysarthria, vertigo, hearing loss, diplopia, or ataxia (Table 4–8). There is controversy as to whether these patients truly represent a clinical or pathophysiologic entity distinct from migraine with aura. Retinal migraine, of course, requires symptoms referable to one eye.

Primary chronic daily headache, defined as headaches on 15 or more days per month (not due to underlying systemic or cranial pathology), is clearly an

Table 4–7 Complications of Migraine (ICHD-II)

1.5.1 Chronic migraine
1.5.2 Status migrainosus
1.5.3 Persistent aura without infarction
1.5.4 Persistent aura without infarction
1.5.5 Migrainous infarction

important public health problem with a surprisingly high prevalence—probably 4% worldwide. This category consists of a mixture of several disorders, including a chronic form of migraine, chronic tension-type headache, hemicrania continua, and new daily persistent headache (NDPH).

The ICHD definition for chronic migraine, 1.5.1, requires that all headaches meet the criteria for migraine. Many have objected to this requirement for chronic migraine since it does not include patients who seem to have evolved from experiencing intermittent migraines to a condition with more frequent but less "migrainous" headaches. This condition was initially termed "transformed migraine" by Mathew in 1982 and was included by Silberstein and Lipton in their commonly accepted classification of chronic daily headache (CDH), which included four basic types of CDH: transformed migraine,

Table 4–8 ICHD-II 1.2.6 Basilar-Type Migraine

A. At least 2 attacks fulfilling criteria B–D
B. Aura consisting of at least two of the following fully reversible symptoms, but no motor weakness:
    1. Dysarthria
    2. Vertigo
    3. Tinnitus
    4. Hypacusia
    5. Diplopia
    6. Visual symptoms simultaneously in both temporal and nasal fields of both eyes
    7. Ataxia
    8. Decreased level of consciousness
    9. Simultaneously bilateral paresthesias
C. At least one of the following:
    1. At least one aura symptom develops gradually over ≥5 minutes and/or different aura symptoms occur in succession over ≥5 minutes
    2. Each aura symptom lasts ≥5 and ≤60 minutes
D. Headache fulfilling criteria B–D for 1.1 Migraine without aura begins during the aura or follows aura within 60 minutes
E. Not attributed to another disorder

Used with permission from the Headache Classification Committee of the International Headache Society. *The International Classification of Headache Disorders*, 2nd edition. *Cephalalgia* 24 Suppl 1(2004):9–160.

**Table 4–9 Proposed Appendix Criteria for a Revised Chronic Migraine
            Category**

A. Headache on 15 or more days each month
B. Diagnosis of Migraine without aura 1.1
C. 8 or more headaches per month meeting criteria for 1.1 Migraine without aura or
   1.2 Migraine with aura, or responsive to migraine-specific medication before
   complete migraine symptomatology develops
D. No medication overuse headache, no chronic tension-type headache, no cluster
   headache, no new daily persistent headache
E. No underlying pathology

Used with permission from the Headache Classification Committee, Olesen, J., Bousser, M-G.,
Diener, H-C., et al. New appendix criteria open for a broader concept of chronic migraine.
Cephalalgia 26(2004):742–747.

chronic tension-type headache, new daily persistent headache, and hemicrania
continua. (See Chapter 5 for a more detailed discussion of CDH.)

The American Headache Society proposed a revised category of chronic
migraine in an attempt to include these patients, with the softened requirement
that only the majority of headaches must meet strict migraine criteria or
respond to migraine-specific medication. The IHS Classification Committee
agreed to include this set of criteria as an appendix diagnosis (Table 4–9).

Status migrainosis 1.5.2, which refers to the uncommon condition of persistent migraine without abatement for at least 72 hours, also requires that the
migraine criteria be met. Here the requirement seems sensible, but the longer the
migraine persists unabated, the more likely some migrainous features will fade,
so here too there may be unnecessary stringency in applying migraine criteria.

Pure menstrual migraine (PMM) and menstrually related migraine (MRM)
are in the appendix (A1.1.1, A1.1.2). Some have recommended including these
subtypes of triggered migraine in the migraine chapter proper.

Three childhood "migraine" syndromes exist in the ICHD-II migraine chapter, ostensibly because they are thought to be precursors of migraine. These
include 1.3.1, cyclical vomiting (spells of nausea and vomiting up to 5 days in
duration), 1.3.2, abdominal migraine (recurrent abdominal pain with varying
degrees of nausea in school-age children), and 1.3.3, benign paroxysmal vertigo
(Table 4–10).

Table 4–10 Childhood Migraine Syndromes

Diagnosis	Nausea&Vomiting	Abd Pain	Vertigo	Duration
Cyclic vomiting	+			1 hr.–5 days
Abdominal migraine	+/–	+		1–72 hr.
Benign paroxysmal vertigo of childhood	+		+	Mins.–hrs.

SUMMARY

The ideal headache classification would be specific, hierarchical, supported by scientific evidence, intuitive, and practical. Unfortunately, the ICHD-II as yet does not fulfill all of these criteria. It is hierarchical, with nesting of diagnostic groups, thereby pleasing both "splitters" and "lumpers." Unfortunately, entities can coexist—like different subtypes of migraine or migraine and tension-type headache, which is not intellectually satisfying. The ICHD-II primary headache portion is really a classification of current headache features rather than of syndromes over time, which is also not entirely satisfactory for certain purposes. Rules are for the most part logical, but not always intuitive. This, as well as the sheer size of the ICHD, makes ease of use a goal rather than a reality. Practicality is arguably the ICHD's biggest shortfall, particularly the primary headache portion. The number of possible diagnoses and diagnostic criteria make use in clinical settings often too time-consuming for most practices, unless single-digit diagnoses are acceptable. Arbitrariness in diagnostic criteria raises concerns when the ICHD is used in research. This, of course, ironically includes those studies designed to add refinement to the ICHD.

However, the ICHD-II must still be considered one of the most important publications in clinical neurology of the past several years. As noted before, it has led to far deeper understanding and authentification of many head and face pain conditions. Moreover, the ICHD-II provides a vehicle for much-needed further study of headaches. This is particularly true for the primary headaches, many of which remain more or less mysterious in terms of etiology, pathophysiology, and treatment.

Review Questions

1. Which is true of the ICHD-II?
   a. Sensitivity is weighted over specificity.
   b. Some primary headaches can be due to known intracranial pathology.
   c. ICHD-II has been linked to ICD9.
   d. Chapter 14 is empty.
2. In the ICHD-II, "chronic" can imply any of the following except:
   a. Lack of remission
   b. Duration of more than 3 months
   c. Intractability
   d. High frequency
3. The appendix of the ICHD-II contains all but:
   a. Disproven headache categories
   b. Suggested criteria for proposed new diagnoses
   c. Previously accepted definitions with questionable support
   d. Alternate criteria for known disorders

4. Which of the following is not a typical aura symptom according to ICHD-II?
   a. Paresthesias
   b. Paresis
   c. Dysphasia
   d. Scintillations

5. Ophthalmoplegic migraine is considered to be most closely related to:
   a. Retinal migraine
   b. Migraine with aura
   c. Hemiplegic migraine
   d. Neuralgia

6. A 45-year-old woman with a long-term history of migraine with aura calls due to persistent patchy left-sided numbness lasting 9 days after her migraine began. The headache lasted only 8 hours. She has no other complaints and an MRI was normal yesterday. The best diagnosis is:
   a. Migrainous infarction
   b. Persistent aura without infarction
   c. Probable migrainous infarction
   d. Status migrainosus

7. An 8-year-old boy has been having episodic moderate to severe abdominal pain accompanied by nausea and occasional vomiting over the past year. His mother describes dizziness and nervousness during these episodes, and recently he had a throbbing headache with one of these episodes. Gastroenterological workup and general exam have been negative. A likely diagnosis at this time is:
   a. Cyclic vomiting
   b. Panic disorder
   c. Celiac disease
   d. Abdominal migraine

8. A 24-year-old graduate student describes recurrent bioccipital or hemicranial headaches accompanied by hemifield visual changes for several years. He occasionally experiences numbness and weakness of the left arm during headache that can last up to 1 hour. A probable diagnosis is:
   a. Migraine with aura
   b. Migrainous infarction
   c. Hemiplegic migraine
   d. Basilar migraine

9. A 35-year-old woman with monthly severe perimenstrual menstrual throbbing headaches accompanied by nausea, blurred vision, photophobia, and phonophobia also has several milder headaches each week, which she treats with acetaminophen–caffeine–aspirin. Which of the following is the best diagnosis?
   a. Migraine without aura
   b. Menstrual migraine

    c. Medication overuse headache

    d. Hormonal headaches

10. A 42-year-old woman describes "headaches on more days than not" for 3 years. There is usually accompanying nausea and she feels best when she goes to a quiet dark room to rest. Previously she had fewer but more severe headaches. The best ICHD diagnosis would be:

    a. Chronic daily headache

    b. Medication overuse headache

    c. Transformed migraine

    d. Chronic migraine

10. d

9. a

8. c

7. d

6. b

5. d

4. b

3. a

2. c

1. d

SUGGESTED READING

Ad Hoc Committee on Classification of Headache of the National Institute of Health. Classification of headache. *JAMA* 179 (1962): 717–718.

Bigal, M.E., Tepper, S.J., Sheftell, F.D., Rapoport, A.M., & Lipton, R.B. Chronic daily headache: Correlation between the 2004 and the 1988 International Headache Society diagnostic criteria. *Headache* 44, no. 7 (2004): 684–691.

Carrera, P., Stenirri, S., Ferrari, M., et al. Familial hemiplegic migraine: An ion channel disorder. *Brain Research Bulletin* 56 (2001): 239–241.

De Fusco, M., Marconi, R., Silvestri, L., et al. Haploinsufficiency of ATP1A2 encoding the Na+/K+ pump alpha2 subunit associated with familial hemiplegic migraine type 2. *Nature Genetics* 33 (2003): 192–196.

Eriksen, M.K., Thomsen, L.L., & Olesen, J. New international classification of migraine with aura (ICHD-2) applied to 362 migraine patients. *European Journal of Neurology* 11, no. 9 (2004): 583–591.

Goadsby, P.J., & Boes, C. New daily persistent headache. *Journal of Neurology, Neurosurgery and Psychiatry* 72 Suppl. 2 (2002):ii6–ii9.

Headache Classification Committee of the International Headache Society. *The International Classification of Headache Disorders*, 2nd edition. *Cephalalgia* 24 Suppl. 1 (2004): 9–160.

Headache Classification Committee, Olesen, J., Bousser, M-G., Diener, H-C., et al. New appendix criteria open for a broader concept of chronic migraine. *Cephalalgia* 26 (2006): 742–747.

International Headache Society Classification Committee. Classification and diagnostic criteria for headache disorders, cranial neuralgias and facial pain. *Cephalalgia* 8, Suppl. 7 (1988): 1–96.

Levin, M. "Classification of primary headaches: Concepts and controversies." In: Headache. *AAN Continuum*. Lifelong Learning Neurology, pp. 32–51, 2006.

Li, D., & Rozen, T.D. The clinical characterisation of new daily persistent headache. *Cephalalgia* 22 (2002); 66–69.

Lipton, R.B., Dodick, D., Sadovsky, R., et al. A self-administered screener for migraine in primary care: The ID Migraine validation study. *Neurology* 61 (2003): 375–382.

Mathew, N.T. Transformed migraine. *Cephalalgia* 13 (1982): 78–83.

Olesen, J., & Rasmussen, B.K. The International Headache Society classification of chronic daily and near-daily headaches: a critique of the criticism. *Cephalalgia* 16 (1996): 407–411.

Pearce, J.M.S. Historical aspects of migraine. *Journal of Neurology, Neurosurgery and Psychiatry* 49 (1986): 1097–1103.

Pearce, J.M.S. Are the International Headache Society criteria for headache useful? *Cephalalgia* 16 (1996): 289–293.

Silberstein, S.D., Lipton, R.B., Solomon, S., & Mathew, N.T. Classification of daily and near-daily headaches: Proposed revision to the IHS criteria. *Headache* 34 (1994): 1–17.

Silberstein, S., et al. Assessment for revised criteria for chronic daily headache. *Neurology* 45 (1995): A394.

Vanast, W.J. New daily persistent headache: Definition of a benign syndrome. *Headache* 26 (1986): 317.

Winner, P., Wasiewski, W., Gladstein, J., et al. Multicenter prospective evaluation of the proposed pediatric migraine revisions to the IHS criteria. *Headache* 48 (1997): 602–607.

5

Classification and Diagnosis of Chronic Daily Headache and Tension-Type Headache

Herbert G. Markley, MD, FAAN, FAHS

Chronic daily headache (CDH) is a common disorder seen in daily medical practice, and it is even more commonly encountered in headache specialty practice. The spectrum of headache disorders producing CDH ranges from chronic migraine through chronic tension-type headache and off to more unusual disorders such as hemicrania continua and new daily persistent headache. Medication overuse headache, a secondary headache disorder, may worsen any of the primary headache types and complicate their management.

Chronic daily headache is not a diagnosis specifically included in ICHD-II; rather, headache disorders that may have daily expression are scattered throughout the classification schema. Most chronic forms of headache also have episodic forms. Primary forms of chronic headache are without known cause—primary disorders in their own right (Table 5–1).

Secondary forms of chronic headache are those attributed to or caused by an underlying pathophysiology (Table 5–2). These are discussed in Part III of this text.

Epidemiology of the primary forms of CDH varies with the disorder, but common to all is the ICHD-II case definition of a frequency of at least 15 headache days per month. Incidence and prevalence vary with the age of subjects studied, even within the same disorder. For example, chronic migraine (1.5.1) prevalence in adults is about 4% of the population (versus 12% for episodic migraine), but only about 2% in children and adolescents. The incidence of chronic migraine is about 2% per year, but the remission rate is about 50% per year.

Even within CDH, there is a wide range of phenotypic expression of the headache pattern, with three patterns being observed: frequent (68%), daily (15%), and continuous (17%).

CHRONIC MIGRAINE

Chronic migraine is classified in ICHD-II as a complication of migraine, not as a disorder in its own right (Table 5–3). In ICHD-I, complications of migraine

Table 5–1 Primary Forms of Chronic Daily Headache (ICHD-II Classification)

Chronic migraine 1.5.1
Chronic tension-type headache 2.3
Trigeminal autonomic cephalalgias (TACs)
    Chronic cluster headache 3.1.2
    Chronic paroxysmal hemicrania 3.2.2
    SUNCT (short-lasting, unilateral neuralgiform headaches with conjunctival injection
       and tearing) 3.3
Other primary headaches
    Primary stabbing headache 4.1
    Hypnic headache 4.5
    Hemicrania continua 4.7
    New daily persistent headache 4.8
Cranial neuralgias (*e.g.*, trigeminal neuralgia) 13

was category 1.6, and it had only two members, status migrainosus and migrainous infarction. The ICHD-II definition, in 2004, stipulated that patients must have 15 or more headaches per month meeting the criteria for migraine without aura.

However, studies performed to validate these criteria failed to demonstrate that most patients with CDH have anywhere near 15 IHS migraines per month. Even before the ICHD-II classification was published, Silberstein and Lipton had published criteria for the diagnosis of chronic migraine that were successfully field-tested (Table 5–4). Even after the 2004 ICHD criteria was published, these so-called Silberstein-Lipton (S-L) criteria continued to be used to define chronic migraine in many clinical trials.

**Table 5–2 Secondary Forms of Chronic Daily Headache (ICHD-II
           Classification)**

Post-traumatic (may mimic any primary headache)
Musculoskeletal
    Cervicogenic (especially C2, C3 upper root entrapment)
    Temporomandibular joint syndrome
Vascular
    Arteriovenous malformation
    Arteritis (including giant cell arteritis)
    Vascular dissection
Raised or lowered intracranial pressure
    Subdural hematoma
    Neoplasm
    Intracranial hypertension
    Intracranial hypotension
Infections
    Sinus disease

Table 5–3 ICHD-II Classification of Chronic Migraine (2004)

1.5 Complications of migraine
    1.5.1 Chronic migraine
        A. Headache fulfilling criteria C and D for 1.1 Migraine without aura on ≥15 d/
           mo for >3 mo
        B. Not attributed to another disorder
    1.5.2 Status migrainosus
    1.5.3 Persistent aura without infarction
    1.5.4 Migrainous infarction
    1.5.5 Migraine-triggered seizures

The S-L criteria were used after the 2004 revision because it was found to be difficult or impossible to prove that headache episodes in these patients could be classified as either migraine without aura or tension-type headache. Efficient early treatment may obscure the characteristics of an attack, so that classification depends upon attacks being untreated or unsuccessfully treated. Most attacks of migraine without aura develop slowly, usually going through a mild phase where they fulfill the criteria for tension-type headache before the headache becomes moderate or severe, becomes unilateral, and has associated symptoms. Early intake of a triptan can abort the attack before features of migraine develop. This would lead to the attack being classified as tension-type headache. When patients suffer from frequent attacks and are very disabled, it is usually not possible to stay medication-free for long. The ICHD-II criterion for chronic migraine stipulates that patients fulfill the criteria for 1.1, migraine without aura, on at least 15 days per month, thereby requiring that patients stay off treatment for an entire month. Furthermore, new evidence has shown that response to triptans is robust when patients with migraine treat attacks that fulfill the criteria for tension-type headache, in contrast to previous studies showing that the effect of triptans is modest or nonexistent for such attacks.

Table 5–4 Silberstein and Lipton Revised Criteria for Transformed Migraine (1996)

A. Daily or almost daily (>15 days/month) head pain for >1 month
B. Average headache duration of 4 hours/day (if untreated)
C. At least one of the following:
    1) History of episodic migraine meeting any IHS criteria 1.1 to 1.6
    2) History of increasing headache frequency with decreasing severity of migrainous features over at least 3 months
    3) Headache at some time meets IHS criteria for migraine 1.1 to 1.6 other than duration
D. Does not meet criteria for new daily persistent headache (4.7) or hemicrania continua (4.8)
E. Not attributed to another disorder

From *Neurology* 47(1996):871–875

These two facts suggest that, in migraineurs, many headaches fulfilling tension-type headache criteria may in fact be mild migraine attacks.

In 2006, the IHS classification committee published an addendum to the 2004 classification specifically addressing these concerns. This revision added new criteria for chronic migraine to a category in the appendix, with the expectation that they would undergo discussion and field-testing over the next few years. Once these criteria have been field-tested, there should be sufficient evidence to allow their inclusion or abolition. They would be introduced into the main body of the classification in a revised edition of the International Headache Classification to be presented in 2009 or 2010. Until then, the International Headache Classification Committee has extended an invitation to the headache community to study these new criteria and to generate clinical trials for this severely affected segment of headache patients. This is currently being done, and modern clinical trials of chronic migraine usually use the appendix 1.5.1 criteria of 2006 rather than the ICHD-II ones of 2004 or the S-L criteria (Table 5–5).

The major change, item C, acknowledges that few patients have ICHD migraine for 15 or more days per month, and also implicitly acknowledges that patients with chronic migraine must have other types of headache to fill out the rest of the 15 minimum days per month required for the definition. These other types of headache usually meet ICHD criteria for probable migraine or tension-type headache, even though they are necessarily included in the definition of chronic migraine. American specialists generally view this nomenclature as

Table 5–5 IHS Criteria for Appendix 1.5.1, Chronic Migraine

A. Headache (tension-type and/or migraine) on ≥15 days per month for at least 3 months

B. Occurring in a patient who has had at least five attacks fulfilling criteria for 1.1, migraine without aura

C. On ≥8 days per month for at least 3 months headache has fulfilled C1 and/or C2 below — that is, has fulfilled criteria for pain and associated symptoms of migraine without aura
  1. Has at least two of a–d
    (a) Unilateral location
    (b) Pulsating quality
    (c) Moderate or severe pain intensity
    (d) Aggravation by or causing avoidance of routine physical activity (*e.g.*, walking or climbing stairs)
  And at least one of a or b
    (a) Nausea and/or vomiting
    (b) Photophobia and phonophobia
  2. Treated and relieved by triptan(s) or ergot before the expected development of C1 above

D. No medication overuse and not attributed to another causative disorder

From *Cephalalgia* 26(2006):742–746

inconsistent, because the criteria require splitting categories and lumping them together at the same time. Chronic migraine is thus conceived of as comprising big migraines, medium-size migraines, and little migraines instead of comprising three different types of headache.

MEDICATION OVERUSE HEADACHES

The phenomenon of headache exacerbation by the overuse of therapeutic medication, formerly referred to as rebound headache, was classified as medication overuse headaches in ICHD-II. These criteria have produced much criticism and discussion since they were introduced, and the criteria have gone through two more revisions. The initial concepts were based upon expert opinion, but these have largely not been sustained by evidence-based clinical trials. Although the concept is very important, many of the initial assumptions, such as that the most common cause for CDH is overuse of symptomatic headache medication, have not stood the test of time and opinion. Several sources, especially Scher and Lipton (2002), have reported that only about a third of all those with CDH (25% to 38%) actually overuse acute medications. Other assumptions, such as that specific types of headache are caused by overuse of specific types of drugs, or the classification "probable medication overuse headache," have had to be again revised or even retracted. Other concepts continue to cause controversy, especially the notion that patients do not respond to prophylactic medication while they are overusing acute medications.

Unlike for the revisions done recently for chronic migraine, the first revision of criteria for medication overuse headache was not placed into the appendix, but in June 2005 it became the full ICHD-II definition (Table 5–6). This revision extended the concept of medication overuse headache beyond that produced by analgesics, ergots, and triptans to include other classes of compounds and even combinations of compounds. The revised criteria stand as the current active definition for medication overuse headache, but nagging problems with the category still remain.

Because of these nagging problems, after further discussion another revision was published in fall 2006. This time, as with the revision to the original definition of chronic migraine, it was relegated to the appendix, pending field trials, discussion, and general acceptance. Reasons for the revision include general dissatisfaction with the concept of making the diagnosis only after the overuse has been discontinued and the patient has improved. In other words, when patients have medication overuse headache, it cannot be diagnosed; it can be diagnosed only after the patient does not have it anymore. Another problem is that not all patients improve after discontinuation of overuse of acute headache medication(s): most studies suggest that only a minority of patients improve after withdrawal. Some headache chronification may happen due to medication overuse, but for many patients the effect seems to be irreversible even after discontinuation of medication overuse. Another change was that the diagnosis

Table 5–6 Medication-Overuse Headache (2005 ICHD-II)

8.2 Medication-overuse headache (MOH)
Previously used terms: Rebound headache, drug-induced headache, medication-misuse headache.
Diagnostic criteria:
>A. Headache present on ≥15 days/month fulfilling criteria C and D.
>B. Regular overuse for >3 months of one or more drugs that can be taken for acute and/or symptomatic treatment of headache.
>C. Headache has developed or markedly worsened during medication overuse.
>D. Headache resolves or reverts to its previous pattern within 2 months after discontinuation of overused medication.

8.2.1 Ergotamine overuse headache
8.2.2 Triptan overuse headache
8.2.3 Analgesic overuse headache
8.2.4 Opioid overuse headache
8.2.5 Combination analgesic overuse headache
8.2.6 Medication overuse headache attributed to combination of acute medications
8.2.7 Headache attributed to other medication overuse
8.2.8 Probable medication overuse headache

From *Cephalalgia* 25(2005):460–465

of probable chronic migraine was deleted. The new appendix criteria for medication overuse headache are listed in Table 5–7.

Most single types of these medications are believed to produce medication overuse headache if they are used for 10 or more days per month, the exceptions being overuse for at least 15 days/month of simple analgesics or multiple agents without overuse of any single class.

There is still the problem that the diagnosis of any medication overuse headache is not confirmed until headaches improve following a period of 2 months' cessation of the suspected substance. If such improvement does not occur

Table 5–7 Revised Criteria for Medication Overuse Headache (2006)

Appendix 8.2 Medication overuse headache
Diagnostic criteria:
>A. Headache present on ≥15 days/month
>B. Regular overuse for >3 months of one or more acute/symptomatic treatment drugs as defined under subforms of 8.2.
>>1. Ergotamine, triptans, opioids, **or** combination analgesic medications on ≥10 days/month on a regular basis for >3 months
>>2. Simple analgesics **or** any combination of ergotamine, triptans, analgesics opioids on ≥15 days/month on a regular basis for >3 months without overuse of any single class alone
>C. Headache has developed or markedly worsened during medication overuse

From *Cephalalgia* 26(2006):742–746

within 2 months, this diagnosis must be discarded. However, patients can be very uncomfortable during this 2-month period due to the withdrawal of medication and use of less-effective rescue medication, and improvement following medication withdrawal is far from certain. In a large recent study, under 50% of those improved within 2 months. Zeeberg and associates studied 337 patients with probable medication overuse headache and found that only 45% had improvement in their headache, 48% had no change, and 7% actually worsened. For the entire sample, only 29% improved, 31% were unchanged, 5% worsened, and 36% dropped out because they could not stay medication-free for 2 months.

A compilation of other such studies shows pretty similar results, with a few outliers. Scher and Lipton summarized nine reports that studied groups from 55 to 400 patients for periods of medication withdrawal from 30 days to 5 years. Three of the studies, including the largest (30-day withdrawal), reported headache improvement in under 50% (range 13% to 46%). Another three reported improvement in about 50% of patients (range 50% to 56%). Only three of the nine studies showed improvement in more than half of the patients withdrawn from frequent medication, and only one showed remarkable improvement (range 62% to 97%).

Another problem with the classification of medication overuse headache, as some specialists see it, is the lack of experimental evidence for the entire concept. Written into the classification is the statement, without evidence, that medication overuse is the most common cause of chronic migraine:

> *8.2 Medication-overuse headache (MOH). Comments:* MOH is an interaction between a therapeutic agent used excessively and a susceptible patient. The best example is overuse of symptomatic headache drugs causing headache in the headache-prone patient. By far the most common cause of migraine-like headache occurring on ≥ 15 days per month and of a mixed picture of migraine-like and tension-type-like headaches on ≥ 15 days per month is overuse of symptomatic antimigraine drugs and/or analgesics.

But what is the evidence that medication overuse is the most likely cause of chronic symptoms? Katsarava's persuasive recent study, described in Table 5–8, is often cited as evidence.

This study appears to validates previous clinical work (by Kudrow, Mathew, Saper, Scher, Rapoport) demonstrating the importance of excessive medication intake as a risk factor for CDH and medication frequency as a cause of transformation of episodic migraine into CDH. To some, it suggests the need for limitation of acute medications as well as the need to implement more aggressive prophylaxis. On the other hand, seven published studies have reported that only 20% to 38% of patients in the population with CDH meet the criteria for medication overuse headache.

There are other, potent additional risk factors for transformation from episodic to chronic migraine besides having frequent migraine and medication overuse: female gender, Caucasian race, low educational level, habitual snoring,

Table 5–8 Risk Factors for Developing Chronic Migraine

532 consecutive patients with episodic migraine (<15 days/mo) prospectively followed for 1 year

Results

Sixty-four patients (14%) developed chronic headache

Odds ratios for developing CDH:

High headache frequency: 20.1 (for patients with HA 10–14 days/month vs. 0–4 days/month)

Medication overuse: 19.4 (for patients ± medication overuse)

Acute medications overused:

Analgesics 53%

Triptans 34%

Ergots 3%

Opioids 1%

None 8%

48% used one medication and 52% used 2 or more.

Conclusions

Overall incidence of CDH within migraine sufferers was 14%.

Odds of developing CDH were 20.1 times higher in those with ≥10 headache days/month.

Odds of developing CDH were 19.4 times higher in those overusing acute medication.

From *Neurology* 62(2004):788–790

obesity (BMI ≥ 30), other painful conditions such arthritis or diabetes, high caffeine intake, or stressful life events such as death of a spouse, friend, or parent, or changing jobs, changing marital status, or moving. Other health risks, such as cigarette smoking, high cholesterol, or sedentary lifestyle, appear to have no effect.

OTHER FORMS OF PRIMARY CHRONIC DAILY HEADACHE

Primary Stabbing Headache

Primary stabbing headache (ICHD-I "idiopathic stabbing headache") is a CDH originally dubbed "ice-pick pains" or "jabs and jolts." The attacks consist of brief, localized stabs of pain in various places in the head that occur spontaneously in the absence of organic disease of underlying structures or of the cranial nerves. Sharp stabbing pains usually last less than 10 seconds, but occasional ones may persist for up to 2 minutes. The ICHD-II classification claims that 80% of stabs last 3 seconds or less and "in rare cases, stabs occur repetitively over days, and there has been one description of *status* lasting one week" (Table 5–9). Our experience is that most patients have multiple attacks per day, not producing disability. The stabs may move around the head in a rather random manner, not being confined to either hemicranium. The bulk of the stabs usually occur in the territory of the first trigeminal division, but sometimes the occipital nerve territory shares in the pain. Surprisingly, the lower trigeminal

Table 5–9 4.1 Primary Stabbing Headache

A. Head pain occurring as a single stab or a series of stabs and fulfilling criteria B–D
B. Exclusively or predominantly felt in the distribution of the first division of the
   trigeminal nerve (orbit, temple and parietal area)
C. Stabs last for up to a few seconds and recur with irregular frequency ranging from one
   to many per day
D. No accompanying symptoms
E. Not attributed to another disorder

and cervical areas are unaffected. Isolated and consistent localization of the pain indicates a structural or secondary cause for the headaches.

Stabbing pains are said to be more commonly experienced by people subject to migraine (about 40%) or cluster headache (about 30%), but a substantial proportion occur in adolescents without any other headache history. The natural history has not been described, but our experience is that about a third of the patients continue to have the pains for many months, another third have spontaneous remission, and the remainder develops more typical primary headaches. It is not infrequent, especially in adolescents, that this benign pattern of brief headaches evolves into continuous pain indistinguishable from new daily persistent headache. Some patients respond to treatment with indomethacin and others to antineuralgia drugs such as topiramate or gabapentin, while others fail to respond to trials of multiple agents.

Hypnic Headache

Hypnic headache awakens the patient from sleep, usually at about the same time every night (hence the other name, "alarm-clock headache") (Table 5–10). The pain is usually mild to moderate, but severe pain is seen in about 20%. Attacks usually begin after age fifty. Two thirds of patients report bilateral pain for 15 to 180 minutes, but longer durations can occur. Caffeine and lithium may be effective in some.

Table 5–10 4.5 Hypnic Headache

A. Dull headache fulfilling criteria B–D
B. Develops only during sleep, and awakens patient
C. At least two of the following characteristics:
   1. Occurs >15 times/mo
   2. Lasts ≥15 min after waking
   3. First occurs after age of 50 y
D. No autonomic symptoms and no more than one of nausea, photophobia or
   phonophobia
E. Not attributed to another disorder

Hemicrania Continua

A continuous, strictly unilateral headache responsive to indomethacin, hemicrania continua is usually unremitting, although occasional spontaneous remissions have been reported (Table 5–11).

New Daily Persistent Headache

New daily persistent headache is the second-most-common type of daily continuous headache seen in tertiary referral centers, representing about 11% of all new patients seen. The diagnosis is practically unknown to non-headache specialists, including most general neurologists. However, the clinical features are so stereotyped that the diagnosis should not be in doubt (Table 5–12). Careful study of papers describing this entity is recommended.

Clinically it is a disorder that starts unexpectedly, usually on awakening. The pain is usually continuous and unremitting from the outset, or it becomes that way in a matter of days. Patients usually recall their exact activity at onset—on awakening, in math class, and so forth. ICHD-II treats new daily persistent headache as a separate entity from 2.3, "chronic tension-type headache," because of its unique onset, typically in individuals without a prior headache history. The headache of new daily persistent headache can have associated features suggestive of either migraine or tension-type headache but usually does not respond to triptans or standard prophylactic medications. Secondary headaches such as low-cerebrospinal-fluid-volume headache, raised-cerebrospinal-fluid-pressure headache, post-traumatic headache, and headache attributed to infection (particularly viral) should be ruled out by appropriate investigations. It is crucial to exclude the syndrome of cerebral venous thrombosis, which mimics the onset of new daily persistent headache but produces headache by reducing cerebrospinal fluid drainage and elevating spinal fluid pressure.

Table 5–11 4.7 Hemicrania Continua

A. Headache for >3 mo fulfilling criteria B–D
B. All of the following characteristics:
    1. Unilateral pain without side shift
    2. Daily and continuous, without pain-free periods
    3. Moderate intensity, with exacerbations of severe pain
C. At least one of the following autonomic features occurs during exacerbations, ipsilateral to the pain:
    1. Conjunctival injection and/or lacrimation
    2. Nasal congestion and/or rhinorrhea
    3. Ptosis and/or miosis
D. Complete response to therapeutic doses of indomethacin
E. Not attributed to another disorder

Table 5–12 4.8 New Daily Persistent Headache (NDPH)

A. Headache for >3 mo fulfilling criteria B–D

B. Headache is daily and unremitting from onset or from <3 d from onset

C. At least two of the following pain characteristics:

    1. Bilateral location

    2. Pressing/tightening (non-pulsating) quality

    3. Mild or moderate intensity

    4. Not aggravated by routine physical activity

D. Both of the following:

    1. Not >1 of photophobia, phonophobia or mild nausea

    2. Neither moderate or severe nausea nor vomiting

E. Not attributed to another disorder

New daily persistent headache may take either of two types: a benign, self-limited type that typically resolves within several months without treatment, and the more common refractory type, which is resistant to aggressive treatments.

TENSION-TYPE HEADACHES

Tension-type headache is reportedly the most common type of primary headache in the population, affecting 30% to 78%, but it is also the least studied of the primary headaches. Its name does not reflect causation by muscular tension (migraine without aura produces more), nor causation by emotional tension (comorbidity of anxiety and depression is higher in migraine). Its relationship to migraine is unclear. It is an integral part of the headache pattern in most patients with chronic migraine, yet it is seldom seen as a pure culture of featureless daily low-level headaches devoid of migraine features. Its pathophysiology is as obscure as its evidence-based treatments. The ICHD-II acknowledges that it was previously considered to be primarily psychogenic. However, a number of studies done after the ICHD-I strongly suggest a neurobiological basis, at least for the more severe subtypes of tension-type headache. Although pathophysiology is not known, peripheral pain mechanisms are most likely to play a role in 2.1, "infrequent episodic tension-type headache," and 2.2, "frequent episodic tension-type headache," whereas central pain mechanisms probably play a more important role in 2.3, "chronic tension-type headache."

The ICHD-II further acknowledges that some patients coded for episodic tension-type headache may include some who have a mild form of migraine without aura, and patients coded for chronic tension-type headache include some who had chronic migraine. This is seen by clinical experience, especially in patients who also have migraine attacks, and some patients may display pathophysiologic features typical of migraine. Because of this confusion, a proposal for new, stricter diagnostic criteria is published under A2, "tension-type headache," in the appendix.

Table 5–13 Classification of Tension-Type Headache (TTH) 2.0

2.1 Infrequent episodic tension-type headache
   2.1.1 Infrequent episodic tension-type headache associated with pericranial tenderness
   2.1.2 Infrequent episodic tension-type headache not associated with pericranial
        tenderness
2.2 Frequent episodic tension-type headache
   2.2.1 Frequent episodic tension-type headache associated with pericranial tenderness
   2.2.2 Frequent episodic tension-type headache not associated with pericranial
        tenderness
2.3 Chronic tension-type headache
   2.3.1 Chronic tension-type headache associated with pericranial tenderness
   2.3.2 Chronic tension-type headache not associated with pericranial tenderness
2.4 Probable tension-type headache
   2.4.1 Probable infrequent episodic tension-type headache
   2.4.2 Probable frequent episodic tension-type headache
   2.4.3 Probable chronic tension-type headache

Tension-type headache has been divided since ICHD-I into episodic and chronic subtypes (Table 5–13). The chronic subtype is a serious disease causing greatly decreased quality of life and high disability. ICHD-II subdivides episodic tension-type headache further, into an infrequent subtype having very little impact on the individual (episodes less than once per month) and a frequent subtype producing considerable disability that may require expensive drugs and prophylactic medication. The first edition arbitrarily separated patients with and without disorder of the pericranial muscles, and this has been continued in the second edition, but the tenderness is now to be judged solely by tenderness on manual palpation.

Patients must have had at least 10 such attacks in the past. Diagnostic criteria for the disorders within the entire class differ only in the frequency of attacks (infrequent, frequent, or chronic), in the presence or absence of pericranial tenderness to manual pressure palpation, and in the degree of adherence to criteria (definite or probable forms of each subtype) (Tables 5–14 and 5–15). Probable subtypes fulfill all but one criterion and do not fulfill criteria for 1.1, "migraine without aura." Probable chronic tension-type headache is associated with medication overuse.

SUMMARY

Chronic daily headache is a common disorder seen in daily medical practice, and it is even more commonly encountered in headache specialty practice. The spectrum of headache disorders producing CDH ranges from chronic migraine through chronic tension-type headache and off to more unusual disorders such as hemicrania continua and new daily persistent headache. These primary

Table 5–14 Types of Tension-Type Headache:
Summary of ICHD II Classification

Type of TTH	Frequency of attacks (number of days/mo or year)	Duration
Infrequent	< 1/month (< 12 days/year)	30 min to 7 d
Frequent	≥1 but <15 d/mo for ≥3 mo (≥12 and <180 d/y)	Not specified
Chronic	≥15 d/mo (≥180 d/y) for >3 mo	Hours to continuous

Table 5–15 2.1 Infrequent Episodic Tension-Type Headache

A. At least 10 episodes occurring on <1 day per month on average (<12 days per year) and fulfilling criteria B–D
B. Headache lasting from 30 minutes to 7 days
C. Headache has at least two of the following characteristics:
    1. Bilateral location
    2. Pressing/tightening (non-pulsating) quality
    3. Mild or moderate intensity
    4. Not aggravated by routine physical activity such as walking or climbing stairs
D. Both of the following:
    1. No nausea or vomiting (anorexia may occur)
    2. No more than one of photophobia or phonophobia
E. Not attributed to another disorder
2.1.1 Infrequent episodic tension-type headache associated with pericranial tenderness
    A. Episodes fulfilling criteria A–E for 2.1, Infrequent episodic tension-type headache
    B. Increased pericranial tenderness on manual palpation
2.1.2 Infrequent episodic tension-type headache not associated with pericranial tenderness
    A. Episodes fulfilling criteria A–E for 2.1, Infrequent episodic tension-type headache
    B. No increased pericranial tenderness
Other types of TTH include:
  2.2 Frequent episodic TTH
    2.2.1 Frequent episodic tension-type headache associated with pericranial tenderness
    2.2.2 Frequent episodic tension-type headache not associated with pericranial tenderness
  2.3 Chronic TTH
    2.3.1 Chronic tension-type headache associated with pericranial tenderness
    2.3.2 Chronic tension-type headache not associated with pericranial tenderness
  2.4 Probable TTH
    2.4.1 Probable infrequent episodic TTH
    2.4.2 Probable frequent episodic TTH
    2.4.3 Probable chronic TTH
As 2.3 except: there is, or has been within the last 2 mo, medication overuse fulfilling criterion B for any of the subforms of 8.2, Medication overuse headache

forms of chronic headache are without known cause—primary disorders in their own right. Medication overuse headache, a secondary headache disorder, may worsen any of the primary headache types and complicate their management. Chronic daily headache is not a diagnosis specifically included in ICHD-II, but headache disorders that may have daily expression are scattered throughout the classification schema. Most chronic forms of headache also have episodic forms. Criteria for diagnosis of several types of primary CDH under the International Headache Society rules have changed in several ways since the publication of the initial ICHD classification. The most changes have been seen in criteria for the diagnosis of chronic migraine and medication overuse headache.

ACKNOWLEDGMENT

Tables, unless otherwise specifically noted, are derived from *The International Classification of Headache Disorders*, 2nd edition (ICHD-II), from the Headache Classification Committee of the International Headache Society. *Cephalalgia* 24, Suppl. 1 (2004). Tables are reproduced by permission of the copyright holders.

Review Questions

1. To meet the diagnosis of chronic migraine under Silberstein-Lipton (revised) criteria for chronic migraine (*Neurology* 1996), how many days of headache per month must meet full criteria for migraine?
   a. 30
   b. 15
   c. 8
   d. Number of days not specified
2. To meet the diagnosis of chronic migraine under the 2006 revision of ICHD-II for chronic migraine (1.5.1) (*Cephalalgia* 2006), how many days of headache per month must meet full criteria for migraine?
   a. 30
   b. 15
   c. 8
   d. Number of days not specified
3. Under the ICHD-II revision for chronic migraine (*Cephalalgia* 2006), what other type or types of headaches are permitted on the non-migraine days, as long as the criterion of a total of 15 or more headache days per month is met?
   a. Tension-type headache
   b. Probable migraine
   c. No headache
   d. All of the above

4. Approximately what percentage of patients with chronic daily headache will improve after withdrawal from their overused medication?
   a. 100%
   b. 75%
   c. 60%
   d. 45%

5. Potent risk factors for transformation from episodic to chronic migraine include which of these?
   a. Obesity
   b. Diabetes
   c. Cigarette smoking
   d. All of the above

6. A 16-year-old cheerleader complains of sharp stabbing pains localized to her forehead. Symptoms started suddenly 3 months before and are sharp enough that she stops, puts her hand to her forehead, and says "Ow!" The pain is quite intense but lasts only a few seconds. A few attacks continue up to 2 minutes. Attacks have been occurring up to four times per hour and involve the right and left sides of her scalp, up to the vertex. Your first diagnosis should be:
   a. New daily persistent headache, 4.8
   b. Hemicrania continua, 4.7
   c. Primary stabbing headache, 4.1
   d. Nummular headache, A13.7.1 (localized scalp neuralgia)

7. A 67-year-old grandmother has begun awakening every night around the same time of night with a moderately severe headache. The headache is bilateral and is not associated with photophobia, phonophobia, nausea, or vomiting. When she gets up and sits for 30 to 45 minutes, she can go back to sleep and not awaken until her usual time of awakening in the morning. She has no headache on awakening in the morning. Your clinical suspicion should fall upon a diagnosis of:
   a. Glioblastoma multiforme
   b. Idiopathic intracranial hypertension
   c. Hypnic headache
   d. Cardiogenic headache

8. A 45-year-old teacher complains that she has developed a continuous daily headache on the left side of her head. It started during her third-period algebra class 3 months ago, and it has never left her. Usually the pain is not bad enough to interfere with her work, but sometimes it becomes severe, and she has had to call in sick twice since the headache started. She used to have migraine in her 20s, but this headache does not have the migraine symptoms she remembers. Several non-prescription and prescription medications have not helped. She also complains of a chronic "sinus infection" in the past 2 months, but only the left side of her nose produces a clear discharge. Maybe her left eye

itches and tears along with it. If you are skillful, or lucky, you can cure her headache with:

a. High-dose gabapentin
b. A lumbar puncture
c. Topiramate
d. Indomethacin

9. Unfortunately, the drug you chose did not help your math teacher patient, so you had best do something else to help her. How about additional history? Fine. Now she says that the pain is really on both sides of her head; it's only worse on the left side. And the sinus infection was just that—her primary care physician cured it with a course of antibiotics, but the headache continues. Her PCP also got an MRI scan, which was normal. Right now she does not have a very high opinion of you and you'd like to do something to salvage your reputation. Which diagnosis would you like to consider now?

a. New daily persistent headache
b. Chronic migraine
c. Chronic tension-type headache not associated with pericranial tenderness
d. Benign intracranial hypertension

10. A 36-year-old accountant complains of intermittently severe pain in the back of his head for the past 6 months. He vaguely recalls being hit in this region with a closing garage door 2 years before. Most of the time the pain is moderate, but sometimes there are sharp jabs. He tells you that the pain is felt only in a small circumscribed area above his right ear, an area "the size of a quarter." When you examine him, you discover an area of alopecia 2.5 cm in diameter. Stroking the scalp lightly produces a disagreeable tingling and pain. What diagnosis would you give this patient?

a. Occipital neuralgia
b. Chronic regional pain syndrome type II
c. Nummular headache
d. Post-traumatic headache

10. c
9. a
8. d
7. c
6. c
5. a
4. d
3. d
2. c
1. d

SUGGESTED READING

Bigal, M.E., Liberman, J.N., & Lipton, R.B. Obesity and migraine: A population study. *Neurology* 66 (2006): 545–550.

Dangond, F., & Spierings, E.L. Idiopathic stabbing headaches lasting a few seconds. *Headache* 33 (1993): 257–258.

Dodick, D.W., Mosek, A.C., & Campbell, I.K. The hypnic ('alarm clock') headache syndrome. *Cephalalgia* 18 (1998): 152–156.

Evans, R.W., & Rozen, T.D. Etiology and treatment of new daily persistent headache. *Headache* 4 (2001): 830–832.

Ghiotto, N., Sances, G., Di Lorenzo, G., Trucco, M., Loi, M., Sandrini, G., & Nappi, G. Report of eight new cases of hypnic headache and a mini-review of the literature. *Functional Neurology* 17 (2002): 211–219.

Goadsby, P.J., & Boes, C. New daily persistent headache. *Journal of Neurology, Neurosurgery & Psychiatry* 72, Suppl. 2 (2002): ii6–ii9.

Headache Classification Committee: Olesen, J., Bousser, M-G., Diener, H-C., Dodick, D., First, M., Goadsby, P.J., Göbel, H., Lainez, M.J.A., Lance, J.W., Lipton, R.B., Nappi, G., Sakai, F., Schoenen, J., Silberstein, S.D., & Steiner, T.J. New appendix criteria open for a broader concept of chronic migraine. *Cephalalgia* 26 (2006): 742–746.

Headache Classification Committee of the International Headache Society. *The International Classification of Headache Disorders*, 2nd edition. *Cephalalgia* 24, Suppl. 1 (2004).

Katsarava, Z., Schneeweiss, S., Kurth, T., Kroener, U., Fritsche, G., Eikermann, A., Diener H-C., & Limmroth, V. Incidence and predictors for chronicity of headache in patients with episodic migraine. *Neurology* 62 (2004): 788–790.

Li, D., & Rozen, T.D. The clinical characterisation of new daily persistent headache. *Cephalalgia* 22 (2002): 66–69.

Limmroth, V., Katsarava, Z., Fritsche, G., Przywara, S., & Diener, H.C. Features of medication overuse headache following overuse of different acute headache drugs. *Neurology* 59 (2002): 1011–1014.

Mathew, N., & Ward, T. "Treatment of primary headache: chronic daily headache." In: *Standards of care for headache diagnosis and treatment.* Chicago: National Headache Foundation, 2004:73–80.

Mathew, N.T., Kurman, R., & Perez, F. Drug-induced refractory headache—clinical features and management. *Headache* 30 (1990): 634–638.

Newman, L.C., Lipton, R.B., & Solomon, S. Hemicrania continua: Ten new cases and a review of the literature. *Neurology* 44 (1994): 2111–2114.

Rapoport, A., Stang, P., Gutterman, D.L., Cady, R., Markley, H., Weeks, R., Saiers, J., & Fox, A.W. Analgesic rebound headache in clinical practice: Data from a physician survey. *Headache* 36 (1996): 14–19.

Rapoport, A.M. Analgesic rebound headache. *Headache* 28 (1988): 662–665.

Rapoport, A.M., & Weeks, R.E. "Characteristics and treatment of analgesic rebound headache." In *Drug-induced headache*, eds. Diener, H.C., & Wilkinson, M. Berlin: Springer-Verlag, 1988:162–167.

Rozen, T.D. New daily persistent headache. *Current Pain and Headache Reports* 7 (2003): 218–223.

Scher, A.I., Lipton, R.B., & Stewart, W. Risk factors for chronic daily headache. *Current Pain and Headache Reports* 6 (2002): 486–491.

Scher, A.I., Stewart, W.F., Liberman, J., & Lipton, R.B. Prevalence of frequent headache in a population sample. *Headache* 38 (1998): 497–506.

Scher, A.I., Stewart, W.F., Ricci, J.A., & Lipton, R.B. Factors associated with the onset and remission of chronic daily headache in a population-based study. *Pain* 106 (2003): 81–89.

Schnider, P., Aull, S., Baumgartner, C., et al. Long-term outcome of patients with headache and drug abuse after inpatient withdrawal: five-year follow-up. *Cephalalgia* 16 (1996): 481–485.

Schnider, P., Aull, S., & Feucht, M. Use and abuse of analgesics in tension-type headache. *Cephalalgia* 14 (1994): 162–167.

Silberstein, S.D., Lipton, R.B., & Sliwinski M. Classification of daily and near-daily headaches: Field trial of revised IHS criteria. *Neurology* 47 (1996): 871–875.

Silberstein, S.D., Lipton, R.B., Solomon, S., & Mathew, N.T. Classification of daily and near-daily headaches: Proposed revisions to the HIS criteria. *Headache* 34 (1994): 1–7.

Silberstein, S.D., Olesen, J., Bousser, M-G., Diener, H-C., Dodick, D., First, M., Goadsby, P.J., Göbel, H., Lainez, M.J.A., Lance, J.W., Lipton, R.B., Nappi, G., Sakai, F., Schoenen, J., & Steiner, T.J., on behalf of the International Headache Society. *The International Classification of Headache Disorders*, 2nd edition (ICHD-II)—revision of criteria for 8.2 *Medication-overuse headache*. *Cephalalgia* 25 (2005): 460–465.

Sjaastad, O., & Spierings, E.L. Hemicrania continua: Another headache absolutely responsive to indomethacin. *Cephalalgia* 4 (1984): 65–70.

Soriani, G., Battistella, P.A., Arnaldi, C., De Carlo, L., Cemetti, R., Corra, S., & Tosato, G. Juvenile idiopathic stabbing headache. *Headache* 36 (1996): 565–567.

Zeeberg, P., Olesen, J., & Jensen, R. Probable medication-overuse headache: The effect of a 2-month drug-free period. *Neurology* June 27;66, no. 12 (2006):1894–1898. Epub May 17, 2006.

6

Classification and Diagnosis of Trigeminal Autonomic Cephalalgias and Other Primary Headaches

Lawrence C. Newman, MD

This chapter will be divided into two sections in which the clinical features of a variety of uncommon headache disorders will be reviewed. In the first part of this chapter, we will discuss a group of headaches that are collectively known as the trigeminal autonomic cephalalgias (TACs) (found in Chapter 3 of the ICHD-II). The TACs are characterized by headaches of excruciating severity accompanied by prominent autonomic features. While the symptomatology of these syndromes may appear similar, they do in fact differ significantly in terms of the frequency and duration of individual attacks. Furthermore, proper treatment of these disorders is predicated upon correct diagnosis; a number of these conditions respond dramatically to therapy with indomethacin but not to agents typically prescribed for cluster, migraine, or tension-type headaches. Although the TACs generally begin during adulthood, adolescent and childhood cases do occur.

The second section of this chapter is devoted to reviewing the clinical features of "other" primary headache disorders. Although the majority of headache sufferers seen in routine clinical practice will have a common primary headache disorder (migraine, tension-type, or cluster), other less common primary headaches exist. Recognition of other less common primary headache syndromes is important as the sufferers tend to be desperate, often misdiagnosed and mismanaged. Furthermore, these disorders (found in Chapter 4 of the ICHD-II) may have secondary mimics and therefore require additional investigations prior to establishing the diagnosis.

TRIGEMINAL AUTONOMIC CEPHALALGIAS

As noted above, headaches in these disorders are severe, relatively brief, and linked by their accompanying autonomic features. They consist of cluster headache, the paroxysmal hemicranias, and short-lasting unilateral neuralgiform headaches with conjunctival injection and tearing (SUNCT).

Cluster Headache

Cluster headache is the most common form of the TACs, yet it is still rare compared to other primary headache disorders. The disorder affects men three to four times as often as women and affects African Americans more often than Caucasians. Cluster headache may demonstrate a familial subtype; the risk of cluster in first-degree relatives has been demonstrated to be between 14- and 39-fold. It appears therefore to be transmitted as an autosomal dominant trait with incomplete penetrance.

Although cluster headaches can begin at any age, the mean age of onset is approximately 28 years. Childhood- and adolescent-onset cluster has been reported, but these early-onset cases appear to be rare: only 18% of patients had their onset of cluster prior to age 18 and 2% began before the age of 10.

Clinical Features

The ICHD-II divides cluster headache into two subtypes, episodic and chronic cluster. The criteria for the diagnosis of cluster headaches are listed in Table 6–1. Patients with cluster headache may demonstrate the following physical traits: heavy facial features, peau d'orange, leonine facies, hazel eyes, and taller-than-average stature.

The majority of patients with cluster headache suffer from the episodic form in which attacks recur for weeks to months at a time (the cluster period) and are then separated by months or years of pain freedom (the remission period). In episodic cluster headache, attacks recur over periods lasting 1 week to 1 year and are separated by pain-free periods lasting 1 month or more. In the ICHD-II guidelines it is noted that the typical cluster cycle lasts 2 weeks to 3 months, and remissions typically last 12 months. When remission periods last less than 1 month or when attacks recur without remission for more than 1 year, the designation "chronic cluster" is given. Approximately 10% to 15% of sufferers never experience remissions. The chronic subtype may evolve from an initially episodic course (previously referred to as *secondary chronic cluster*) or may begin de novo (previously referred to as *primary chronic*). Approximately 27% of patients experience only a single cluster period; in these instances they should be coded as per the ICHD-II as 3.1, "cluster headache (not episodic or chronic)."

Cluster headache is so named because attacks occur in groups or clusters separated by periods of pain-free remissions. During the cluster period, attacks may recur from once every other day to eight attacks per day. Most patients experience one or two attacks daily. The individual attacks are usually brief, lasting from 15 to 180 minutes each (mean 45 minutes). Attacks tend to recur at the same time each day and are notable in that they often occur at night, awakening the patient from a sound sleep. A seasonal preponderance may be present so that the cluster phase often occurs in the spring or autumn months.

Table 6–1 Criteria for Cluster Headache (ICHD-II)

3.1 Cluster Headache

Diagnostic criteria:

    A. At least 5 attacks fulfilling criteria B–D

    B. Severe or very severe unilateral orbital, supraorbital and/or temporal pain lasting 15–180 minutes if untreated[1]

    C. Headache accompanied by at least one of the following:

        1. Ipsilateral conjunctival injection and/or lacrimation

        2. Ipsilateral nasal congestion and/or rhinorrhea

        3. Ipsilateral eyelid edema

        4. Ipsilateral forehead and facial sweating

        5. Ipsilateral miosis and/or ptosis

        6. A sense of restlessness or agitation

    D. Attacks have a frequency from one every other day to 8 per day[2]

    E. Not attributed to another disorder[3]

Notes:

    1. During part (but less than half) of the time-course of cluster headache, attacks may be less severe and/or of shorter or longer duration.

    2. During part (but less than half) of the time-course of cluster headache, attacks may be less frequent.

    3. History and physical and neurological examinations do not suggest any of the disorders listed in groups 5–12 and/or neurological examinations do suggest such disorder but it is ruled out by appropriate investigations, or such disorder is present but attacks do not occur for the first time in close temporal relation to the disorder.

3.1.1 Episodic Cluster Headache

Diagnostic criteria:

    A. Attacks fulfilling criteria A–F for 3.1 Cluster headache

    B. At least two cluster periods lasting 7–365 days[1] and separated by pain-free remission periods of ≥1 month

Note:

    1. Cluster periods usually last between 2 weeks and 3 months.

3.1.2 Chronic Cluster Headache

Diagnostic criteria:

    A. Attacks fulfilling criteria A–F for 3.1 Cluster headache

    B. Attacks recur over >1 year without remission or with remission periods lasting <1 month

Attacks of cluster are excruciatingly severe, unilateral, and of maximal intensity in, around, or behind the eye. The pain may radiate into the ipsilateral temple, neck, jaw, or upper teeth, resulting in a misdiagnosis of sinus or dental disease. Most sufferers report that headaches always affect the same side; however, 14% of patients report side-shift during cluster cycles and 18% report side-shift with subsequent cycles. The pain is typically described as boring or stabbing and has been likened to a "hot poker in the eye." The onset of pain is usually rapid, peaking within 5 to 10 minutes. Whereas migraine sufferers prefer to lie in a darkened, quiet room, sufferers of cluster headache are restless; in fact, lying down often exacerbates the pain. Not uncommonly, patients will pace during an attack, sit upright in a chair holding their heads in their hands, or bang their heads against a wall. During acute attacks of pain, sufferers experience one or more autonomic features ipsilateral to the headache. These autonomic signs and symptoms include ptosis, miosis, lacrimation, conjunctival injection, nasal congestion, and rhinorrhea. These accompanying features are brief, lasting only for the duration of the acute pain. Recently, patients with typical cluster headaches preceded by visual auras have been described.

The repetitive nature of these headaches, together with the intense pain and dramatic associated autonomic disturbances, would seem to present an easily diagnosable condition. Nonetheless, the mean time to appropriate diagnosis ranges from 7 to 16 years.

Secondary mimics of cluster headaches have been reported and include vascular lesions such as vertebral artery dissection, pseudoaneurysm of the intracavernous carotid, aneurysms of the anterior communicating, carotid, and vertebral arteries, arteriovenous malformations of the occipital lobe or middle cerebral artery, and giant cell arteritis; spinal cord lesions such as cervical meningiomas and infarction; pituitary adenomas, sphenoid wing meningiomas, facial trauma, Tolosa-Hunt syndrome, and maxillary sinusitis.

Two other primary headache disorders, the paroxysmal hemicranias and the SUNCT syndrome, are considered TACs and are often mistaken for cluster headaches. These headaches differ from cluster headache primarily in their frequency, duration, and treatment response.

Paroxysmal Hemicranias

The paroxysmal hemicranias are a group of rare, benign headache disorders that clinically resemble cluster headache, fail to remit with standard anti-cluster therapies, and respond dramatically to treatment with indomethacin.

Although only chronic paroxysmal hemicrania was recognized in the first edition, an episodic form now also appears in the ICHD-II. The diagnostic criteria for the paroxysmal hemicranias are listed in Table 6–2.

Clinically, it appears that the chronic form is more common than the episodic form. Unlike cluster headache, chronic paroxysmal hemicrania demonstrates a female preponderance, with a sex ratio of approximately 2:1, whereas there is no gender preference noted for the episodic form. The age of onset ranges from 1 to 81 years, with a mean of approximately 34 years. No family history of chronic or episodic paroxysmal hemicrania was found in any of the reported cases. A documented family history of migraine was evident in 21% of reported cases, whereas only one prior report documented a positive family history of cluster headaches.

Table 6–2 Criteria for the Paroxysmal Hemicranias (ICHD-II)

3.2 Paroxysmal Hemicrania

Diagnostic Criteria:

A. At least 20 attacks fulfilling B–E

B. Attacks of severe unilateral orbital, supraorbital and/or temporal pain always on the same side lasting 2–30 minutes

C. Headache is accompanied by at least one of the following:

1. Ipsilateral conjunctival injection and/or lacrimation
2. Ipsilateral nasal congestion and/or rhinorrhea
3. Ipsilateral eyelid edema
4. Ipsilateral forehead and facial sweating
5. Ipsilateral miosis and/or ptosis

D. Attacks have a frequency above 5 per day for more than half the time, although periods with lower frequency may occur

E. Attacks are prevented completely by therapeutic doses of indomethacin[1]

F. Not attributed to another disorder[2]

Notes:

1. In order to rule out incomplete response, indomethacin should be used in a dose of ≥150 mg daily orally or rectally, or ≥100 mg by injection, but for maintenance smaller doses are often sufficient.

2. History and physical and neurological examinations do not suggest any of the disorders listed in groups 5–12 and/or neurological examinations do suggest such disorder but it is ruled out by appropriate investigations, or such disorder is present but attacks do not occur for the first time in close temporal relation to the disorder.

3.2.1 Episodic Paroxysmal Hemicrania (EPH)

A. Attacks fulfilling A–F for 3.2, *Paroxysmal hemicrania*

B. At least 2 attack periods lasting 7–365 days and separated by pain-free remission periods of ≥1 month

3.2.2 Chronic Paroxysmal Hemicrania (CPH)

A. Attacks fulfilling A–F for 3.2 *Paroxysmal hemicrania*

B. Attacks recur over ≥1 year without remission periods or with remission periods lasting <1 month

Clinical Features

As the clinical profiles of both the episodic and chronic forms are essentially identical, they will be discussed together. As with the diagnostic criteria for cluster headache, episodic paroxysmal hemicrania is diagnosed when attacks occur in periods lasting from 1 week to 1 year separated by pain-free remission periods of 1 month or longer. The chronic form is diagnosed when attacks occur for longer than 1 year without a remission period, or if the remission lasts less than 1 month.

In both forms of the disorder the pain is strictly unilateral and without side-shift in the vast majority of sufferers. The maximal pain is experienced in the ocular, temporal, maxillary, and frontal regions; nuchal and retro-orbital pain has less often been described. At times, the pain has been reported to radiate into the ipsilateral shoulder and arm.

The pain is usually reported to be a throbbing, boring, pulsatile, or stabbing sensation that ranges from moderate to excruciating in severity. On occasion, a mild discomfort at the usual site of pain is present interictally. During acute attacks, sufferers act more like those with migraine, preferring to sit quietly or lie in bed in the fetal position; only in rare reports do the patients assume the pacing activity usually seen in cluster headache. In fact the ICHD-II criteria do not list restlessness or pacing for these disorders.

In chronic paroxysmal hemicrania, attacks recur from 1 to 40 times daily. Most patients experience 15 or more attacks per day. There is, however, a marked variability in attack frequency. Mild attacks recur from 2 to 14 times per day; severe attacks recur 6 to 40 times per day. In the ICHD-II classification, attacks should have a frequency greater than five per day for more than half of the time.

Individual headaches usually last between 2 and 30 minutes, with a range of 2 to 120 minutes. In episodic paroxysmal hemicrania, the daily attack frequency ranges from 2 to 30, with attacks lasting 3 to 30 minutes each. The headache phase lasts from 2 weeks to 4.5 months; remissions range from 1 to 36 months. As with cluster headaches, attacks of chronic and episodic paroxysmal hemicrania recur throughout the day and night; nocturnal attacks have also been reported to occur in association with REM sleep.

Unlike patients with migraine or cluster headache, some patients with paroxysmal hemicrania report that attacks may be triggered by bending or rotating their head, pressing on the transverse process of C4-C5, C2 root, or greater occipital nerve. These features do not appear in the ICHD-II classification.

During acute attacks, one or more ipsilateral autonomic symptoms are usually present. Approximately 60% of sufferers report ipsilateral lacrimation. Homolateral ptosis (33%), conjunctival injection (36%), nasal congestion (42%), and rhinorrhea (36%) also may accompany the headaches. Unlike cluster headache, Horner's syndrome does not appear to accompany attacks of chronic or episodic paroxysmal hemicrania.

Cases of symptomatic paroxysmal hemicrania have been reported as well. Disorders that have mimicked the paroxysmal hemicranias have included aneurysms within the circle of Willis, arteriovenous malformations and cerebrovascular accidents, collagen vascular disease, Pancoast tumor, tumors of the frontal lobe, sella turcica, and cavernous sinus, intracranial hypertension, and thrombocythemia. A single post-traumatic case of chronic paroxysmal hemicrania with typical migrainous aura has also been described.

Because of the possibility of secondary mimics of the paroxysmal hemicranias, a prudent workup might include blood tests to screen for thrombocythemia and vasculitis, and brain imaging to exclude intracranial lesions.

Indomethacin is the treatment of choice for the paroxysmal hemicranias and has been deemed the sine qua non for establishing the diagnosis.

Short-Lasting Unilateral Neuralgiform Headaches with Conjunctival Injection and Tearing (SUNCT Syndrome)

The SUNCT syndrome is one of the rarest of the unusual primary headache disorders and has the most dramatic and variable clinical presentation. The syndrome was first described in 1978 and more fully characterized in 1989. Similarly to cluster headache, SUNCT has a male predominance, with a sex ratio of 1.2:1. The ICHD-II criteria for the diagnosis of SUNCT are listed in Table 6–3.

Clinical Features

SUNCT is characterized by very brief headache episodes that recur multiple times per day. The age of onset ranges from 10 to 77 years (mean 51). The pain is usually felt along the ophthalmic distribution of the trigeminal nerve, with maximal involvement in the orbital and periorbital regions. Pain may radiate to the ipsilateral forehead, temple, nose, cheek, and palate and at times into the ear and occiput. Attacks are typically unilateral; in three patients, however, pain was also simultaneously experienced on the opposite side. The pain quality is usually described as burning, stabbing, or electric-like. Paroxysms begin and end abruptly, reaching maximum intensity within 2 to 3 seconds. Individual headache attacks last between 5 and 250 seconds each (mean 49 seconds), although attacks lasting 2 hours each have been described. Some patients describe a dull interictal discomfort that persists between acute episodes, although most patients report being totally pain-free between attacks. Four patients experienced a "status-like" pattern in which painful paroxysms persisted from 1 to 3 days.

Table 6-3 3.3 Short-Lasting Unilateral Neuralgiform headache attacks with Conjunctival Injection and Tearing (SUNCT)

Description:
This syndrome is characterized by short-lasting attacks of unilateral pain that are much briefer than those seen in any other TAC and very often accompanied by prominent lacrimation and redness of the ipsilateral eye.
Diagnostic criteria:
A. At least 20 attacks fulfilling criteria B–D
B. Attacks of unilateral orbital, supraorbital or temporal stabbing or pulsating pain lasting 5–240 seconds
C. Pain is accompanied by ipsilateral conjunctival injection and lacrimation
D. Attacks occur with a frequency from 3 to 200 per day
E. Not attributed to another disorder[1]

Note:
1. History and physical and neurological examinations do not suggest any of the disorders listed in groups 5–12 and/or neurological examinations do suggest such disorder but it is ruled out by appropriate investigations, or such disorder is present but attacks do not occur for the first time in close temporal relation to the disorder.

The temporal pattern is also quite variable, with symptomatic periods alternating with periods of pain-free remissions occurring in an erratic fashion. Symptomatic periods generally last from a few days to several months and occur once or twice yearly. Remissions range from 1 week to 7 years but usually are of a few months' duration. During the symptomatic phase, daily attacks recur from 6 to 77 times (mean 28); however, tremendous variability occurs between different patients and within the same patient. Attacks may be as infrequent as once per day or less to more than 30 attacks per hour. In one patient, attacks would recur in a repetitive and overlapping fashion for 1 to 3 hours at a time, twice daily. Although attacks recur throughout the day, a bimodal distribution with increased attack frequency occurring in the morning and afternoon/evening hours has been described. Nocturnal attacks were experienced by 12 patients.

The acute attacks of headache in the SUNCT syndrome are accompanied by a variety of associated symptoms, the most prominent of which are ipsilateral conjunctival injection and lacrimation. Ipsilateral nasal congestion, rhinorrhea, and eyelid edema are less commonly reported. In some patients, the accompanying autonomic phenomena were bilateral although more pronounced on the side of the headache. The associated tearing and conjunctival injection usually begin 1 to 2 seconds following the acute episodes of pain and may persist for a few seconds longer than the painful episodes. In two patients, the associated symptoms remained from 30 to 60 seconds following headache resolution, and in one patient, eyelid edema persisted for 5 to 10 minutes. Rhinorrhea, when present, is delayed, occurring relatively late during the course of the headache.

Many patients can precipitate acute attacks by touching certain trigger zones within the territory of V1–V3. Other precipitating maneuvers include touching the hair, forehead, face, nose, and lip on the symptomatic side. Washing, shaving, eating, chewing, tooth brushing, talking, and coughing were also reported as headache triggers. Mechanical movements of the neck can also precipitate attacks, although some patients could lessen or abort attacks by continuously rotating their neck. Unlike trigeminal neuralgia, most patients have no refractory period.

Secondary causes of SUNCT have been reported in 18 patients and lesions are typically located within the pituitary gland or posterior fossa. Because of the rarity of this disorder and the frequent association with pituitary and posterior fossa lesions, brain imaging should be performed in all patients prior to initiating therapy.

The TACs are relatively rare but probably are more common than previously thought. As these disorders cause significant pain and disability, recognition is essential as treatment response differs from that of migraine, tension-type, and cluster headaches. Table 6–4 reviews the important clinical features of these syndromes.

Table 6–4 Clinical Features

	Chronic Paroxysmal Hemicrania	Episodic Paroxysmal Hemicrania	SUNCT	Cluster
Sex (F:M)	2:1	1:1	1:2.1–6.7	1:3–4
Pain quality	Throbbing, boring, stabbing	Throbbing, boring, stabbing	Stabbing, throbbing	Stabbing, boring
Pain severity	Very severe	Very severe	Moderate	Very severe
Site of maximal pain	Orbit, temple	Orbit, temple	Orbital, supraorbital, temporal	Orbit, temple
Attacks per day	1–40 (more than 5/day for more than half the time)	2–30 (more than 5/day for more than half the time)	3–200	1 every 2nd day–8
Attack duration	2–30 minutes	2–30 minutes	5–240 seconds	15–180 minutes
Autonomic features	Present	Present	Present	Present
Triggers	Alcohol, bending head, pressing C4-5, C2, occipital nerve	Alcohol, bending head, pressing C4-5, C2, occipital nerve	Neck movements, touching face	Alcohol
Nocturnal attacks	Yes	Yes	Yes	Yes
Prior attacks needed for diagnosis	20	20	20	5

OTHER PRIMARY HEADACHES

While included under the rubric of primary headache disorders, some of the syndromes listed within this classification may in fact have secondary etiologies. As noted in the ICHD-II criteria for these disorders, the diagnosis of the primary headache can be given only after secondary causes have been excluded. Furthermore, the proper treatment of these disorders can begin only after establishing the correct diagnosis; like the TACs, some of the conditions described in this section also respond dramatically to therapy with indomethacin but not to agents typically prescribed for the other more common primary headaches.

Primary Stabbing Headache

Primary stabbing headache is the new ICHD-II term for idiopathic stabbing/ ice pick headache. The disorder has been reported to have a lifetime prevalence of 2%. The age at onset ranges from 12 to 70 years, with a mean of approximately 47 years. Primary stabbing headache has a female predominance, with a sex ratio that has ranges from 1.49:1 to 6.6:1. Primary stabbing headache is characterized by spontaneous, paroxysmal attacks of fleeting head pain. The pain is moderate to severe in intensity and usually maximal in the ophthalmic distribution of the trigeminal nerve, particularly the orbital region. Less commonly affected sites of pain include the facial, temporal, parietal, retroauricular, and occipital regions of the head. Attacks are typically unilateral, but may be bilateral, and vary in location. The pain is often sharp, pricking, or stabbing in nature. Individual attacks are very brief and generally last between 1 and 10 seconds, with more than two thirds of reported attacks lasting 1 second. The frequency of attacks is quite variable, ranging from 1 attack per year to 50 attacks daily. Most attacks are distributed throughout the day and evening and may recur at irregular intervals. The pattern and frequency of attacks are quite variable and in more than 50% of cases, this headache is associated with other headache disorders, such as migraine, hemicrania continua, chronic paroxysmal hemicrania, and cluster. The diagnostic criteria for this primary headache disorder are listed in Table 6–5.

Indomethacin 25 to 50 mg three times a day brings relief in most but not all cases. Secondary stabbing headache has been associated with intracerebral meningiomas and giant cell arteritis.

Primary Cough Headache

Primary cough headache typically affects men over 40 years of age and while often described as a severe headache of sudden onset, it is by definition benign. Within seconds of coughing, sneezing, straining, or other Valsalva maneuvers, an immediate headache is experienced. The headache usually subsides within minutes; however, some sufferers may continue to experience a dull ache for several hours afterward. Often bilateral in location, the throbbing pain is

Table 6–5 Primary Stabbing Headache

Description:
Transient and localized stabs of pain in the head that occur spontaneously in the absence
  of organic disease of underlying structures of the cranial nerves.
Diagnostic criteria:
A. Head pain occurring as a single stab or a series of stabs and fulfilling criteria B and C
B. Exclusively or predominantly felt in the distribution of the first division of the
   trigeminal nerve
C. Stabs last for up to a few seconds and recur with irregular frequency ranging from one
   to many per day
D. No accompanying symptoms
E. Not attributed to another disorder[1]

Note:
1. History and physical and neurological examinations do not suggest any of the disorders listed in
    groups 5–12 and/or neurological examinations do suggest such disorder but it is ruled out by
    appropriate investigations, or such disorder is present but attacks do not occur for the first time in
    close temporal relation to the disorder

maximally felt at the vertex, frontal, occipital, or temporal areas, and associated
neurologic features or nausea and vomiting are absent. While the precise etiology is unknown, it may relate to a sudden increase in intracranial pressure with
traction on pain-sensitive structures from a downward displacement of cerebellar tonsils.

When cough headache occurs in a younger patient, is of long duration, is
strictly unilateral, or is associated with other features, the diagnosis must be
questioned. Secondary cough headache has been described in Chiari malformation; brain tumors, both malignant and benign (meningioma/acoustic neu-
roma); cerebral aneurysm; and carotid or vertebrobasilar disease. Neuroimaging
is important in distinguishing the secondary causes from primary cough
headache.

Indomethacin is the treatment of choice in patients who frequently experience cough headache. A positive response to indomethacin may be seen in secondary cases and is therefore not diagnostic of primary cough headache. The
diagnostic criteria for primary cough headache are listed in Table 6–6.

Primary Exertional Headache

Primary exertional headache, not surprisingly, occurs with exertional effort as
may occur during physical exercise, weight-lifting, straining, or bending over.
While cough and exertional headache are often linked as "Valsalva maneuver
headache," they remain distinct entities in the ICHD-II classification. The
headache is of sudden onset and often bilateral in location, but unlike
cough headache the pain is often pulsatile and of longer duration (5 minutes to
48 hours).

Table 6–6 Primary Cough Headache

Previously used terms: benign cough headache, Valsalva-maneuver headache
Description:
Headache precipitated by coughing or straining in the absence of any intracranial disorder
Diagnostic Criteria:
  A. Headache fulfilling criteria B and C
  B. Sudden onset, lasting one second to 30 minutes
  C. Brought on by and occurring only in association with coughing, straining and/or Valsalva maneuver
  D. Not attributed to another disorder[1]

Note:
1. Cough headache is symptomatic in about 40% of cases and the large majority of these present Arnold-Chiari malformation type I. Other reported causes of symptomatic cough headache include carotid or vertebrobasilar diseases and cerebral aneurysms. Diagnostic neuroimaging plays an important role in differentiating secondary cough headache from 4.2, Primary cough headache.

As in cough headache, neuroimaging to rule out a posterior fossa or craniocervical junction abnormality should be undertaken in a patient presenting with new exertional headache, particularly when the headache is unilateral. In addition to unilaterality, secondary exertional headache often begins later in life and lasts longer (24 hours to weeks), and in cases of subarachnoid hemorrhage, the headache is associated with neurologic features such as meningismus.

Other secondary causes include Chiari malformation, subdural hematoma, neoplasm (primary and metastatic), and platybasia. A first-ever presentation of exertional headache requires a workup to rule out subarachnoid hemorrhage or arterial dissection.

While the pathophysiology of primary exertional headache is unknown, it is theorized that venous distention following exercise or arterial distention as a result of exercise (especially in a warm environment) may be at the root of the cause, with subsequent release of vasoactive peptides leading to downstream neurogenic inflammation. Table 6–7 lists the diagnostic criteria for this disorder.

Primary Headaches Associated with Sexual Activity

Headaches with sexual activity affect men more often than women. These headaches have also been referred to as benign sex headache, coital cephalalgia, benign vascular sexual headache, or benign orgasmic headaches. As they are not solely precipitated by sexual intercourse (similar headaches provoked by masturbation and during nocturnal emissions have been reported) or orgasm, the ICHD-II has classified these as primary headaches associated with sexual activity. Three varieties of these headaches were described in the first edition of the ICHD: a dull type, an explosive type, and a postural type. In ICHD-II, however, these subtypes are not classified as such. Rather, primary headache

Table 6–7 Primary Exertional Headache

Description:
Headache precipitated by any form of exercise
Diagnostic criteria:
A. Pulsating headache fulfilling B and C
B. Lasting 5 minutes to 48 hours
C. Brought on by and occurring only during or physical exertion
D. Not attributed to another disorder[1]

Note:
1. On first occurrence of this headache type it is mandatory to exclude subarachnoid hemorrhage and arterial dissection.

associated with sexual activity is now separated into preorgasmic and orgasmic headaches. The criteria for these headaches are listed in Table 6–8.

Preorgasmic headaches (previously classified as the dull subtype) occur in approximately 20% of sufferers. These headaches resemble tension-type headaches in that they are characterized by a dull ache in the muscles of the head and neck. Some patients describe an awareness of tightness of the muscles of the jaw and neck occurring during sexual activity. Preorgasmic headaches are bilateral, beginning as sexual excitement builds, and can be prevented or reduced by deliberate muscle relaxation.

Orgasmic headaches (previously called the explosive subtype) are the most common, accounting for approximately 75% of cases. It is estimated that 50% of these sufferers also have pre-existing migraine headaches. These headaches begin abruptly, at the moment of orgasm, and may be caused by an increase in

Table 6–8 IHS Criteria of Primary Headache Associated with Sexual Activity

Description:
Headache precipitated by sexual activity, usually starting as a dull bilateral ache as sexual excitement increases and suddenly becoming intense at orgasm, in the absence of any intracranial disorder.

Preorgasmic headache
A. Dull ache in the head and neck associated with awareness of neck and/or jaw muscle contraction and fulfilling criterion B
B. Occurs during sexual activity and increases with sexual excitement
C. Not attributed to another disorder

Orgasmic headache
A. Sudden severe ('explosive') headache fulfilling criterion B
B. Occurs at orgasm
C. Not attributed to another disorder[1]

Note:
1. On first onset of orgasmic headache it is mandatory to exclude conditions such as subarachnoid hemorrhage.

blood pressure. The pain is excruciatingly severe, most often described as explosive or throbbing, and may be frontal, occipital, or generalized. On occasion this type of headache may be associated with nausea and vomiting. These headaches typically last from 1 minute to 3 hours.

The postural variety is the least common subtype, affecting approximately 5% of sufferers. This headache resembles the headache that follows lumbar puncture in that it worsens with sitting or standing and is relieved by recumbency. It may be caused by a rent in the dura that spontaneously develops during sexual activity. This rare subtype is no longer included in the ICHD classification of headaches associated with sexual activity. Instead, these headaches are now classified as headaches attributed to spontaneous low cerebrospinal fluid pressure.

The diagnosis of primary headache associated with sexual activity can be made only after excluding secondary causes such as subarachnoid hemorrhage, arterial dissection, and lesions of the posterior fossa, cerebrospinal fluid pathways, and cervical spine. The mainstay of treatment of the primary forms of headaches associated with sexual activity is reassurance, both of the patient and his or her partner. For most patients, these are self-limited disorders; however, the course may be unpredictable. Headaches often recur during several encounters over a brief period of time and never return again, while other patients experience them at infrequent intervals throughout their lifetime. Often patients can lessen the severity of an impending attack by stopping the sexual activity as soon as the headache begins. For patients who suffer from frequent, recurrent episodes, preventive strategies should be employed.

Hypnic Headache Syndrome

The hypnic headache syndrome is a rare, recurrent, sleep-related, primary headache disorder that usually begins after 50 years of age. Raskin first described the disorder in 1988; more than 90 cases have been subsequently reported. In the largest case study hypnic headache was diagnosed in 0.07% of all headache patients assessed annually at a specialty clinic, reflecting the rarity of this syndrome.

Hypnic headache usually begins late in life, with a mean age at onset of 61 ± 10 years (range 30 to 83 years). A case of a 9-year-old girl with probable hypnic headache has been reported, although the headache frequency did not meet IHS criteria. The condition is more prevalent in women (65%) than in men.

The headaches occur at a consistent time each night, usually between 1 and 3 a.m., and may on rare instances occur during a daytime nap. The headaches begin abruptly, are diffuse and throbbing, and spontaneously resolve in 15 to 180 minutes. Rarely, the headache is hemicranial. The pain is usually localized anteriorly and less often involves the lateral aspects of the head or is felt as a diffuse headache. On occasion it involves the occiput or radiates into the neck.

The duration of an untreated attack varies among the patients and between attacks. Usually the pain resolves within 1 to 2 hours (range 15 to 180 minutes), but longer attacks of up to 10 hours have been reported. The frequency of the attacks is high: more than four attacks per week occurred in 70% of the cases and about half of these patients had daily attacks (range one per week to six per night). No associated autonomic symptoms accompany the pain, but nausea, photophobia, and phonophobia may rarely be present. Diagnostic criteria are listed in Table 6–9.

Two reports of probable secondary hypnic headache have been described. In one, the patient had a 9-month history of typical hypnic headache but also reported brief episodes of giddiness. A brain MRI revealed a large posterior-fossa meningioma. Following tumor resection, there was complete resolution of the headache. In the second report, hypnic-like headaches occurred in the setting of intracranial hypotension. Headaches remitted following a spinal blood patch.

Primary Thunderclap Headache

Primary thunderclap headache is a severe headache of sudden onset that may persist for several hours. Severe headaches with abrupt onset are often associated with a sinister underlying secondary cause; that thunderclap headache exists as a primary subtype is controversial, but criteria have been suggested in the ICHD-II (Table 6–10).

The disorder was first described in 1984. In 1986 Day and Raskin coined the term "thunderclap headache" when describing a patient with a severe, rapidly developing headache who had a normal computed tomography scan of the brain and lumbar puncture, but in whom angiography revealed an unruptured aneurysm with diffuse vasospasm. Patients often describe thunderclap headache as the worst headache of their life. It comes on suddenly, peaks in intensity

---

Table 6–9 IHS Criteria for Hypnic Headache

Description:
Attacks of dull headache that always awaken the patient from sleep.
Diagnostic Criteria:
A. Dull headache fulfilling criteria B–D
B. Develops only during sleep, and awakens patient
C. At least two of the following characteristics:
1. Occurs >15 times per month
2. Lasts ≥15 minutes after waking
3. First occurs after age of 50 years
D. No autonomic symptoms and no more than one of nausea, photophobia or phonophobia
E. Not attributed to another disorder[1]

Note:
1. Intracranial disorders must be excluded. Distinction from one of the trigeminal autonomic cephalgias is necessary for effective management.

Table 6–10 Diagnostic Criteria for Thunderclap Headache

A. Severe head pain fulfilling criteria B and C
B. Both of the following characteristics:
   1. Sudden onset, reaching maximum intensity in <1 minute
   2. Lasting from 1 hour to 10 days
C. Does not recur regularly over subsequent weeks or months[1]
D. Not attributed to another disorder[2]

Notes:
1. Headache may recur within the first week after onset.
2. Normal CSF and normal brain imagining are required.

within 1 minute and typically lasts several hours. Patients may experience repeated bouts in the first 2 weeks; rarely, the headache may linger at a lower level. Primary thunderclap headache is often self-limiting, although one third of patients may experience recurrent episodes over the following months to years. It may occur spontaneously, while at rest, although in one third of reported cases the headache was precipitated by exertion.

Primary thunderclap headache may be part of the migraine continuum. Some patients have a prior history of migraine; in others it may presage the development of migraine. Clinically, a consistent location or quality of pain has not been described. The headache may be associated with light and sound sensitivity, neck stiffness, and nausea and/or vomiting. Usually patients have a normal neurologic examination, although focal neurologic deficits have been described.

According to the ICHD-II criteria, cerebrospinal fluid and brain imaging must be normal. These criteria make no mention of the need for angiography, yet two subtypes of primary thunderclap headache may exist: one with no angiographic abnormalities and a second subtype with diffuse segmental vasospasm.

As mandated by the ICHD-II criteria, this is a diagnosis of exclusion. Secondary causes should be aggressively sought. The differential diagnosis includes subarachnoid hemorrhage (12% of patients with subarachnoid hemorrhage present with the worst headache of their life), cerebral venous sinus thrombosis, pituitary apoplexy, and arterial dissection, among others. In patients with angiographic evidence of segmental vasospasm, central nervous system vasculitis should be considered. Initial workup should include a head CT, lumbar puncture, and when appropriate magnetic resonance imaging and conventional, CT, or magnetic resonance angiography of the brain.

Since primary thunderclap headache is usually a self-limited disorder, there are no treatment recommendations. Long-term follow-up in patients with primary thunderclap headache and unruptured aneurysms thus far has not revealed a tendency to bleed, but this remains controversial. Recurrent thunderclap headache with vasospasm leading to stroke has been reported; nimodipine may lessen the risk.

Hemicrania Continua

Hemicrania continua is another primary headache that is responsive to treatment with indomethacin. The disorder was first described in 1981 and officially named in 1984. There are now more than 100 reports in the literature. It was not included in the first edition of the ICHD guidelines. Because of the presence of autonomic features that accompany the painful exacerbations, hemicrania continua was considered to be one of the TACs. However, the ICHD-II includes hemicrania continua within the other primary headaches section (Table 6–11).

Hemicrania continua is thought to be underrecognized in the general population but is a common cause of refractory, unilateral, chronic daily headaches in subspecialty practices. The disorder demonstrates a female predominance, with a female-to-male ratio of approximately 2:1. The age of onset ranges from 11 to 58 years (mean 34 years). Clinically, it is characterized by a unilateral, continuous headache of mild to moderate intensity. Patients usually describe this baseline discomfort as dull, aching, or pressing, and it is not associated with other symptoms. The pain is maximal in the ocular, temporal, and maxillary regions. Superimposed upon this background discomfort, exacerbations of more severe pain, lasting 20 minutes to several days, are experienced by the majority of sufferers. Although significantly more intense than the baseline pain, these painful exacerbations never reach the level experienced by cluster headache sufferers. During these flare-ups, one or more autonomic symptoms (ptosis, conjunctival injection, lacrimation, and nasal congestion) occur

---

Table 6–11 Diagnostic Criteria for Hemicrania Continua

A. Headache for >3 months fulfilling criteria B–D
B. All of the following characteristics:
   1. Unilateral pain without side-shift
   2. Daily and continuous, without pain-free periods
   3. Moderate intensity, but with exacerbations of severe pain
C. At least one of the following autonomic features occurs during exacerbations and ipsilateral to the side of pain:
   1. Conjunctival injection and/or lacrimation
   2. Nasal congestion and/or rhinorrhea
   3. Ptosis and/or miosis
D. Complete response to therapeutic doses of indomethacin
E. Not attributed to another disorder[1]

Note:
1. History and physical and neurological examinations do not suggest any of the disorders listed in groups 5–12, or history and/or physical and/or neurological examinations do suggest such disorder but it is ruled out by appropriate investigations, or such disorder is present but headache does not occur for the first time in close temporal relation to the disorder.

ipsilateral to the pain. These exacerbations may occur at any time and frequently awaken the patient from sleep. Migrainous symptoms, such as nausea, vomiting, photophobia, and phonophobia, may also accompany the exacerbations of pain. Many patients report primary stabbing headaches (stabs and jabs) and a feeling of sand or an eyelash in the affected eye (foreign body sensation). Most patients experience strictly unilateral headaches without side-shift, although three patients in whom attacks alternated sides and three bilateral cases have been described.

Two temporal profiles of hemicrania continua exist: an episodic form with distinct headache phases separated by pain-free remissions, and a chronic form in which headaches persist without remissions. Hemicrania continua is chronic from onset in 53% of patients; in 35% the disorder began as the episodic subtype and evolved into the chronic form; in 12% it begins and remains episodic. Two atypical presentations have been described: in one patient an initially chronic course evolved into the episodic form, and another patient had episodic hemicrania continua with a clear seasonal pattern.

Hemicrania continua is frequently misdiagnosed as another primary headache syndrome. If the physician focuses on the ipsilateral autonomic features that accompany the painful exacerbations, the disorder may be incorrectly diagnosed as cluster headache. Similarly, by focusing on the associated photophobia, phonophobia, nausea, and vomiting that may occur during exacerbations, it may be misdiagnosed as migraine. Hemicrania continua is distinguished from cluster and migraine by the presence of a continuous baseline headache of mild to moderate severity; neither the ipsilateral autonomic features of cluster nor the associated phenomena typically reported with migraine accompany this baseline pain.

Organic mimics of hemicrania continua have been reported: a mesenchymal tumor involving the sphenoid bone, clinoid process, and skull base created symptoms of hemicrania continua. The diagnosis may be masked by medication overuse headache; with discontinuation of the overused agents, an unremitting headache will remain, and the diagnosis of hemicrania continua can then be made.

Indomethacin is the treatment of choice, and response to therapy with indomethacin is necessary for establishing the diagnosis.

New Daily Persistent Headache

New daily persistent headache (NDPH) is a headache that develops de novo, either acutely or over a maximum of 3 days, and then persists as a daily, unremitting headache. It has features of both migraine and tension-type headache: it is usually bilateral, pressure-like, and of mild to moderate intensity without worsening by physical activity, and it may be accompanied by photophobia, phonophobia, or mild nausea. The patient typically can recall the day of onset;

Table 6–12 Diagnostic Criteria for New Persistent Daily Headache

A. Headache for >3 months fulfilling criteria B–D
B. Headache is daily and unremitting from onset or from <3 days from onset[1]
C. At least two of the following pain characteristics:
   1. Bilateral location
   2. Pressing/tightening (non-pulsating) quality
   3. Mild or moderate intensity
   4. Not aggravated by routine physical activity such as walking or climbing stairs
D. Both of the following:
   1. No more than one of photophobia, phonophobia or mild nausea
   2. Neither moderate or severe nausea nor vomiting
E. Not attributed to another disorder[2]

Notes:

1. Headache may be unremitting from the moment of onset or very rapidly build up to continuous and unremitting pain. Such onset or rapid development must be clearly recalled and unambiguously described by the patient. Otherwise code as 2.3, Chronic tension-type headache.
2. History and physical and neurological examinations do not suggest any of the disorders listed in groups 5–12 (including 8.2, Medication overuse headache and its subforms), or history and/or physical and/or neurological examinations do suggest such a disorder but it is ruled out by appropriate investigations, or such disorder is present but headache does not occur for the first time in close temporal relation to the disorder.

in fact, an unambiguous description of this recollection is part of the criteria. Table 6–12 lists the diagnostic criteria for NDPH.

NDPH was first described in 1986. The initial report described 45 patients with no previous headache history who developed daily headaches from onset. These headaches were usually bilateral, continuous, and associated with nausea, vomiting, and photophobia and phonophobia. Over subsequent years, further cases were identified and various investigators published proposed criteria.

NDPH appears to be a relatively rare disorder with a female predominance. The age of onset in women ranges from 13 to 73, with the peak age in the second to fourth decades. In men, the age of onset ranges from 14 to 67, with the peak age in the third to fifth decades. Additionally, a significant number of adolescents with chronic daily headache have been found to meet criteria for NDPH. No consistent pain location is described in the reported cases of NDPH. A high percentage of patients have features typical of migraine. Neck pain, lightheadedness, blurred vision, and concentration difficulties are also described.

There are some data suggesting an infectious etiology to the disorder. Two studies have found elevated Epstein-Barr virus titers in these patients, invoking a possible autoimmune etiology or even perhaps direct, virally induced trigeminal nerve damage. Secondary mimics of NDPH include low- or high-pressure cerebrospinal fluid headaches, cerebral venous sinus thrombosis, post-infectious headache, post-traumatic headache, subarachnoid hemorrhage, chronic meningitis, neoplasm, and giant cell arteritis.

Whereas the initial report of NDPH suggested a benign outcome, with most patients becoming headache-free regardless of treatment, subsequent descriptions suggest a more intractable course. Indeed, there may be two forms of NDPH: a self-limited subtype and a refractory, persistent subtype.

SUMMARY

This chapter reviewed the clinical features of several less common primary headache disorders, including the trigeminal autonomic cephalalgias, exertional headaches, and a variety of other types. Many of these disorders share features with the more common conditions; others have more ominous secondary mimics. The clinician needs to be aware of these less common primary headaches as they are disabling and respond to different therapeutic agents than the more common headache syndromes.

Review Questions

1. All of the following disorders are considered TACs except:
   a. Cluster
   b. Episodic paroxysmal hemicrania
   c. Hemicrania continua
   d. SUNCT
   e. Chronic paroxysmal hemicrania
2. A 53-year-old man presents with recurrent attacks of severe, lancinating left eye, temple, and cheek pain lasting 10 seconds each. Attacks recur 30 times daily and are associated with ipsilateral tearing and reddening of the eye. This disorder:
   a. Occurs more frequently in women
   b. Requires five prior attacks
   c. Is responsive to treatment with indomethacin
   d. May be mimicked by posterior fossa lesions
   e. Is triggered by alcohol
3. A 43-year-old man reports that for the past 3 weeks he experiences a sudden, severe headache that occurs whenever he coughs. The headache lasts 5 to 10 seconds and then spontaneously resolves. His neurologic exam and brain MRI are normal. The condition in question:
   a. Commonly affects young women
   b. Commonly affects young men
   c. May be associated with nausea
   d. Is often unilateral
   e. Lasts up to 30 minutes

4. Which is true regarding cluster headache and the paroxysmal hemicranias?
   a. Similar number of prior headaches needed for diagnosis
   b. Only cluster is triggered by ETOH
   c. Male predominance for both
   d. Restlessness/pacing frequent
   e. Usually begin in adulthood

5. Which of the following is true regarding cluster headache?
   a. Episodic implies remission periods of more than 2 weeks
   b. About one quarter of patients have only a single cluster period
   c. Decreased CGRP and VIP is seen ipsilaterally
   d. May be transmitted as an autosomal recessive trait
   e. Occurs eight times more often in men

6. Primary thunderclap headache:
   a. Is usually self-limited
   b. Lasts up to 10 days
   c. Reaches peak intensity in less than 10 seconds
   d. Can be due to pituitary apoplexy
   e. a and b only

7. New daily persistent headache:
   a. May be self-limited
   b. Typically begins in 20s
   c. Is usually moderate to severe
   d. Is occasionally associated with vomiting
   e. Develops over 3 months

8. A 35-year-old woman complains of sharp, stabbing pains that recur 1 to 30 times daily without precipitant. Her neurologic exam and brain MRI are normal. This condition:
   a. Occurs in V2 most often
   b. May occur as part of a secondary headache disorder
   c. May accompany another primary headache disorder
   d. Is associated with photophobia/phonophobia
   e. Always responds to indomethacin

9. A 28-year-old man reports a 5-year history of a constant left-sided mild headache. Twice weekly the pain worsens and persists for 6 hours. During this time his left nostril stuffs. The disorder described:
   a. Is a form of TAC
   b. Occurs equally in both sexes
   c. Has no nocturnal attack pattern
   d. Responds to treatment with indomethacin
   e. Often begins in childhood

10. A 67-year-old woman presents with a 2-month history of global headaches that have been awakening her from sleep at 3 a.m. She denies associated autonomic features, nausea, vomiting, or

photophobia. Attacks last 1 hour each. Her neurologic exam and brain MRI are normal. The headache syndrome described in this case:

a. Occurs only during sleep
b. Occurs on a nightly basis
c. Is associated with ipsilateral autonomic signs
d. Is triggered by alcohol
e. Is often familial

10. a

9. d

8. c

7. a

6. e

5. b

4. e

3. e

2. d

1. c

SUGGESTED READING

Goadsby, P.J., & Lipton, R.B. A review of paroxysmal hemicranias, SUNCT syndrome and other short-lasting headaches with autonomic features, including new cases. *Brain* 120 (1997): 193–209.

Mathew NT. Transformed migraine. *Cephalalgia* 13 (1993): 78–83.

Rozen, T.D. New daily persistent headache. *Current Pain Headache Reports* 7 (2003): 218–223.

Sheftell, F.D., & Bigal, M.E. Medication overuse headache. *Continuum* 12 (2006): 153–169.

Silberstein, S.D., Lipton, R.B., & Goadsby, P.J., eds. *Headache in clinical practice*, 2nd edition. London: Martin Dunitz Ltd., 2002:147–180.

III

Diagnosis of Secondary Headache Disorders

7

Classification and Diagnosis of Secondary Headaches due to Traumatic and Vascular Causes

Alan M. Rapoport, MD, and Mark J. Rapoport, MD

Trauma to the head and neck occurs frequently and is a common cause of headache and neck pain. *Vascular disease* of the head and neck is a major cause of headache throughout the lifetime and more so in older age. Making an early diagnosis can be vital to the successful treatment of a patient.

This chapter is divided into two sections: part 1 is devoted to trauma and part 2 to vascular causes of headache. Each part is composed of a listing of the ICHD-II criteria, with some authors' comments about certain categories. Comments from the ICHD-II are in *italics*. There are plain films, MRIs, and CT scans interspersed, which the reader should be able to recognize as confirming particular diagnoses.

HEADACHES DUE TO HEAD AND NECK TRAUMA

Trauma causes headache via multiple mechanisms, some unknown. Head trauma, neck trauma, and "whiplash" injuries are all recognized causes of acute and chronic headache presentations. The ICHD-II classification of these is shown in Table 7–1.

After head and neck trauma, patients often develop headache and the post–head trauma syndrome consisting of dizziness, depression, other psychological symptoms, cognitive changes, and insomnia. If the trauma is severe, patients can become comatose and even develop neurologic changes on examination, which may become permanent.

There is often much emphasis on concussion when discussing head trauma, but there is no current consensus on what constitutes concussion. In a recent article by Ropper and Gorson in the *New England Journal of Medicine*, concussion was described as an "immediate and transient loss of consciousness accompanied by a brief period of amnesia after a blow to the head." But the authors go on to say that being "starstruck" or dazed after head injury without loss of consciousness may be considered the mildest form of concussion. We agree and feel that if a patient sustains head or neck trauma followed by some immediate

Table 7–1 Headache Attributed to Head and/or Neck Trauma (ICHD-II Classification)

5.1 Acute post-traumatic headache
    5.1.1 Acute post-traumatic headache attributed to moderate or severe head injury
    5.1.2 Acute post-traumatic headache attributed to mild head injury
5.2 Chronic post-traumatic headache
    5.2.1 Chronic post-traumatic headache attributed to moderate or severe head injury
    5.2.2 Chronic post-traumatic headache attributed to mild head injury
5.3 Acute headache attributed to whiplash injury
5.4 Chronic headache attributed to whiplash injury
5.5 Headache attributed to traumatic intracranial haematoma
    5.5.1 Headache attributed to epidural haematoma
    5.5.2 Headache attributed to subdural haematoma
5.6 Headache attributed to other head and/or neck trauma
    5.6.1 Acute headache attributed to other head and/or neck trauma
    5.6.2 Chronic headache attributed to other head and/or neck trauma
5.7 Post-craniotomy headache
    5.7.1 Acute post-craniotomy headache
    5.7.2 Chronic post-craniotomy headache

symptomatology such as dizziness, confusion, or any mild neurologic symptoms, that can be considered a concussion, even without actual loss of consciousness or amnesia. Cervical spine injury, even without direct trauma to the skull or spine, is sufficient to produce all these symptoms.

At times, very mild trauma causes severe symptoms. The same article suggests that the mechanism of concussion is due to "rotational motion of the cerebral hemispheres in the anterior-posterior plane, around the fulcrum of the fixed-in-place upper brainstem (the midbrain). Young children have the highest rates of concussion. Sports and bicycle accidents account for the majority of cases among 5- to 14-year-olds, whereas falls and vehicular accidents are the most common causes of concussion in adults." Concussion is more common in children, usually due to sporting and biking accidents. In adults, falls and auto accidents account for most head injuries that might lead to concussion.

Today most neurologists believe that concussion is due to disruption of the reticular activating system in the upper brain stem and thalamus. It is here that maximal rotational forces occur after trauma (Fig. 7–1).

The typical headache that occurs after trauma can take many forms, but it is usually phenotypically similar to tension-type headache and occasionally migraine and sometimes even cluster headache. Therefore, we do not specify the type of post-traumatic headache in terms of its headache characteristics. If trauma results in a recognizable type of headache, we might unofficially call

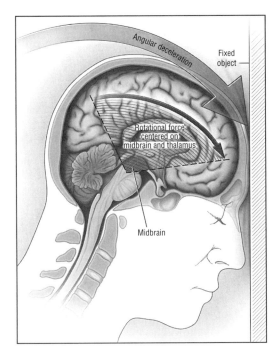

Figure 7–1 Mechanism of concussion. (Courtesy of the *New England Journal of Medicine*)

such a headache either post-traumatic migraine or cluster headache, but this is not an official IHS term. Although we see patients developing headache more than 1 week after the trauma, the IHS recognizes headaches as post-traumatic only when they begin within 1 week after the trauma. We believe that the official criteria should be changed to "between 1 and 3 months after trauma."

Women have a greater chance of developing post-traumatic headache. Older individuals tend to have more permanent headaches after trauma than younger ones or children. Children usually experience very brief headaches after trauma and are headache-free in 24 to 48 hours.

In some countries where there are limited chances to litigate injuries after accidents, there are fewer reports of post-traumatic headache. In a poster presented at the International Headache Congress in Stockholm in June 2007, Stovner concluded, "Headache after concussion did not differ significantly from headache after non-head injury 1–3 years after the trauma, neither by frequency, severity, prevalence of different headache diagnoses or prevalence of accompanying symptoms."

Acute Post-traumatic Headache

The ICHD divides the post-traumatic headaches into those resulting from severe head injury and those resulting from mild head injury. This is true for

Table 7–2 Criteria for Acute Post-traumatic Headache Attributed to Moderate or Severe Head Injury

5.1.1 Acute post-traumatic headache attributed to moderate or severe head injury
Diagnostic criteria:
A. Headache, no typical characteristics known, fulfilling criteria C and D
B. Head trauma with at least one of the following:
    1. Loss of consciousness for >30 minutes
    2. Glasgow Coma Scale (GCS) <13
    3. Post-traumatic amnesia for >48 hours
    4. Imaging demonstration of a traumatic brain lesion (cerebral haematoma, intracerebral and/or subarachnoid haemorrhage, brain contusion and/or skull fracture)
C. Headache develops within 7 days after head trauma or after regaining consciousness following head trauma
D. One or other of the following:
    1. Headache resolves within 3 months after head trauma
    2. Headache persists but 3 months have not yet passed since head trauma

both the acute forms and chronic forms. The acute post-traumatic headache criteria are listed in Table 7–2.

This could be any type of headache occurring right after severe head trauma. The patient should have an obvious history or examination or imaging results suggestive of significant brain trauma.

Acute post-traumatic headache attributed to mild head injury is described in Table 7–3. This could be any type of headache due to mild head trauma after which the patient rapidly develops mild symptoms or signs of cerebral injury; test results may or may not be abnormal (e.g., MRI, CT, EEG).

Figure 7–2 shows a CT scan done after head injury producing an acute post-traumatic headache attributable to mild head injury.

Table 7–3 Criteria for Acute Post-traumatic Headache Attributed to Mild Head Injury

5.1.2 Acute post-traumatic headache attributed to mild head injury
Diagnostic criteria:
A. Headache, no typical characteristics known, fulfilling criteria C and D
B. Head trauma with all the following:
    1. Either no loss of consciousness, or loss of consciousness of <30 minutes' duration
    2. Glasgow Coma Scale (GCS) >13
    3. Symptoms and/or signs diagnostic of concussion
C. Headache develops within 7 days after head trauma
D. One or other of the following:
    1. Headache resolves within 3 months after head trauma
    2. Headache persists but 3 months have not yet passed since head trauma

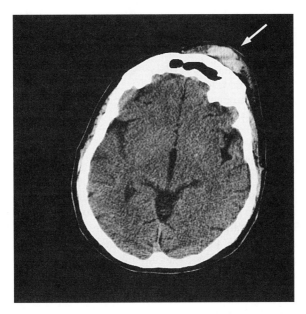

Figure 7–2 CT of left frontal subgaleal hemorrhage not affecting the skull contents. (Courtesy of Mark J. Rapoport, MD)

Chronic Post-traumatic Headache

Chronic post-traumatic headache is any headache that occurs within 7 days of an injury and persists for at least 3 months. The patient often has post–head trauma syndrome with cognitive dysfunction, irritability, poor concentration, and sleep disorder (Tables 7–4 and 7–5).

Table 7–4 Chronic Post-traumatic Headache Attributed to Moderate or Severe Head Injury

5.2.1 Chronic post-traumatic headache attributed to moderate or severe head injury
Diagnostic criteria:
A. Headache, no typical characteristics known, fulfilling criteria C and D
B. Head trauma with at least one of the following:
  1. Loss of consciousness for >30 minutes
  2. Glasgow Coma Scale (GCS) <13
  3. Post-traumatic amnesia for >48 hours
  4. Imaging demonstration of a traumatic brain lesion (cerebral haematoma, intracerebral and/or subarachnoid haemorrhage, brain contusion and/or skull fracture)
C. Headache develops within 7 days after head trauma or after regaining consciousness following head trauma
D. Headache persists for >3 months after head trauma

Table 7–5 Chronic Post-Traumatic Headache Attributed to Mild Head Injury

5.2.2 Chronic post-traumatic headache attributed to mild head injury
Diagnostic criteria:
A. Headache, no typical characteristics known, fulfilling criteria C and D
B. Head trauma with all the following:
    1. Either no loss of consciousness, or loss of consciousness of <30 minutes' duration
    2. Glasgow Coma Scale (GCS) >13
    3. Symptoms and/or signs diagnostic of concussion
C. Headache develops within 7 days after head trauma
D. Headache persists for >3 months after head trauma

These patients have a milder head injury, with few neurologic symptoms and signs. They often have post–head trauma syndrome. Although performing a brain CT or MRI scan is not considered routine after mild head trauma, if there is a concussion or any significant symptoms or any change in the Glasgow Coma Scale score or neurologic examination, most neurologists would do at least a CT scan looking for acute hemorrhage, and possibly an MRI of the head. If the non-contrast CT is unrevealing, further workup is often negative.

Headaches Attributed to Whiplash Injury

Although still controversial, most headache specialists believe that whiplash can produce headache. The ICHD divides these into the acute form (lasting less than 3 months) (Table 7–6) and the chronic form (longer than 3 months) (Table 7–7).

Table 7–6 Acute Headache Attributed to Whiplash Injury

5.3 Acute headache attributed to whiplash injury
Diagnostic criteria:
A. Headache, no typical characteristics known, fulfilling criteria C and D
B. History of whiplash (sudden and significant acceleration/deceleration movement of the neck) associated at the time with neck pain
C. Headache develops within 7 days after whiplash injury
D. One or other of the following:
    1. Headache resolves within 3 months after whiplash injury
    2. Headache persists but 3 months have not yet passed since whiplash injury
ICHD-2 Comments:
The term whiplash commonly refers to a sudden acceleration and/or deceleration of the neck (in the majority of cases due to a road accident). The clinical manifestations include symptoms and signs that relate to the neck, as well as somatic extracervical, neurosensory, behavioural, cognitive and affective disorders whose appearance and modes of expression and evolution can vary widely over time. Headache is very common in this post-whiplash syndrome. The Quebec Task Force on Whiplash-Associated Disorders has proposed a classification in five categories that may be useful in prospective studies.
There are important differences in the incidence of post-whiplash syndrome in different countries, perhaps related to expectations for compensation.

Table 7–7 Chronic Headache Attributed to Whiplash Injury

5.4 Chronic headache attributed to whiplash injury
Diagnostic criteria:
A. Headache, no typical characteristics known, fulfilling criteria C and D
B. History of whiplash (sudden and significant acceleration/deceleration movement of the neck) associated at the time with neck pain
C. Headache develops within 7 days after whiplash injury
D. Headache persists for >3 months after whiplash injury

In the United States the term "whiplash" has been used more by chiropractors than neurologists, but headache specialists should now adopt this term to mean someone with cervical spine acceleration or deceleration injury resulting in headache and symptoms of the post–head trauma syndrome. It is possible that many headaches, especially after head and neck trauma, may stem from abnormalities of the cervical cord, roots, and nerves. Special anesthetic blocking techniques may be helpful diagnostic procedures.

Chronic patients are the ones who often get involved in litigation as the trauma occurs during a motor vehicle accident and the symptoms are chronic and often disabling. The history is strongly positive, but the examination and all test results are usually negative. In addition to the headache, the patient often has a significant post–head trauma syndrome. In our experience, although some patients may exaggerate their symptoms, they are not usually malingering. Figure 7–3 shows a plain film from a patient who may have undergone significant cervical trauma with neck pain and ended up with a subluxation and possible small fracture of C1.

Headaches Attributed to Traumatic Hematoma

Post-traumatic intracranial hemorrhage is an obvious cause of headache, presumably related to increased intracranial pressure with dural stretching, and/or meningeal irritation by blood products. Key diagnostic entities are listed in Table 7–8.

Epidural hematoma (Table 7–9) usually occurs shortly after direct skull trauma and is most commonly related to tearing of a middle meningeal artery. It is somewhat more common in children, and there is often a lucid period followed by deterioration in the level of consciousness. The focal signs and symptoms may be more significant than the headache. They are certainly more worrisome to the clinician.

The patient whose CT scan is seen in Figure 7–4 had a left epidural hematoma and probably had weakness of the right face, arm and leg with decreased sensation and increased reflexes on the right in addition to headaches. Emergency surgery is usually indicated when a fresh epidural hematoma is found that causes significant neurologic signs and symptoms.

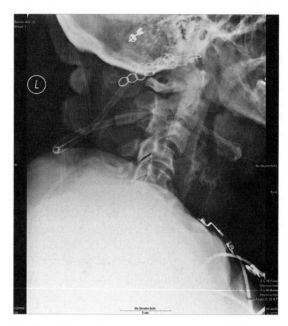

Figure 7–3 Plain film of cervical spine trauma with anterior subluxation of C3 on C4 and possible fracture of the arch of the atlas. (Courtesy of Mark J. Rapoport, MD)

Table 7–8 Headache Attributed to Traumatic Intracranial Hematoma

5.5 Headache attributed to traumatic intracranial haematoma
Coded elsewhere:
Headache attributed to traumatic intracerebral and/or subarachnoid haemorrhage or to traumatic intracerebral haematoma is coded as 5.1.1 *Acute post-traumatic headache attributed to moderate or severe head injury* or 5.2.1 *Chronic post-traumatic headache attributed to moderate or severe head injury.*

Table 7–9 Headache Attributed to Epidural Hematoma

5.5.1 Headache attributed to epidural haematoma
Diagnostic criteria:
A. Acute-onset headache, no other typical characteristics known, fulfilling criteria C and D
B. Neuroimaging evidence of epidural haematoma
C. Headache develops within minutes to 24 hours after development of the haematoma
D. One or other of the following:
    1. Headache resolves within 3 months after evacuation of the haematoma
    2. Headache persists but 3 months have not yet passed since evacuation of the haematoma

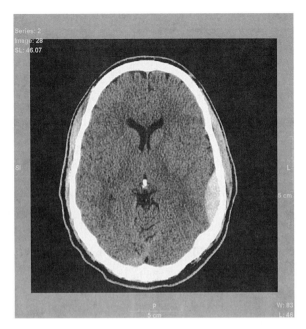

Figure 7–4 CT of small left epidural hematoma. (Courtesy of Mark J. Rapoport, MD)

Acute subdural hematoma produces a headache that is usually minor compared to the neurologic signs and symptoms the patient develops (Table 7–10).
In chronic subdural hematomas, headache is very common, but the patient
often does not recall the mild head trauma that may have caused it. Whenever
an older person, with or without a history of trauma, has increasing headache,
weakness, and cognitive problems, a chronic subdural hematoma should be
considered.

Table 7–10 Headache Attributed to Subdural Hematoma

5.5.2 Headache attributed to subdural haematoma
Diagnostic criteria:
A. Acute or progressive headache, no other typical characteristics known, fulfilling criteria
   C and D
B. Neuroimaging evidence of subdural haematoma
C. Headache develops within 24–72 hours after development of the haematoma
D. One or other of the following:
   1. Headache resolves within 3 months after evacuation of the haematoma
   2. Headache persists but 3 months have not yet passed since evacuation of the
      haematoma

Bilateral subdural hematomas may be a complication of cerebrospinal fluid hypotension with low spinal fluid pressure. These headaches are usually initially postural and may either remain predominantly postural or become continuous.

In an elderly patient, a subdural hematoma can occur with very mild trauma or even spontaneously. On a CT scan, a subdural will show up clearly acutely with blood appearing dense; it shows up less clearly at 1 week after trauma and it may well be isodense with brain at 2 weeks after trauma. This can make it hard to see. Small bilateral subdural hematomas, 2 weeks after trauma, can be missed on CT with cursory evaluation as the density is the same as brain and shift will not be apparent.

The CT in Figure 7–5 is of a middle-aged patient who probably developed a gradual-onset headache with motor symptoms on the left side.

HEADACHES DUE TO CRANIAL OR CERVICAL VASCULAR DISORDER

A number of vascular conditions of the head and neck cause head pain. This is related to the extensive nociceptive innervation of arterial and venous structures in these tissues. Table 7–11 lists the ICHD-II classification schema covering cranial and cervical vascular causes of headaches.

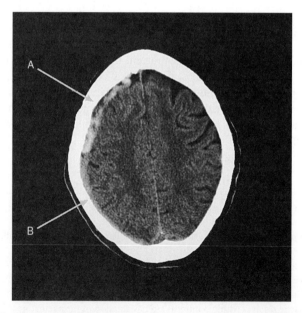

Figure 7–5 CT of right holohemispheric subdural hematoma with mass effect. Acute hemorrhage is seen anteriorly (A), while subacute hematoma is present posteriorly (B). (Courtesy of Mark J. Rapoport, MD)

Table 7–11 ICHD-2 Classification of Headache Attributed to Cranial or Cervical Vascular Disorder

6.1 Headache attributed to ischaemic stroke or transient ischaemic attack
    6.1.1 Headache attributed to ischaemic stroke (cerebral infarction)
    6.1.2 Headache attributed to transient ischaemic attack (TIA)
6.2 Headache attributed to non-traumatic intracranial haemorrhage
    6.2.1 Headache attributed to intracerebral haemorrhage
    6.2.2 Headache attributed to subarachnoid haemorrhage (SAH)
6.3 Headache attributed to unruptured vascular malformation
    6.3.1 Headache attributed to saccular aneurysm
    6.3.2 Headache attributed to arteriovenous malformation (AVM)
    6.3.3 Headache attributed to dural arteriovenous fistula
    6.3.4 Headache attributed to cavernous angioma
    6.3.5 Headache attributed to encephalotrigeminal or leptomeningeal angiomatosis (Sturge-Weber syndrome)
6.4 Headache attributed to arteritis
    6.4.1 Headache attributed to giant cell arteritis (GCA)
    6.4.2 Headache attributed to primary central nervous system (CNS) angiitis
    6.4.3 Headache attributed to secondary central nervous system (CNS) angiitis
6.5 Carotid or vertebral artery pain
    6.5.1 Headache or facial or neck pain attributed to arterial dissection
    6.5.2 Post-endarterectomy headache
    6.5.3 Carotid angioplasty headache
    6.5.4 Headache attributed to intracranial endovascular procedures
    6.5.5 Angiography headache
6.6 Headache attributed to cerebral venous thrombosis (CVT)
6.7 Headache attributed to other intracranial vascular disorder
    6.7.1 CADASIL (Cerebral Autosomal Dominant Arteriopathy with Subcortical Infarcts and Leukoencephalopathy)
    6.7.2 MELAS (Mitochondrial Encephalopathy, Lactic Acidosis and Stroke-like Episodes)
    6.7.3 Headache attributed to benign angiopathy of the central nervous system
    6.7.4 Headache attributed to pituitary apoplexy

Introduction from ICHD-2

The diagnosis of headache and its causal link is easy in most of the vascular conditions listed below because the headache presents both acutely and with neurological signs and because it often remits rapidly. The close temporal relationship between the headache and these neurological signs is therefore crucial to establishing causation.

In many of these conditions, such as ischaemic or haemorrhagic stroke, headache is overshadowed by focal signs and/or disorders of consciousness. In others, such as subarachnoid haemorrhage, headache is usually the prominent symptom. In a number of other conditions that can induce both headache and stroke, such as dissections, cerebral venous thrombosis, giant cell arteritis and central nervous system angiitis, headache is often an initial warning symptom. It is therefore crucial to recognise the association of headache with these disorders in order to diagnose correctly the underlying vascular disease and start appropriate treatment as early as possible, thus preventing potentially devastating neurological consequences.

Continued

Table 7–11 *(Continued)*

All of these conditions can occur in patients who have previously suffered a primary headache of any type. A clue that points to an underlying vascular condition is the onset, usually sudden, of a new headache, so far unknown to the patient. Whenever this occurs, vascular conditions should urgently be looked for.

For all vascular disorders listed here, the diagnostic criteria include whenever possible:

A. *Headache with one (or more) of the stated characteristics (if any are known) and fulfilling criteria C and D*

B. *Major diagnostic criteria of the vascular disorder*

C. *The temporal relationship of the association with, and/or other evidence of causation by, the vascular disorder*

D. *Improvement or disappearance of headache within a defined period[1] after its onset or after the vascular disorder has remitted or after its acute phase*

Note:

1. For headache attributed to some vascular disorders, criterion D is not indicated because there are not enough data to give any time limit for improvement or disappearance of the headache.

Headache from Ischemia

The headache of ischemic stroke is sudden or stuttering in onset and is associated with specific focal signs and symptoms and at times even loss of consciousness (Table 7–12). The headache can be moderately severe and associated with specific neurologic syndromes. Headaches occur with stroke up to one third of the time and much more often in strokes involving the posterior circulation. Headaches are also more common in strokes involving the large arteries of the cortex, such as the left middle cerebral artery (MCA) stroke seen in Figure 7–6, and are uncommon in lacunar strokes. The patient in Figure 7–6 probably had a sudden weakness on the right with eyes deviated to the left.

Headache attributed to migrainous infarction is classified as 1.5.4, not in Chapter 5 of ICHD-II, and consists of one or more migrainous aura symptoms associated with an ischemic brain lesion in the appropriate territory demonstrated by neuroimaging. The neurologic presentation must be identical to the

Table 7–12 Headache Attributed to Ischemic Stroke (Cerebral Infarction)

6.1.1 Headache attributed to ischaemic stroke (cerebral infarction)

Diagnostic criteria:

A. Any new acute headache fulfilling criterion C

B. Neurological signs and/or neuroimaging evidence of a recent ischaemic stroke

C. Headache develops simultaneously with or in very close temporal relationship to signs or other evidence of ischaemic stroke

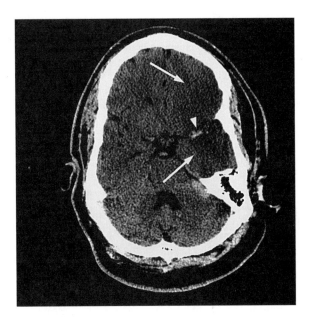

Figure 7–6 CT of a left cerebral ischemic stroke (*arrows*) with dense clot in the left middle cerebral artery (*arrowhead*). (Courtesy of Mark J. Rapoport, MD)

typical aura the patient has, and imaging shows a lesion in the appropriate territory (see Chapter 4).

Table 7–13 gives the ICHD-II criteria for headache attributed to transient ischemic attack.

Headache Attributed to Nontraumatic Intracranial Hemorrhage

Like traumatic intracranial hemorrhages, atraumatic hemorrhages from aneurysm rupture, arteriovenous malformation rupture, hypertension, or unknown cause(s) can lead to headaches, which can be important early clues to aid diagnosis and proper treatment. Table 7–14 gives the criteria for headache attributed to intracerebral hemorrhage.

The patient whose CT scan is seen in Figure 7–7 probably had a thunderclap headache with right-sided numbness and maybe some difficulty speaking.

A thunderclap headache comes on in seconds and is severe. It is always cause for concern and must be worked up completely. It may be due to hemorrhage, stroke, cerebral vein thrombosis, or other serious causes. In rare cases it can be simply due to migraine.

Thunderclap headache is commonly caused by a hemorrhage into the subarachnoid space; this is a very serious condition with a 50% mortality rate within hours (Table 7–15). Half of those who survive are permanently disabled with cognitive and motor deficits. The great majority of these hemorrhages are

Table 7–13 Headache Attributed to Transient Ischemic Attack (TIA)

6.1.2 Headache attributed to transient ischaemic attack (TIA)
Diagnostic criteria:
A. Any new acute headache fulfilling criteria C and D
B. Focal neurological deficit of ischaemic origin lasting <24 hours
C. Headache develops simultaneously with onset of focal deficit
D. Headache resolves within 24 hours
ICHD-2 Comment:
Whilst more common with basilar- than carotid-territory TIA, headache is very rarely a prominent symptom of TIA. The differential diagnosis between TIA with headache and an attack of migraine with aura may be particularly difficult. The mode of onset is crucial: the focal deficit is typically sudden in a TIA and more frequently progressive in a migrainous aura. Furthermore, positive phenomena (eg, scintillating scotoma) are far more common in migrainous aura than in TIA whereas negative phenomena are more usual in TIA.

caused by ruptured saccular aneurysms at the base of the brain. The headache lasts for many days but slowly resolves over one month. It may start out unilaterally but becomes holocephalic and associated with nausea, vomiting, nuchal rigidity, and cardiac arrhythmias. It can be responsible for severe vasospasm in the major cerebral arteries, leading to various territory strokes. Nimodipine therapy may be helpful in preventing stroke.

The diagnosis is easily confirmed by a CT scan done without contrast enhancement or an MRI with FLAIR sequences. If imaging is negative, a lumbar puncture should be performed. Figure 7–9 shows a CT scan with a typical diffuse subarachnoid hemorrhage.

Table 7–14 Headache Attributed to Intracerebral Hemorrhage

6.2.1 Headache attributed to intracerebral haemorrhage
Diagnostic criteria:
A. Any new acute headache fulfilling criterion C
B. Neurological signs or neuroimaging evidence of recent non-traumatic intracerebral haemorrhage
C. Headache develops simultaneously with or in very close temporal relation to intracerebral haemorrhage
ICHD-2 Comments:
Through usage, the term intracerebral is taken in this context to include intracerebellar. Headache is more frequent and more severe in haemorrhagic than in ischaemic stroke. It is usually overshadowed by focal deficits or coma, but it can be the prominent early feature of cerebellar haemorrhage which may require emergency surgical decompression.
6.2.1 Headache attributed to intracerebral haemorrhage is more often due to associated subarachnoid blood and to local compression than to intracranial hypertension. It can occasionally present as thunderclap headache.

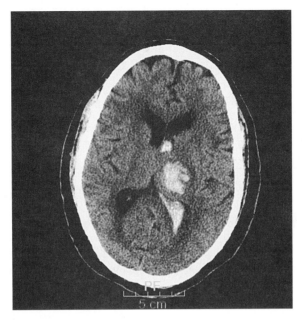

Figure 7–7 CT of left thalamic hemorrhage with blood in the left ventricle. (Courtesy of Mark J. Rapoport, MD)

Subarachnoid hemorrhage is a neurosurgical emergency, and today angiography is performed more quickly than it was years ago.

Headache Attributed to Vascular Malformations

Nonhemorrhagic (unruptured) vascular malformations can also lead to headache. Timing patterns usually, but not always, suggest chronic conditions rather than the sudden presentation of intracranial hemorrhage. Table 7–16 gives the criteria for diagnosis of headache attributed to saccular aneurysm, and Table 7–17 gives the criteria for diagnosis of headache attributed to arteriovenous malformation.

Table 7–15 Headache Attributed to Subarachnoid Hemorrhage

6.2.2 Headache attributed to subarachnoid haemorrhage (SAH)
Diagnostic criteria:
A. Severe headache of sudden onset fulfilling criteria C and D
B. Neuroimaging (CT or MRI T2 or FLAIR) or CSF evidence of non-traumatic subarachnoid haemorrhage with or without other clinical signs
C. Headache develops simultaneously with haemorrhage
D. Headache resolves within 1 month

Table 7–16 Headache Attributed to Saccular Aneurysm

6.3.1 Headache attributed to saccular aneurysm
Diagnostic criteria:
A. Any new acute headache including thunderclap headache and/or painful third nerve palsy fulfilling criteria C and D
B. Neuroimaging evidence of saccular aneurysm
C. Evidence exists of causation by the saccular aneurysm
D. Headache resolves within 72 hours
E. Subarachnoid haemorrhage, intracerebral haemorrhage and other causes of headache ruled out by appropriate investigations

Figure 7–8, a diagram from an article on aneurysms in the *New England Journal of Medicine*, shows the most common areas where they are found. Figure 7–9 is a CT scan of a patient who may have gone into coma after a thunderclap headache due to a subarachnoid hemorrhage secondary to a bleeding aneurysm.

Sometimes aneurysms are small, 4 mm or less, and although they do not rupture they can cause headache in up to 18% of such patients. In rare cases, the same syndrome is seen with ptosis, limited movement of the eye, and a

Table 7–17 Headache Attributed to Arteriovenous Malformation (AVM)

6.3.2 Headache attributed to arteriovenous malformation (AVM)
Diagnostic criteria:
A. Any new acute headache fulfilling criteria C and D
B. Neuroimaging evidence of arteriovenous malformation
C. Evidence exists of causation by the arteriovenous malformation
D. Headache resolves within 72 hours
E. Subarachnoid haemorrhage, intracerebral haemorrhage and other causes of headache ruled out by appropriate investigations
ICHD-2 Comments:
Cases have been reported highlighting the association of AVM with a variety of headaches such as cluster headache, chronic paroxysmal hemicrania (CPH) and short-lasting unilateral neuralgiform headache with conjunctival injection and tearing (SUNCT), but these cases had atypical features. There is no good evidence of a relationship between AVM and these primary headaches when they are typical.
Migraine with aura has been reported in up to 58% of women with AVM. A strong argument in favour of a causal relationship is the overwhelming correlation between the side of the headache or of the aura and the side of the AVM. There is thus a strong suggestion that AVM can cause attacks of migraine with aura (symptomatic migraine). Yet in large AVM series, migraine as a presenting symptom is rare, much less common than haemorrhage, epilepsy or focal deficits.

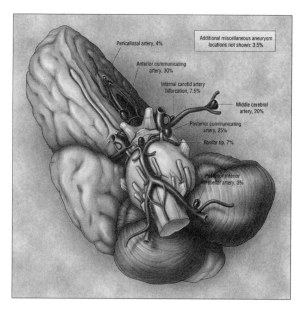

Figure 7–8 Percentage of aneurysms at different locations. (Courtesy of the *New England Journal of Medicine*)

normal pupil. We had a patient who had the sudden onset of moderately severe pain on the right side of the head. She gradually developed complete ptosis on the right. One week later, when first seen by author A.R., she had unilateral headache on the right and ptosis, and the right eye was abducted and otherwise plegic. However, her pupils were equal and reactive. She had been examined 6 months previously by a neurologist for recent right-sided headache and had a normal exam, lumbar puncture, MRI, and MRA. On this second occasion she had a CT scan, which was normal. We did an emergency cerebral angiogram that showed a small, unruptured posterior communicating artery aneurysm, which was clipped successfully the next day. She had severe postoperative pain for a month, but her eye signs improved rapidly and were gone in 4 weeks.

Figure 7–10 is an MRI showing a right carotid aneurysm at the base of the brain. Aneurysms occur in 5% of the population, and they may be familial. If headache symptoms are present in a patient with two family members who have intracranial aneurysms, four-vessel angiography or at least MRA or CTA should be considered. Up to 10% to 20% of angiograms in patients with aneurysms are negative.

The patient with the MRI seen in Figure 7–11 and the angiogram in Figure 7–12 could have a left frontal headache, or focal findings on the right,

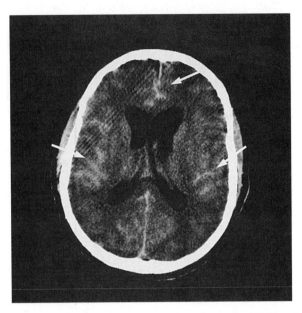

Figure 7–9 CT of diffuse subarachnoid hemorrhage (*arrows*) with dilated ventricles. (Courtesy of Mark J. Rapoport, MD)

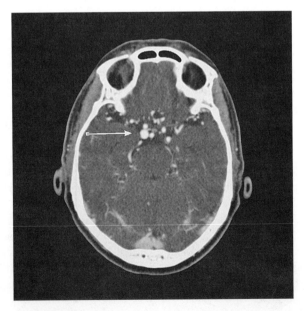

Figure 7–10 CTA showing a right carotid aneurysm (*arrow*) at the base of the brain. (Courtesy of Mark J. Rapoport, MD)

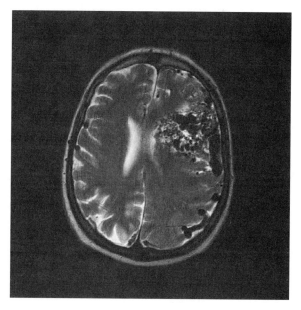

Figure 7–11 MRI of left frontal arteriovenous malformation. (Courtesy of Mark J. Rapoport, MD)

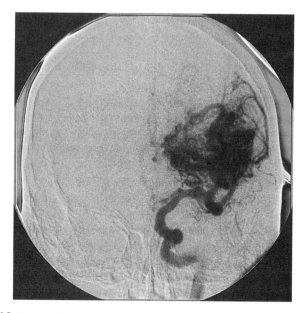

Figure 7–12 Conventional angiogram of a left frontal arteriovenous malformation. (Courtesy of Mark J. Rapoport, MD)

or just a nondescript headache. The treatment would be based on size, the feeding arteries, whether or not it is in the dominant hemisphere, and the patient's symptoms.

Table 7–18 gives the criteria for diagnosis of a headache attributed to a dural arteriovenous fistula and Table 7–19 gives the criteria for diagnosis of a headache attributed to cavernous angioma. Because of the contents of the cavernous sinus, suspect a fistula in this area if there are signs of dysfunction in the third, fourth, and sixth cranial nerves, plus V1 and V2 plus the sympathetic innervation to the eye. Tolosa-Hunt syndrome must be suspected if the patient has painful ophthalmoplegia; it is easy to diagnose with a CT of the orbits and cavernous sinus and easier to treat with steroids.

The patient whose MRI is shown in Figure 7–13 could have a new-onset headache due to this small cavernous angioma seen on a post-contrast T1 view. The same lesion is seen to be more benign-looking on the CT scan in Figure 7–14.

Table 7–20 gives the criteria for a headache attributed to encephalotrigeminal or leptomeningeal angiomatosis (Sturge Weber syndrome).

Headache Attributed to Arteritis

Inflammation of the cranial arteries is generally very painful. There are a number of arteritides that affect only the cranial or pericranial arteries (see below), but many systemic vasculitic conditions, such as polyarteritis nodosa and Wegener's granulomatosis, affect cerebral and pericranial arterial structures and may also produce headache as a cardinal symptom.

Table 7–21 gives the criteria for diagnosis of headache attributed to giant cell arteritis. Classic features of giant cell arteritis are tenderness of one or both temporal arteries, elevated ESR and/or CRP, symptoms of general disease such as fever, anemia, proximal weakness, and aches and pains proximally and in the joints, jaw claudication, night sweats, visual problems, and a positive biopsy.

Table 7–18 Headache Attributed to Dural Arteriovenous Fistula

6.3.3 Headache attributed to dural arteriovenous fistula
Diagnostic criteria:
A. Any new acute headache fulfilling criterion C
B. Neuroimaging evidence of dural arteriovenous fistula
C. Evidence exists of causation by the fistula
D. Subarachnoid haemorrhage, intracerebral haemorrhage and other causes of headache ruled out by appropriate investigations
ICHD-2 Comment:
Studies devoted to headache with dural arteriovenous fistula are lacking. A painful pulsatile tinnitus can be a presenting symptom, as well as headache with other signs of intracranial hypertension due to decrease in venous outflow and sometimes to sinus thrombosis. Carotid-cavernous fistulae may present as painful ophthalmoplegia.

Table 7–19 Headache Attributed to Cavernous Angioma

6.3.4 Headache attributed to cavernous angioma
Coded elsewhere:
Headache attributed to cerebral haemorrhage or seizure secondary to cavernous angioma
is coded as 6.2.1 *Headache attributed to intracerebral haemorrhage* or 7.6 *Headache attributed to epileptic seizure.*
Diagnostic criteria:
A. Any new acute headache fulfilling criterion C
B. Neuroimaging evidence of cavernous angioma
C. Evidence exists of causation by the cavernous angioma
D. Subarachnoid haemorrhage, intracerebral haemorrhage and other causes of headache ruled out by appropriate investigations
ICHD-2 Comment:
Cavernous angiomas are increasingly recognised on MRI. There is no good study devoted to headache associated with these malformations. Headache is commonly reported as a consequence of cerebral haemorrhage or of seizures due to cavernous angioma; and should be coded to these accordingly.

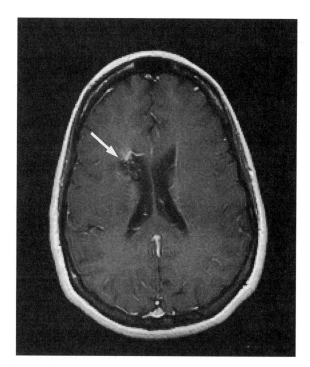

Figure 7–13 MRI of right frontal cavernous angioma. (Courtesy of Mark J. Rapoport, MD)

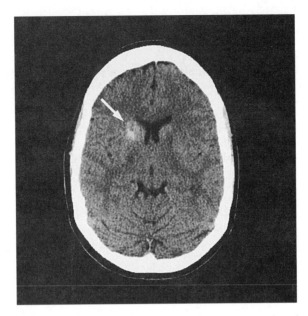

Figure 7–14 CT of a right frontal cavernous angioma. (Courtesy of Mark J. Rapoport, MD)

Treatment is a true medical emergency to prevent blindness and should be started with prednisone 80 mg per day or higher. Treatment can begin before the biopsy is done. Response to steroids usually occurs quickly (within 3 days).

Tables 7–22 and 7–23 give the criteria for diagnosis of headache attributed to primary and secondary central nervous system angiitis, respectively.

Table 7–20 Headache Attributed to Encephalotrigeminal or Leptomeningeal Angiomatosis (Sturge-Weber Syndrome)

6.3.5 Headache attributed to encephalotrigeminal or leptomeningeal angiomatosis (Sturge-Weber syndrome)

Diagnostic criteria:

A. Any new acute headache fulfilling criterion C
B. Facial angioma, seizures and neuroimaging evidence of meningeal angioma ipsilateral to the facial angioma
C. Evidence exists of causation by the angiomas
D. Other causes of headache ruled out by appropriate investigations

ICHD-2 Comment:

Headache is commonly reported in this condition but poorly documented. Isolated cases suggest that encephalotrigeminal or leptomeningeal angiomatosis may be a cause of symptomatic migraine, particularly of attacks with prolonged auras (possibly related to chronic oligaemia).

Table 7–21 Headache Attributed to Giant Cell Arteritis (GCA)

6.4.1 Headache attributed to giant cell arteritis (GCA)
Previously used terms:
Temporal arteritis, Horton's disease
Diagnostic criteria:
A. Any new persisting headache fulfilling criteria C and D
B. At least one of the following:
    1. Swollen tender scalp artery with elevated erythrocyte sedimentation rate (ESR) and/or C-reactive protein (CRP)
    2. Temporal artery biopsy demonstrating giant cell arteritis
C. Headache develops in close temporal relation to other symptoms and signs of giant cell arteritis
D. Headache resolves or greatly improves within 3 days of high-dose steroid treatment
ICHD-2 Comments:
Of all arteritides and collagen vascular diseases, giant cell arteritis is the disease most conspicuously associated with headache (which is due to inflammation of head arteries, mostly branches of the external carotid artery). The following points should be stressed:
- the variability in the characteristics of headache and other associated symptoms of GCA (polymyalgia rheumatica, jaw claudication) are such that any recent persisting headache in a patient over 60 years of age should suggest GCA and lead to appropriate investigations;
- recent repeated attacks of amaurosis fugax associated with headache are very suggestive of GCA and should prompt urgent investigations;
- the major risk is of blindness due to anterior ischaemic optic neuropathy, which can be prevented by immediate steroid treatment;
- the time interval between visual loss in one eye and in the other is usually less than 1 week;
- there are also risks of cerebral ischaemic events and of dementia;
- on histological examination, the temporal artery may appear uninvolved in some areas (skip lesions) pointing to the necessity of serial sectioning;
- duplex scanning of the temporal arteries may visualise the thickened arterial wall (as a halo on axial sections) and may help to select the site for biopsy.

Carotid or Vertebral Artery Pain

It has been demonstrated (by Raskin and others) not only that the cervical carotid and vertebral arteries are sensitive to pain, but that they can also lead to referred pain in a number of areas, including the eyes, face, and virtually any region of the head. Thus, conditions that alter the usual anatomy of these vessels or produce irritation in them may produce head, neck, or facial pain. Important entities are described below.

Table 7–24 gives the criteria for diagnosis of headache or facial or neck pain attributed to arterial dissection. Carotid artery dissection typically produces headache. Key features include fronto-orbital ipsilateral headache preceding ischemic symptoms (headache in 55% to 100% of series); painful Horner's syndrome, pulsatile tinnitus; and carotid bruit, dysgeusia, ipsilateral neck pain,

Table 7–22 Headache Attributed to Primary Central Nervous System (CNS) Angiitis

6.4.2 Headache attributed to primary central nervous system (CNS) angiitis
Previously used terms:
Isolated CNS angiitis, granulomatous CNS angiitis
Diagnostic criteria:
A. Any new persisting headache fulfilling criteria D and E
B. Encephalic signs of any type (e.g., stroke, seizures, disorders of cognition or consciousness)
C. CNS angiitis proven by cerebral or meningeal biopsy or suspected on angiographic signs in the absence of systemic arteritis
D. Headache develops in close temporal relation to encephalic signs
E. Headache improves within 1 month of steroid and/or immunosuppressive treatment
ICHD-2 Comments:
Headache is the dominant symptom in CNS angiitis (either primary or secondary). It is present in 50–80% of cases according to the diagnostic methods used, respectively angiography and histology. Nevertheless it has no specific features and is therefore of little diagnostic value until other signs are present such as focal deficits, seizures, altered cognition or disorders of consciousness. However, the absence of both headache and CSF pleocytosis makes CNS angiitis unlikely.
The pathogenesis of the headache is multifactorial: inflammation, stroke (ischaemic or haemorrhagic), raised intracranial pressure and/or SAH.
The effect of treatment is far less dramatic than in 6.4.1. Headache attributed to giant cell arteritis. Histologically proven primary CNS angiitis remains a serious and not infrequently lethal condition.

cerebral or retinal ischemia. It usually occurs in middle-aged patients. It affects the cervical section of the carotid. Triggers are cough, sneeze, or trauma. Risks are lues, Marfan syndrome, Ehlers-Danlos, cystic medial necrosis, and fibromuscular dysplasia. 60% of cases resolve spontaneously and 85% of patients do well.

The patient whose CTA is seen in Figure 7–15 probably had left neck pain, headache, and a left Horner's syndrome. He might have been treated with Coumadin.

The most common symptom of carotid artery dissection is orbital or peri-orbital headache associated with neck pain. A Horner's syndrome is commonly observed, and the patient can look like a cluster patient with longer-lasting, continual pain. There may be a bruit in the neck and the patient might complain of tinnitus. Complete occlusion of the artery could lead to a transient ischemic attack or stroke. Investigation should cover the entire length of the carotid and vertebral arteries both in the neck and the skull. Migraineurs are more susceptible to spontaneous dissection that non-migraineurs.

Table 7–25 gives the criteria for post-endarterectomy headache and Table 7–26 for angiography headache.

Table 7–23 Headache Attributed to Secondary Central Nervous System (CNS) Angiitis

6.4.3 Headache attributed to secondary central nervous system (CNS) angiitis
Diagnostic criteria:
A. Any new persisting headache fulfilling criteria D and E
B. Encephalic signs of any type (e.g., stroke, seizures, disorders of cognition or consciousness)
C. Evidence of systemic arteritis
D. Headache develops in close temporal relation to encephalic signs
E. Headache improves within 1 month of steroid and/or immunosuppressive treatment
ICHD-2 Comments:
Headache is the dominant symptom in CNS angiitis (either primary or secondary). It is present in 50–80% of cases according to the diagnostic methods used, respectively angiography and histology. Nevertheless it has no specific features and is therefore of little diagnostic value until other signs are present such as focal deficits, seizures, altered cognition or disorders of consciousness. However, the absence of both headache and CSF pleocytosis makes CNS angiitis unlikely.

The difficulty here is two-fold: 1) diagnosing CNS angiitis in a patient known to have one of the many conditions that can cause angiitis; 2) finding the underlying condition (inflammatory, infectious, malignant, toxic) in a patient presenting with CNS angiitis. The pathogenesis of the headache is multifactorial: inflammation, stroke (ischaemic or haemorrhagic), raised intracranial pressure and/or subarachnoid haemorrhage.

Table 7–24 Headache or Facial or Neck Pain Attributed to Arterial Dissection

6.5.1 Headache or facial or neck pain attributed to arterial dissection
Diagnostic criteria:
A. Any new headache, facial pain or neck pain of acute onset, with or without other neurological symptoms or signs and fulfilling criteria C and D
B. Dissection demonstrated by appropriate vascular and/or neuroimaging investigations
C. Pain develops in close temporal relation to and on the same side as the dissection
D. Pain resolves within 1 month
ICHD-II Comments:
Headache with or without neck pain can be the only manifestation of cervical artery dissection. It is by far the most frequent symptom (55–100% of cases) and it is also the most frequent inaugural symptom (33–86% of cases).

Headache and facial and neck pain are usually unilateral (ipsilateral to the dissected artery), severe and persistent (for a mean of 4 days). However, it has no constant specific pattern and it can sometimes be very misleading, mimicking other headaches such as migraine, cluster headache, primary thunderclap headache and SAH (particularly since intracranial vertebral artery dissection can itself present with SAH). Associated signs are frequent: signs of cerebral or retinal ischaemia and local signs. A painful Horner's syndrome or a painful tinnitus of sudden onset are highly suggestive of carotid dissection.

Continued

Table 7–24 *(Continued)*

Headache usually precedes the onset of ischaemic signs and therefore requires early diagnosis and treatment. Diagnosis is based on Duplex scanning, MRI, MRA and/or helical CT and, in doubtful cases, conventional angiography. Several of these investigations are commonly needed since any of them can be normal. There have been no randomised trials of treatment but there is a consensus in favour of heparin followed by warfarin for 3–6 months according to the quality of the arterial recovery.

Cerebral Venous Thrombosis

Cerebral venous thrombosis can cause serious cerebral pathology, including intracranial hypertension, which can mimic idiopathic intracranial hypertension. It can become progressive over days to weeks. Patients may develop papilledema and sixth-nerve palsies bilaterally with horizontal diplopia and transient visual obscurations. Patients can also develop venous infarction with focal signs. This can acutely mimic arterial stroke or be chronic and progressive, looking like a tumor or abscess. It can present with a thunderclap headache. Lastly, patients can develop subacute encephalopathy with diffuse headache and a decreased level of consciousness.

Focal neurologic signs occur in 50% of patients and seizures in 40%. Papilledema is usually absent. Patients with cavernous sinus thrombosis develop

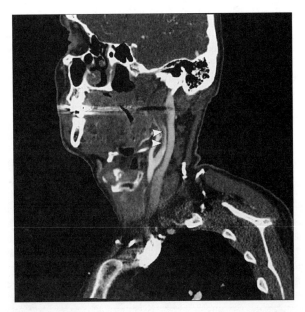

Figure 7–15 CTA of a left internal carotid artery dissection (*arrowheads*). (Courtesy of Mark J. Rapoport, MD)

Table 7–25 Post-endarterectomy Headache

6.5.2 Post-endarterectomy headache
Diagnostic criteria:
A. Acute headache with one of the following sets of characteristics and fulfilling criteria C and D:
   1. Diffuse mild pain
   2. Unilateral cluster-like pain occurring once or twice a day in attacks lasting 2–3 hours
   3. Unilateral pulsating severe pain
B. Carotid endarterectomy has been performed
C. Headache, in the absence of dissection, develops within 1 week of surgery
D. Headache resolves within 1 month after surgery
ICHD-2 Comment:
Three subforms of headache have been described after carotid endarterectomy. The most frequent (up to 60% of cases) is a diffuse, mild isolated headache occurring in the first few days after surgery. It is a benign self-limiting condition. The second type (reported in up to 38% of cases) is a unilateral cluster-like pain with attacks, lasting 2–3 hours, occurring once or twice a day. It resolves in about 2 weeks. The third type is part of the rare hyperperfusion syndrome with a unilateral pulsating and severe pain occurring after an interval of 3 days after surgery. It often precedes a rise in blood pressure and the onset of seizures or neurological deficits on about the 7th day. Urgent treatment is required since these symptoms can herald cerebral haemorrhage.

a frontal headache, chemosis, proptosis, ophthalmoparesis, and signs due to disruptions of the third, fourth, and sixth cranial nerves and the first two divisions of the fifth nerve plus sympathetic fibers.

There are many secondary causes of cerebral venous thrombosis, and these include hypercoagulable states (factor V Leiden, protein C and S deficiency), cancer, sepsis, Behçet's syndrome, lupus, and estrogen therapy.

Table 7–26 Angiography Headache

6.5.5 Angiography headache
Diagnostic criteria:
A. Acute headache with one of the following sets of characteristics and fulfilling criteria C and D
   1. Diffuse burning severe headache
   2. Headache, in a patient with migraine, having the features of migraine
B. Intra-arterial carotid or vertebral angiography has been performed
C. Headache develops during angiography
D. Headache resolves within 72 hours
ICHD-2 Comment:
The intracarotid or intravertebral injection of contrast induces a diffuse severe headache with a burning sensation which resolves spontaneously. The injection can also trigger a migraine attack in a person who has migraine. This should be coded both under 1. Migraine (as the appropriate subtype) and as 6.5.5 Angiography headache.

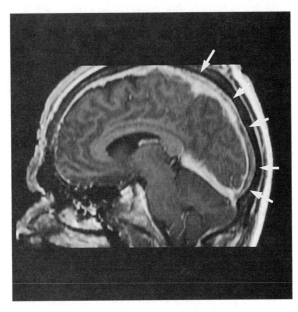

Figure 7–16 MR venography of superior sagittal thrombosis (*arrows*). (Courtesy of
Mark J. Rapoport, MD)

The patient whose scan is seen in Figure 7–16 with a superior sagittal sinus
thrombosis probably has a diffuse headache and multiple neurologic findings.

Headache Attributed to Other Intracranial Vascular Disorders

The conditions described in Tables 7–27, 7–28, 7–29, and 7–30 (CADASIL,
MELAS, reversible angiopathy, and pituitary apoplexy) are rare but serious and
should be kept in mind when evaluating headache patients.

Migraine with aura with a prolonged aura phase is present in one third of
patients with CADASIL, and in those cases it may precede MRI changes by up
to 15 years. The pathologic hallmark of this disease is a marked thickening of
the media by a deposit of electron-dense granular extracellular material located
in the media. There is marked vessel wall damage, smooth muscle cell degen-
eration, and abnormal endothelium. The destruction of vascular smooth muscle cells leads to progressive, fibrotic wall thickening, and luminal narrowing.
This weakens the vessel wall in small/medium arteries of almost all organs;
however, brain vessel pathology predominates.

Benign (or reversible) angiopathy of the central nervous system causes a diffuse, severe headache that can present as a thunderclap headache. Neurologically
the patient has fluctuating signs and symptoms, and seizures are possible.
Angiography is diagnostic and shows "strings and beads" and intermittent constriction. Cerebrospinal fluid is usually normal. This syndrome is often seen

Table 7–27 Cerebral Autosomal Dominant Arteriopathy with Subcortical Infarcts and Leukoencephalopathy (CADASIL)

6.7.1 Cerebral Autosomal Dominant Arteriopathy with Subcortical Infarcts and
      Leukoencephalopathy (CADASIL)

Diagnostic criteria:

A. Attacks of migraine with aura, with or without other neurological signs
B. Typical white matter changes on MRI T2WI
C. Diagnostic confirmation from skin biopsy evidence or genetic testing (notch 3
    mutations on chromosome 19)

Table 7–28 Mitochondrial Encephalopathy, Lactic Acidosis and Stroke-like Episodes (MELAS)

6.7.2 Mitochondrial Encephalopathy, Lactic Acidosis and Stroke-like episodes (MELAS)

Diagnostic criteria:

A. Attacks of migraine with or without aura
B. Stroke-like episodes and seizures
C. Genetic abnormality (3243 point mitochondrial DNA mutation in the tRNA Leu gene
or other DNA MELAS point mutation)

ICHD-2 Comment:

Migraine attacks are frequent in MELAS and this has led to the hypothesis that mitochondrial mutations could play a role in migraine with aura but the 3243 mutation was not detected in two groups of subjects with migraine with aura. Other yet-undetected mutations may play a role in both migraine and ischaemic stroke since migraine attacks, mostly with aura, also occur in other mitochondrial disorders.

Table 7–29 Headache Attributed to Benign (or Reversible) Angiopathy of the Central Nervous System (Previously Termed Call-Fleming Syndrome)

6.7.3 Headache attributed to benign (or reversible) angiopathy of the central nervous
      system *(previously termed Call-Fleming syndrome)*

Diagnostic criteria:

A. Diffuse, severe headache of abrupt or progressive onset, with or without focal
    neurological deficits and/or seizures and fulfilling criteria C and D
B. "Strings and beads" appearance on angiography and subarachnoid haemorrhage ruled
    out by appropriate investigations
C. One or both of the following:
    1. Headache develops simultaneously with neurological deficits and/or seizures
    2. Headache leads to angiography and discovery of "strings and beads" appearance
D. Headache (and neurological deficits, if present) resolves spontaneously within
    2 months

Table 7–30 Headache Attributed to Pituitary Apoplexy

6.7.4 Headache attributed to pituitary apoplexy

Diagnostic criteria:

A. Severe acute retro-orbital, frontal or diffuse headache accompanied by at least one of the following and fulfilling criteria C and D:
   1. Nausea and vomiting
   2. Fever
   3. Diminished level of consciousness
   4. Hypopituitarism
   5. Hypotension
   6. Ophthalmoplegia or impaired visual acuity
B. Neuroimaging evidence of acute haemorrhagic pituitary infarction
C. Headache develops simultaneously with acute haemorrhagic pituitary infarction
D. Headache and other symptoms and/or signs resolve within 1 month

ICHD-2 Comment:

This rare clinical syndrome is an acute, life-threatening condition, characterised by spontaneous haemorrhagic infarction of the pituitary gland. It is one of the causes of thunderclap headache.

Magnetic resonance imaging is more sensitive than CT scan for detecting intrasellar pathology.

postpartum and can be caused by the use of bromocriptine. The entire syndrome is self-limited and disappears in 1 to 2 months. Because of the diagnostic difficulty with separation from primary central nervous system angiitis, a course of high-dose steroids is sometimes given.

SUMMARY

Mild head injury may lead to mild concussion with no loss of consciousness but some dizziness, drowsiness, or cognitive impairment. Headache has to begin within 1 week after head or neck trauma to be considered post-traumatic. It becomes chronic if it lasts more than 3 months. To diagnose post-traumatic headache, the patient does not need to have a direct blow to the head, as acute or chronic whiplash injury can be due to acceleration or deceleration trauma to the neck.

A transient ischemic attack does not usually cause headache, but a stroke may have headache associated with posterior circulation disease about 30% of the time. A migrainous infarction is a stroke that occurs during an aura and leaves the patient with a deficit in the same distribution as his or her typical aura. It is not listed in the vascular disease section but rather as a complication of migraine, a primary headache disorder.

A number of vascular anomalies can produce headache without rupture, including aneurysms, arteriovenous malformations, fistulas, and angiomas.

Anterior and posterior communicating aneurysms make up 55% of saccular aneurysms. Cerebral venous thrombosis is sometimes overlooked as the cause of headache due to the challenges in finding evidence for it on standard neuroimaging. Some secondary causes of cerebral venous thrombosis are cancer, hypercoagulable state (factor V Leiden, protein C and S deficiency), sepsis, Behçet's syndrome, lupus, and estrogen therapy.

CADASIL is caused by an abnormality in the notch 3 gene on chromosome 19. MELAS is due to a mitochondrial DNA mutation in the tRNA gene. The typical headache in both CADASIL and MELAS is migraine with aura.

Review Questions

1. A 34-year-old man was stopped at a traffic light in his car and was hit from behind by a car going 25 m.p.h. that did not brake. He was not belted in and had no airbags, and his head hit the windshield. He had a questionable 1-minute loss of consciousness and was dazed and dizzy. He had a normal Glasgow Coma Scale score and his CT was normal. He denied neck pain. He developed a holocephalic headache 6 days later that was moderately severe, constant, and associated with dizziness and depression. This headache lasted over 1 year. When seen by his neurologist at 4 months after trauma, what was his initial diagnosis?
   a. 5.2.1 Chronic post-traumatic headache attributed to moderate or severe head injury
   b. 5.2.2 Chronic post-traumatic headache attributed to mild head injury
   c. 5.3 Acute headache attributed to whiplash injury
   d. 5.4 Chronic headache attributed to whiplash injury
   e. 5.5.2 Headache attributed to subdural hematoma
2. What would the diagnosis have been if the headache had been present for only 2 months and the patient did not strike his head?
   a. 5.2.1 Chronic post-traumatic headache attributed to moderate or severe head injury
   b. 5.2.2 Chronic post-traumatic headache attributed to mild head injury
   c. 5.3 Acute headache attributed to whiplash injury
   d. 5.4 Chronic headache attributed to whiplash injury
   e. 5.5.2 Headache attributed to subdural hematoma
3. A 77-year-old woman slips on the last step and twists her ankle. She has trouble getting off the floor and is taken to the emergency department, where she is given a good report and sent home. She gradually develops a mild bilateral headache lasting for several hours each day. She denies any visual symptoms or weakness and her examination is normal. Two weeks after this fall, with progressive headache, she

undergoes a non-contrast CT, which is read as normal. Her headache is now severe and she is slightly confused. What is the most appropriate next test?

- a. An ESR
- b. A carotid Doppler
- c. A CT of the head with contrast
- d. An MRI of the head
- e. A cerebral angiogram

4. This patient probably has:
   - a. Nothing seen on any test
   - b. Carotid dissection
   - c. Primary central nervous system angiitis
   - d. Bilateral subdural hematomas
   - e. Giant cell arteritis

5. A 49-year-old woman comes to the office with a 1-week history of right-sided headache and drooping eyelid. She gives a history of a right-sided headache without other symptoms 6 months before that lasted 2 weeks and resolved; she had a full workup, including neurologic evaluation, lumbar puncture, CT, MRI and MRA, all normal. On examination she has right ptosis and the right eye does not adduct or move well up or down but can abduct. The pupils are normal in size and they react. There is no eye tenderness. The following test should be done:
   - a. ESR
   - b. CT of the right orbit
   - c. Cerebral angiogram
   - d. Lumbar puncture
   - e. Carotid Doppler

6. The most likely diagnosis on this patient is:
   - a. Glaucoma
   - b. Meningitis
   - c. Occipital arteriovenous malformation
   - d. Right posterior communicating artery aneurysm
   - e. Right glioblastoma

7. A 62-year-old woman without a history of headache has brief attacks of loss of vision in one eye. She then develops difficulty combing her hair. On further questioning she admits to pain in her jaw when she chews, a low-grade fever, and a frontotemporal throbbing pain. Her treatment should be:
   - a. 80 mg prednisone per day
   - b. Sumatriptan tablets100 mg
   - c. Topiramate 100 mg per day
   - d. Heparin IV
   - e. Butalbital medication PO

8. A 49-year-old physician is dancing and develops right neck pain and temporal headache. He is taken to the emergency department, where he has a Horner's syndrome, right eye tearing, and periorbital pain. The diagnosis is cluster headache, but the pain does not relent for 3 days. The most likely diagnosis is:
   a. Subdural hematoma
   b. Migraine
   c. Tension-type headache
   d. MELAS
   e. Carotid artery dissection
9. Patients with CADASIL often have headaches. The type they usually have is:
   a. Cluster headache
   b. SUNCT
   c. Migraine with aura
   d. Migraine without aura
   e. Tension-type headache
10. CADASIL is associated with an abnormality in:
    a. A chromosome 19 Ca channel gene
    b. A chromosome 1 Na/K ATPase pump gene
    c. A chromosome 2 Na channel gene
    d. A glutamate transporter gene
    e. A chromosome 19 notch 3 gene

10. e
9. c
8. e
7. a
6. d
5. c
4. d
3. d
2. c
1. b

SUGGESTED READING

Brisman, J.L., Song, J.K., & Newell, D.W. Cerebral aneurysms. *New England Journal of Medicine* 355 (2006): 928–939.

Ropper, A.H., & Gorson, K.C. Concussion. *New England Journal of Medicine* 356 (2007):166–172.

Stovner, L.J., Schrader, H., Mickeviciene, D., et al. Headache after concussion. *Cephalalgia* 27 (2007): 575–579.

8

Classification and Diagnosis of Secondary Headaches: Altered Intracranial Pressure, Neoplasm, and Infection

Brian E. McGeeney, MD, MPH

A thorough familiarity with secondary headache etiologies is needed as the practitioner is faced with a multitude of secondary headache causes. The following chapter covers the secondary headaches in Sections 7 and 9 of the International Classification of Headache Disorders (ICHD), second edition. This chapter defines headaches from altered intracranial pressure and inflammatory, neoplastic, and infectious etiologies. Images are provided and diagnostic criteria from the ICHD are presented. It is worth keeping in mind that patients with an underlying primary headache disorder are often more likely to develop headache as part of other etiologies.

HEADACHE ATTRIBUTED TO IDIOPATHIC INTRACRANIAL HYPERTENSION

Idiopathic intracranial hypertension (IIH), otherwise known as pseudotumor cerebri, has an incidence between 2 and 5 per 100,000 in the population and is much more common in obese women. The typical age range is 20 to 45 years old, but it can occur outside of this, such as childhood presentation. Idiopathic intracranial hypertension is a disorder of abnormal cerebrospinal fluid (CSF) mechanics, but the exact abnormality is unknown. Raised intracranial pressure may be associated with obstructive sleep apnea, polycystic ovary syndrome, antiphospholipid antibody syndrome, HIV infection, and cerebral venous thrombosis or stenosis, among other secondary causes that should be considered. Oral contraceptive use or pregnancy is not a risk factor for IIH. Evidence supports the association of IIH with use of tetracyclines, vitamin A and retinoids, nalidixic acid, leuprorelin acetate, and the *withdrawal* of corticosteroids.

It is possible to fulfil the diagnostic criteria (Table 8–1) with no papilledema. In such cases one needs to be particularly careful about the CSF pressure measurement and carefully consider other causes. The diagnosis of IIH may be made

Table 8–1 Idiopathic Intracranial Hypertension

Diagnostic criteria:

A. Progressive headache with at least one of the following characteristics and fulfilling criteria C and D:
1. Daily occurrence
2. Diffuse and/or constant (non-pulsating) pain
3. Aggravated by coughing or straining

B. Intracranial hypertension fulfilling the following criteria:
1. Alert patient with neurological examination that either is normal or demonstrates any of the following abnormalities:
   a) Papilloedema
   b) Enlarged blind spot
   c) Visual field defect (progressive if untreated)
   d) Sixth nerve palsy
2. Increased CSF pressure (>200 mm H_2O in the non-obese, >250 mm H_2O in the obese) measured by lumbar puncture in the recumbent position or by epidural or intraventricular pressure monitoring
3. Normal CSF chemistry (low CSF protein is acceptable) and cellularity
4. Intracranial diseases (including venous sinus thrombosis) ruled out by appropriate investigations
5. No metabolic, toxic or hormonal cause of intracranial hypertension

C. Headache develops in close temporal relation to increased intracranial pressure

D. Headache improves after withdrawal of CSF to reduce pressure to 120–170 mm H_2O and resolves within 72 hours of persistent normalisation of intracranial pressure

without symptoms (no headache), usually by opthalmologists noting papilledema. Associated features similar to migraine may accompany the headache. Transient visual obscurations occur in approximately 75% of patients; they last less than 60 seconds and are associated with papilledema. Tinnitus is common also. The biggest complication is visual loss, which can be permanent.

Workup involves imaging the brain, magnetic resonance venography, and consideration of secondary causes. The brain appears normal on most imaging studies and there is no ventriculomegaly. An empty sella is commonly seen (Fig. 8–1) and reverse cupping of the optic disk may be seen also on MRI. The use of corticosteroids in subjects with IIH should be avoided if possible due to the potential for weight gain and withdrawal associated worsening. Of note, normal-pressure hydrocephalus does not cause headache.

Treatment

There is no FDA-approved treatment for IIH, and the lack of controlled treatment trials precludes evidence-based decision making. Weight loss is advocated for those who are overweight, and treatment is primarily to protect vision. Most patients are started on acetazolamide, a carbonic anhydrase inhibitor that decreases CSF production. Patients taking acetazolamide will be expected to

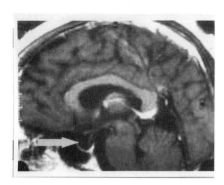

Figure 8–1 Sagittal MR image demonstrating an empty sella, a radiologic sign for a sella turcica partially or completely filled with CSF. This occurs in normal adults 5% to 15% of the time and in approximately 70% of those with idiopathic intracranial hypertension. (Used with permission from www.endotext.org, Neuroendocrinology Section, Chapter 11b, Pituitary-Hypothalamic Tumor Syndromes: Adults. von Werder K, Clayton R, version 23 June 2007)

experience paresthesias, often dysgeusia (altered taste sensation), and much less commonly renal stones. A low bicarbonate level often occurs.

Methazolamide is an alternative carbonic anhydrase inhibitor, and other medications sometimes used for IIH include topiramate, furosemide, spironolactone, steroids and triamterine. Surgical options to reduce CSF pressure include fenestration of the optic nerve sheath and a lumboperito-neal shunt. Vision loss is a complication of optic nerve fenestration that occurs in less than 10% of subjects, and the procedure should not be done unless there is papilledema. Lumboperitoneal shunts are more likely to require revision, and complications include acquired type 1 Chiari due to the low-pressure state.

HEADACHE ATTRIBUTED TO INTRACRANIAL HYPERTENSION SECONDARY TO METABOLIC, TOXIC, OR HORMONAL CAUSES

Hypervitaminosis A causing intracranial hypertension and headache would properly fall into this category. Table 8–2 lists the diagnostic criteria for head-ache attributed to intracranial hypertension secondary to metabolic, toxic or hormonal causes.

POST-DURAL (POST-LUMBAR) PUNCTURE HEADACHE

Headache and backache continue to be common adverse events of a lumbar puncture (LP). Headache occurs in as many as 60% of patients who undergo LP, although there is a wide variation in reported series since Bier in 1898 first reported post-LP headaches. Most post-LP headaches are gone in a week or two; they commonly occur the day after the LP. Risk factors for post-LP head-ache include headache before LP, patients with a lower body mass index (BMI), and younger female patients. Length of recumbency following LP

Table 8–2 Headache Attributed to Intracranial Hypertension Secondary to Metabolic, Toxic, or Hormonal Causes

Diagnostic criteria:
A. Headache with at least one of the following characteristics and fulfilling criteria C and D:
   1. Daily occurrence
   2. Diffuse and/or constant (non-pulsating) pain
   3. Aggravated by coughing or straining
B. Intracranial hypertension fulfilling the following criteria:
   1. Alert patient with neurological examination that either is normal or demonstrates any of the following abnormalities:
      a) Papilloedema
      b) Enlarged blind spot
      c) Visual field defect (progressive if untreated)
      d) Sixth nerve palsy
   2. Increased CSF pressure (>200 mm H_2O in the non-obese, >250 mm H_2O in the obese) measured by lumbar puncture in the recumbent position or by epidural or intraventricular pressure monitoring
   3. Normal CSF chemistry (low CSF protein is acceptable) and cellularity
   4. Intracranial diseases (including venous sinus thrombosis) ruled out by appropriate investigations
C. Headache develops after weeks or months of endocrine disorder, hypervitaminosis A or intake of substances (other than medications) that can elevate CSF pressure
D. Headache resolves within 3 months after removal of the cause

does not appear to influence the chance of a post-LP headache, and neither does opening pressure, LP position, and the amount of CSF removed. Small-gauge atraumatic needles do appear to reduce the risk of post-LP headache. Table 8–3 lists the diagnostic criteria for post-LP headache (Figs. 8–2 and 8–3).

Table 8–3 Post-dural (Post-lumbar) Puncture Headache

Diagnostic criteria:
A. Headache that worsens within 15 minutes after sitting or standing and improves within 15 minutes after lying, with at least one of the following and fulfilling criteria C and D:
   1. Neck stiffness
   2. Tinnitus
   3. Hypacusia
   4. Photophobia
   5. Nausea
B. Dural puncture has been performed
C. Headache develops within 5 days after dural puncture
D. Headache resolves either:
   1. Spontaneously within 1 week
   2. Within 48 hours after effective treatment of the spinal fluid leak (usually by epidural blood patch)

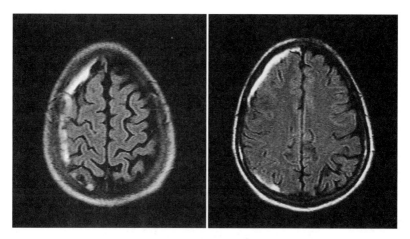

Figures 8–2 and 8–3 These FLAIR MR images are from a young man who had an LP for what turned out to be a migraine attack. He developed a post-LP headache and the low pressure syndrome. The intracranial hypotension and a high NSAID intake resulted in a right subdural hematoma, a recognized rare complication of low-pressure headache. The extra-axial high signal is blood on the images.

CSF FISTULA HEADACHE

Sinus surgery or spinal surgery may be complicated by a CSF fistula. Table 8–4 lists the diagnostic criteria for CSF fistula headache.

HEADACHE ATTRIBUTED TO SPONTANEOUS (OR IDIOPATHIC) LOW CSF PRESSURE

Idiopathic low-pressure headache typically results from a CSF leak, often at the thoracic spine or lower cervical spine, and is commonly attributed to minor trauma or weakness of the meninges. Headache is orthostatic and bilateral, often occipital predominant. With time the orthostatic feature may fade. Other symptoms include changes in hearing, dizziness, and diplopia. Visual symptoms have been attributed to traction of the optic nerve. In common with low pressure from known causes, a frequent feature on MR imaging is diffuse enhancement of the pachymeninges. The great majority of patients improve spontaneously, although it can take many months. Imaging appearance also includes descent of the posterior fossa structures, giving a type 1 Chiari appearance. If the diagnosis of low pressure is not made, the patient is at risk for surgery to correct the apparent posterior fossa crowding. Other imaging abnormalities include engorgement of venous sinuses and subdural fluid collections. Pituitary hyperemia may result in pituitary enlargement, and increased prolactin may be noted, likely as a result of traction on the pituitary stalk.

Table 8–4 CSF Fistula Headache

Diagnostic criteria:

A. Headache that worsens within 15 minutes after sitting or standing, with at least one of the following and fulfilling criteria C and D:
   1. Neck stiffness
   2. Tinnitus
   3. Hypacusia
   4. Photophobia
   5. Nausea
B. A known procedure or trauma has caused persistent CSF leakage with at least one of the following:
   1. Evidence of low CSF pressure on MRI (*eg*, pachymeningeal enhancement)
   2. Evidence of CSF leakage on conventional myelography, CT myelography or cisternography
   3. CSF opening pressure <60 mm H_2O in sitting position
C. Headache develops in close temporal relation to CSF leakage
D. Headache resolves within 7 days of sealing the CSF leak

High CSF protein may be found. Investigation with cisternography using indium-111 is occasionally used. It may demonstrate a source of the leak, early appearance in the kidneys suggesting early passage into soft tissues and lack of appearance on the cerebral convexities. Myelography with CT is the most reliable way to detect meningeal diverticula.

Treatment

Proposed treatment options include bed rest, analgesics, caffeine (no good reason for intravenous over oral!), steroids, hydration, epidural saline infusion, and blood patch. Caffeine and theophylline are advocated but not particularly useful. There is no evidence supporting use of steroids. The epidural blood patch, which is often very useful and acts immediately by volume replacement, effectively reduces the subarachnoid space volume and can act to seal the dural defect also. It does not have to be given at the same level of the presumed leak. Table 8–5 lists the diagnostic criteria for headache attributed to spontaneous (or idiopathic) low CSF pressure (Figs. 8–4 and 8–5).

HEADACHE ATTRIBUTED TO NON-INFECTIOUS INFLAMMATORY DISEASE

Headache Attributed to Neurosarcoidosis

Approximately 5% of those with sarcoid will have neurologic involvement, either peripheral or central. Headache from involvement of the brain is not invariable, and when present it has no particular characteristics. Table 8–6 lists the diagnostic criteria for headache attributed to neurosarcoidosis.

Table 8–5 Headache Attributed to Spontaneous (or Idiopathic) Low CSF Pressure

Diagnostic criteria:
A. Diffuse and/or dull headache that worsens within 15 minutes after sitting or standing, with at least one of the following and fulfilling criterion D:
 1. Neck stiffness
 2. Tinnitus
 3. Hypacusia
 4. Photophobia
 5. Nausea
B. At least one of the following:
 1. Evidence of low CSF pressure on MRI (*eg*, pachymeningeal enhancement)
 2. Evidence of CSF leakage on conventional myelography, CT myelography or cisternography
 3. CSF opening pressure <60 mm H_2O in sitting position
C. No history of dural puncture or other cause of CSF fistula
D. Headache resolves within 72 hours after epidural blood patching

Headache Attributed to Aseptic (Non-infectious) Meningitis

This category is for drug-induced aseptic meningitis (DIAM). Drug-induced aseptic meningitis is associated with the use of nonsteroidal anti-inflammatory drugs (NSAIDs), intravenous immunoglobulins, antibiotics, and OKT3 monoclonal antibodies, which are used in the setting of transplant rejection. Therapy with high-dose intravenous immunoglobulins induces aseptic meningitis,

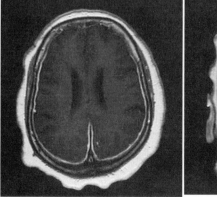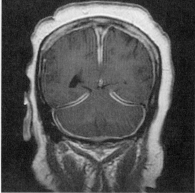

Figures 8–4 and 8–5 Axial and coronal T1-weighted MRI post-gadolinium images from a 60-year-old woman with a history of chronic low-pressure headache. Note the diffusely enhancing pachymeninges.

Table 8–6 Headache Attributed to Neurosarcoidosis

Diagnostic criteria:
A. Headache, no typical characteristics known, fulfilling criteria C and D
B. Evidence of neurosarcoidosis
C. Headache develops in temporal relation to neurosarcoidosis
D. Headache resolves within 3 months after successful treatment of neurosarcoidosis

with focal symptoms in up to 10% of patients. The pathophysiology is thought to involve hypersensitivity reactions or cytokine release. The clinical presentation is similar to infectious meningitis, with headache, meningismus, and mental status changes. The CSF picture is of elevated protein values, normal-low glucose values, and several hundred to several thousand white cells per cubic millimeter. Eosinophils are noted in some patients, but neurtrophils still predominate. Systemic lupus erythematosus is the most common underlying disorder associated with DIAM, and HIV infection is also noted. Migraine is likely not a predisposing condition. Pseudomigraine with pleocytosis syndrome, known in the classification as the "syndrome of transient headache and neurological deficits with CSF lymphocytosis" (HaNDL), may be confused with DIAM, but the large majority of patients with HaNDL syndrome have focal deficits. Table 8–7 lists the diagnostic criteria for headache attributed to aseptic (non-infectious) meningitis.

HEADACHE ATTRIBUTED TO OTHER NON-INFECTIOUS INFLAMMATORY DISEASE

This category includes headache associated with systemic lupus erythematosus, antiphospholipid antibody syndrome, and Behçet's syndrome. Aseptic meningitis from lupus would be included here. Table 8–8 lists the diagnostic criteria for headache attributed to other non-infectious inflammatory disease (Figs. 8–6 and 8–7).

Headache Attributed to Lymphocytic Hypophysitis

Lymphocytic hypophysitis is a rare disorder that has made its way into the classification. This disorder affects women predominantly and results in headache,

Table 8–7 Headache Attributed to Aseptic (Non-infectious) Meningitis

Diagnostic criteria:
A. Diffuse headache fulfilling criterion D
B. Examination of CSF shows lymphocytic pleocytosis, mildly elevated protein and normal glucose in the absence of infectious organisms
C. Use of one of the following: ibuprofen, immunoglobulins, penicillin or trimethoprim, intrathecal injections, or insufflations
D. Headache resolves within 3 months after withdrawal of the offending substance

Table 8–8 Headache Attributed to Other Non-infectious Inflammatory Disease

Diagnostic criteria:
A. Headache, no typical characteristics known, fulfilling criteria C and D
B. Evidence of one of the inflammatory diseases known to be associated with headache
C. Headache develops in close temporal relation to the inflammatory disorder
D. Headache resolves within 3 months after successful treatment of the inflammatory disorder

hypopituitarism, and visual field defects and requires a biopsy for definitive diagnosis. Half of such patients have hyperprolactinemia. Steroids have been used to treat this inflammatory disorder and the natural history is not clear. Table 8–9 lists the diagnostic criteria for headache attributed to lymphocytic hypophysitis.

HEADACHE ATTRIBUTED TO INTRACRANIAL NEOPLASM

Table 8–10 lists the mechanisms of headache in brain tumors (Figs. 8–8 and 8–9). Headache occurs in 50% to 70% of those with brain tumors, but the presence of early morning severe headache with nausea and vomiting occurs in no more than 20% of patients. Rapidly growing tumors and those located in the posterior fossa are more likely to be associated with headache. Approximately one third of patents with supratentorial tumors present with headache, and at

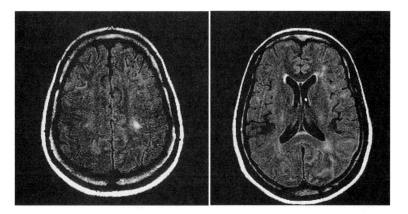

Figures 8–6 and 8–7 This is a 45-year-old woman with a third episode of aseptic meningitis. A diagnosis of lupus was made. Two FLAIR MRI images are shown to demonstrate small hyperintensities, which were predominantly subcortical and periventricular with a small amount of cortical involvement. This picture is nonspecific for a meningoencephalitis of many etiologies.

Table 8-9 Headache Attributed to Lymphocytic Hypophysitis

Diagnostic criteria:
A. Headache, no typical characteristics known, fulfilling criterion C
B. Hypopituitarism fulfilling the following criteria:
　　1. MRI demonstrates symmetrical pituitary enlargement with homogeneous contrast-enhancement
　　2. Biopsy confirmation of lymphocytic hypophysitis
C. Headache develops in close temporal relation to hypopituitarism

least a half of those with an infratentorial tumor present with headache. Those with underlying primary headache are more likely to have headache problems with the development of a brain tumor. The characteristics of the headache are not generally helpful, and brain tumor headache can easily be mistaken for primary headache and respond to mild analgesics. Ipsilateral headache in those with a supratentorial tumor without papilledema has some lateralizing diagnostic specificity.

Headache Attributed to Increased Intracranial Pressure or Hydrocephalus Caused by Neoplasm

Raised intracranial pressure commonly occurs with brain neoplasms with or without obstruction of the CSF system and hydrocephalus (Fig. 8–10). Headache does not always occur and in this situation the patient may present only with papilledema and visual symptoms. Table 8–11 lists the diagnostic criteria for headache attributed to increased intracranial pressure or hydrocephalus caused by neoplasm.

Headache Attributed Directly to Neoplasm

Table 8–12 lists the diagnostic criteria for headache attributed directly to neoplasm.

Headache Attributed to Carcinomatous Meningitis

This headache may improve temporarily with chemotherapy or steroids. Table 8–13 lists the diagnostic criteria for headache attributed to carcinomatous meningitis.

Table 8-10 Mechanisms of Headache in Brain Tumors

Traction of dura and large vessels
Direct pressure on cranial and cervical nerve fibers
The release of inflammatory/hormonal mediators
Raised intracranial pressure

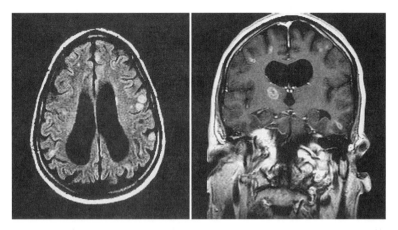

Figures 8–8 and 8–9 Axial FLAIR MRI image on the left and coronal T1 post-gadolinium image on the right demonstrating multiple lesions from metastatic disease in a patient who presented with headache and left leg weakness.

Headache Attributed to Hypothalamic or Pituitary Hyper- or Hyposecretion

The ability of pituitary tumors to cause headache goes beyond any local structural affects and suggests a hormonal explanation. The likelihood of significant headache due to pituitary tumors is high: in one study 48% of patients had MIDAS (disability assessment) scores within the severe range. Attributing headache to a

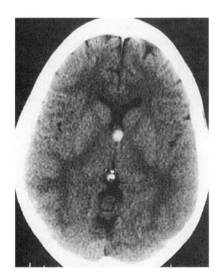

Figure 8–10 A CT scan demonstrating a colloid cyst. Colloid cysts arise in the anterior part of the third ventricle near the foramen of Monro. By intermittent CSF obstruction they can cause positional headaches and an acute rise in pressure. Hydrocephalus may result. The lesion is usually hyperdense on CT due to a high protein concentration, which often results in high signal on T1-weighted images on MRI also. (Used with permission from Leonard Tyminski, MD, California)

160 Diagnosis of Secondary Headache Disorders

Table 8–11 Headache Attributed to Increased Intracranial Pressure or Hydrocephalus Caused by Neoplasm

Diagnostic criteria:

A. Diffuse non-pulsating headache with at least one of the following characteristics and fulfilling criteria C and D:
  1. Associated with nausea and/or vomiting
  2. Worsened by physical activity and/or manoeuvres known to increase intracranial pressure (such as Valsalva manoeuvre, coughing or sneezing)
  3. Occurring in attack-like episodes
B. Space-occupying intracranial tumour demonstrated by CT or MRI and causing hydrocephalus
C. Headache develops and/or deteriorates in close temporal relation to the hydrocephalus
D. Headache improves within 7 days after surgical removal or volume-reduction of tumour

pituitary tumor, especially a small tumor, is furthered by the observation that headache improves after surgery in about half of such patients. There are no special characteristics of pituitary tumors. In one study of 84 patients with pituitary tumor and bothersome headache, 76% fulfilled criteria for migraine, along with three cases of cluster headache and four cases of short-lasting unilateral neuralgiform headache with conjunctival injection and tearing (SUNCT). Clearly the cluster and SUNCT patients were overrepresented in this group, reminding us that trigeminal autonomic cephalalgias may have secondary causes. Only two of the three cluster cases in that study had cavernous sinus invasion. Table 8–14 lists the diagnostic criteria for headache attributed to hypothalamic or pituitary hyper- or hyposecretion.

HEADACHE ATTRIBUTED TO EPILEPTIC SEIZURE

The term "migralepsy" refers to a migraine aura triggering a seizure, followed by a migraine attack, a rare event. A more common occurrence is simply a seizure followed by a migraine-like headache. Both migraine and epilepsy

Table 8–12 Headache Attributed Directly to Neoplasm

Diagnostic criteria:

A. Headache with at least one of the following characteristics and fulfilling criteria C and D:
  1. Progressive
  2. Localized
  3. Worse in the morning
  4. Aggravated by coughing or bending forward
B. Intracranial neoplasm shown by imaging
C. Headache develops in temporal (and usually spatial) relation to the neoplasm
D. Headache resolves within 7 days after surgical removal or volume-reduction of neoplasm or treatment with corticosteroids

Table 8–13 Headache Attributed to Carcinomatous Meningitis

Diagnostic criteria:
A. Diffuse or localised headache fulfilling criterion C
B. Carcinomatous meningitis proven by (repeated) CSF examination and/or dural enhancement on MRI
C. Headache develops and/or deteriorates with advancing disease

may occur together without interaction. There does appear to be a higher prevalence of migraine in certain seizure types, such as benign occipital epilepsy and benign rolandic epilepsy, suggesting some shared predisposing factors. The mitochondrial disorder MELAS is associated with migraine and seizure disorder. Structural brain lesions may result in seizures and migrainous headache.

Approximately 50% of patients with a seizure disorder have postictal headache, which is migrainous in character. It is much more common after tonic–clonic generalized seizures and also said to be common in those with occipital lobe seizures.

Hemicrania Epileptica

Hemicrania epileptica is a rare syndrome requiring the simultaneous onset of headache with seizure discharge. Table 8–15 lists the diagnostic criteria for hemicrania epileptica.

Postictal Headache

Seizures are commonly followed by headache. Table 8–16 lists the diagnostic criteria for postictal headache.

HEADACHE ATTRIBUTED TO CHIARI MALFORMATION TYPE I

Headache is the most common symptom of Chiari malformation type 1 (Figs. 8–11 and 8–12a). It is important to scrutinize not just the descent of the

Table 8–14 Headache Attributed to Hypothalamic or Pituitary Hyper- or Hyposecretion

Diagnostic criteria:
A. Bilateral, frontotemporal and/or retro-orbital headache fulfilling criteria C and D
B. At least one of the following:
 1. Prolactin, growth hormone (GH) and adrenocorticotropic hormone (ACTH) hypersecretion associated with microadenomas <10 mm in diameter
 2. Disorder of temperature regulation, abnormal emotional state, altered thirst and appetite and change in level of consciousness associated with hypothalamic tumour
C. Headache develops during endocrine abnormality
D. Headache resolves within 3 months after surgical resection or specific and effective medical therapy

Table 8–15 Hemicrania Epileptica

Diagnostic criteria:
A. Headache lasting seconds to minutes, with features of migraine, fulfilling criteria C and D
B. The patient is having a partial epileptic seizure
C. Headache develops synchronously with the seizure and is ipsilateral to the ictal discharge
D. Headache resolves immediately after the seizure

posterior fossa structures but also the amount of posterior fossa crowding. Axial views (see Figure 8–12a) can be very helpful in that regard. Patients without posterior predominance of pain and cough exacerbation in headache do not do well with surgery. Cough headache is common with headache attributed to Chiari I. There are plenty of patients who are borderline diagnostically, and they generally do not do as well with surgical decompression. Chiari headache can be mistaken for primary headache. Symptoms may also include lower cranial nerve palsies, long tract signs, and an associated syrinx, which may contribute to the symptom and sign complex considerably. The cough headache component may respond to indomethacin, but clearly definitive treatment is surgical decompression. Table 8–17 lists the diagnostic criteria for headache attributed to Chiari malformation type I.

SYNDROME OF TRANSIENT HEADACHE AND NEUROLOGICAL DEFICITS WITH CEREBROSPINAL FLUID LYMPHOCYTOSIS (HANDL)

Also known as pseudomigraine with lymphocytic pleocytosis, this is an uncommon syndrome. In contrast to migraine, HaNDL is more commonly seen in men and occurs between 15 and 40 years of age. The incidence and prevalence are unknown, and approximately 100 cases have been reported in the literature. The neurologic deficit typically lasts a couple of hours, and fever may occur. In a series of 50 cases, the neurologic deficits lasted from 5 minutes to 3 days, and in contrast to migraine aura, only 12% of episodes involved visual symptoms. Seizures occurred in only 2% of HaNDL cases. The CSF pressure is often elevated, but CSF glucose is always normal. Cerebrospinal fluid protein levels are increased

Table 8–16 Postictal Headache

Diagnostic criteria:
A. Headache with features of tension-type headache or, in a patient with migraine, of migraine headache and fulfilling criteria C and D
B. The patient has had a partial or generalised epileptic seizure
C. Headache develops within 3 hours following the seizure
D. Headache resolves within 72 hours after the seizure

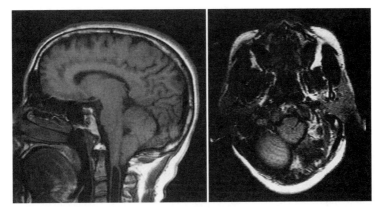

Figures 8–11 and 8–12a FLAIR MRI images. On the left, a sagittal image
demonstrating a Chiari malformation with a syrinx. On the right, an axial image below
the foramen magnum with cerebellar tonsillar tissue crowding the upper cervical cord.
(Courtesy of Jimmy Wang, MD, Dept. of Radiology, Boston University)

in more than 90% of cases. Other diagnoses should be carefully considered, such
as hemiplegic migraine, Lyme, HIV infection, mycoplasma, granulomatous disease, neoplastic meningitis, and lupus. The main theories on etiology are autoimmune and infectious rather than migraine: in migraine or hemiplegic migraine
we do not see a CSF pleocytosis of over 15 cells/mm^3. Treatment is supportive,
with a good prognosis. Table 8–18 lists the diagnostic criteria for HaNDL.

HEADACHE ATTRIBUTED TO OTHER NONVASCULAR INTRACRANIAL DISORDER

This is a wastebasket final category! Table 8–19 lists the diagnostic criteria for
headache attributed to other nonvascular intracranial disorder.

HEADACHE AND INFECTION

Headache is a typical accompaniment to intracranial infection and a common
symptom of systemic infection. Those with an underlying primary headache
disorder are more likely to develop headache as part of systemic infection and
more likely to be severely affected by headache as part of the symptom complex
of systemic infection. These points are separate to any direct infection of the
central nervous system. This section follows the IHC classification outline for
headaches attributed to infection. When a new headache develops for the first
time in close association with an infection it is coded as a secondary headache,
even if the characteristics are consistent with migraine, as such symptoms are
not specific to primary headaches.

Table 8–17 Headache Attributed to Chiari Malformation Type I (CM1)

Diagnostic criteria:

A. Headache characterized by at least one of the following and fulfilling criterion D:
   1. Precipitated by cough and/or Valsalva maneuver
   2. Protracted (hours to days) occipital and/or sub-occipital headache
   3. Associated with symptoms and/or signs of brainstem, cerebellar and/or cervical cord dysfunction
B. Cerebellar tonsillar herniation as defined by one of the following on craniocervical MRI:
   1. ≥5 mm caudal descent of the cerebellar tonsils
   2. ≥3 mm caudal descent of the cerebellar tonsils plus at least one of the following indicators of crowding of the subarachnoid space in the area of the craniocervical junction:
      a) Compression of the CSF spaces posterior and lateral to the cerebellum
      b) Reduced height of the supraocciput
      c) Increased slope of the tentorium
      d) Kinking of the medulla oblongata
C. Evidence of posterior fossa dysfunction, based on at least two of the following:
   1. Otoneurological symptoms and/or signs (*eg*, dizziness, dysequilibrium, sensations of alteration in ear pressure, hypacusia or hyperacusia, vertigo, down-beat nystagmus, oscillopsia)
   2. Transient visual symptoms (spark photopsias, visual blurring, diplopia or transient visual field deficits)
   3. Demonstration of clinical signs relevant to cervical cord, brainstem or lower cranial nerves or of ataxia or dysmetria
D. Headache resolves within 3 months after successful treatment of the Chiari malformation

A lymphocytic meningitis clinical picture, sometimes referred to as aseptic meningitis, may have infective or just inflammatory etiologies. A neutrophilic predominance may be seen early in viral meningitis. Cerebrospinal fluid glucose may occasionally be low in viral infections.

Table 8–18 Syndrome of Transient Headache and Neurological Deficits with Cerebrospinal Fluid Lymphocytosis (HaNDL)

Diagnostic criteria:

A. Episodes of moderate or severe headache lasting hours before resolving fully and fulfilling criteria C and D
B. Cerebrospinal fluid pleocytosis with lymphocytic predominance (>15 cells/µl) and normal neuroimaging, CSF culture and other tests for etiology
C. Episodes of headache are accompanied by or shortly follow transient neurological deficits and commence in close temporal relation to the development of CSF pleocytosis
D. Episodes of headache and neurological deficits recur over <3 months

Table 8–19 Headache Attributed to Other Nonvascular Intracranial Disorder

Diagnostic criteria:
A. Headache with at least one of the following characteristics and fulfilling criteria C and D:
   1. Daily occurrence
   2. Diffuse pain
   3. Aggravated by Valsalva manoeuvre
B. Evidence of an intracranial disorder other than those described above
C. Headache develops in close temporal relation to the intracranial disorder
D. Headache resolves within 3 months after cure or spontaneous remission of the
   intracranial disorder

Headache Attributed to Intracranial Infection

Headache Attributed to Bacterial Meningitis

When headache persists after 3 months, it is coded as *Chronic post-bacterial meningitis headache.* Headache may be the first symptom of intracranial infection, before meningismus or fever. Direct stimulation of the sensory terminals located in the meninges by bacterial infection causes the onset of headache. Bacterial products (toxins), mediators of inflammation such as bradykinin, prostaglandins, and cytokines, and other agents released by inflammation not only directly cause pain but also induce pain sensitization and neuropeptide release. Headache and meningismus can occur with systemic infection in the absence of intracranial infection, so CSF examination is needed for definite diagnosis. Table 8–20 lists the diagnostic criteria for headache attributed to bacterial meningitis (see Figs. 8–12b and 8–12c).

Table 8–20 Headache Attributed to Bacterial Meningitis

Diagnostic criteria:
A. Headache with at least one of the following characteristics and fulfilling criteria C and D:
   1. Diffuse pain
   2. Intensity increasing to severe
   3. Associated with nausea, photophobia and/or phonophobia
B. Evidence of bacterial meningitis from examination of CSF
C. Headache develops during the meningitis
D. One or other of the following:
   1. Headache resolves within 3 months after relief from meningitis
   2. Headache persists but 3 months have not yet passed since relief from meningitis

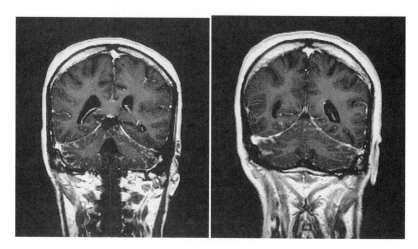

Figures 8–12b and 8–12c Axial T1 images post-gadolinium in a patient with tuberculosis meningitis, demonstrating leptomeningeal enhancement along the tentorium and bilateral cerebellar hemispheres. Note the enhancement goes into the folds of the cerebellum. (Courtesy of Jimmy Wang, MD, Dept. of Radiology, Boston University)

Headache Attributed to Lymphocytic Meningitis

This category covers headache from viral meningitis, tuberculosis, and fungal infections such as cryptococci, among other pathogens (Figs. 8–13, 8–14, 8–15, and 8–16). Enteroviruses account for most viral cases of meningoencephalitis. Herpes simplex, adenovirus, mumps, and others may also be responsible. Lymphocytic meningitis is the result of many situations that vary greatly. Cryptococcal meningitis characteristically causes a high intracranial pressure and may mimic primary intracranial hypertension. There is no separation of viral lymphocytic meningitis from granulomatous etiologies in the classification. Recurrent aseptic meningitis is predominantly caused by herpes simplex virus-2 infection and is indistinguishable from "Mollaret's meningitis," a term that should be reserved for idiopathic cases of recurrent aseptic meningitis.

Table 8–21 lists the diagnostic criteria for headache attributed to lymphocytic meningitis.

Headache Attributed to Encephalitis

The classification separates headache due to meningitis from encephalitis, when in clinical practice there is often a mixture of both. Herpes simplex virus (HSV), arbovirus, and mumps are known causes of encephalitis. Except for HSV encephalitis (in which 95% of cases are identifiable with polymerase chain reaction [PCR]), the causative virus is identified in fewer than half of cases of encephalitis. Headache with behavioral change is a neurologic emergency

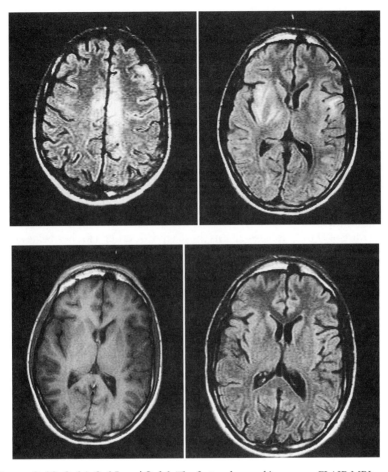

Figures 8–13, 8–14, 8–15 and 8–16 The first and second images are FLAIR MRI images of a young man with Eastern equine encephalitis, demonstrating bilateral insular and cortical hyperintensities. The third image is a post-gadolinium axial T1-weighted image demonstrating no contrast enhancement. The patient became comatose but survived and had a very good outcome. The lesions are not marked but are good examples of what encephalitis looks like on MRI. Finally, a follow-up FLAIR MRI study months later with resolution of lesions is shown.

warranting imaging and CSF examination. Herpes simplex encephalitis accounts for 10% to 20% of all cases of acute encephalitis, is equally prevalent in men and women, and has no seasonal preference. The temporal and orbitofrontal lobes of the brain are typically more severely affected, and the prognosis depends on when treatment is started. Focal neurologic signs are present in many patients with herpes simplex encephalitis, and MRI is the imaging

Table 8–21 Headache Attributed to Lymphocytic Meningitis

Diagnostic criteria:
A. Headache with at least one of the following characteristics and fulfilling criteria C and D:
   1. Acute onset
   2. Severe intensity
   3. Associated with nuchal rigidity, fever, nausea, photophobia and/or phonophobia
B. Examination of CSF shows lymphocytic pleocytosis, mildly elevated protein and normal glucose
C. Headache develops in close temporal association to meningitis
D. Headache resolves within 3 months after successful treatment or spontaneous remission of infection

procedure of choice. Table 8–22 lists the diagnostic criteria for headache attributed to encephalitis.

HEADACHE ATTRIBUTED TO BRAIN ABSCESS

Extension of sinus infection is often found, and abscess is not invariably associated with headache (Figs. 8–17 and 8–18). Table 8–23 lists the diagnostic criteria for headache attributed to brain abscess.

HEADACHE ATTRIBUTED TO SUBDURAL EMPYEMA

Headache is caused by meningeal irritation, increased intracranial pressure, and/or fever. Table 8–24 lists the diagnostic criteria for headache attributed to subdural empyema.

Table 8–22 Headache Attributed to Encephalitis

Diagnostic criteria:
A. Headache with at least one of the following characteristics and fulfilling criteria C and D:
   1. Diffuse pain
   2. Intensity increasing to severe
   3. Associated with nausea, photophobia or phonophobia
B. Neurological symptoms and signs of acute encephalitis, and diagnosis confirmed by EEG, CSF examination, neuroimaging and/or other laboratory investigations
C. Headache develops during encephalitis
D. Headache resolves within 3 months after successful treatment or spontaneous remission of the infection

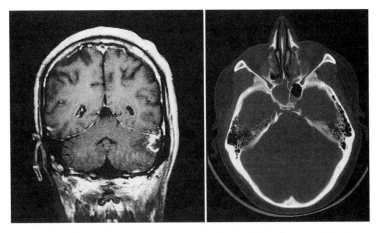

Figures 8–17 and 8–18 First image is a coronal T1-weighted post-gadolinium MRI of a left-sided posterior fossa abscess. The contrast produces ring enhancement. The second image is a CT with bone views showing an occluded right sphenoid and partially filled left sphenoid sinus in a patient with sinusitis. Sphenoid involvement is a risk for extension into the cranial cavity, which is what happened to this patient.

HEADACHE ATTRIBUTED TO SYSTEMIC INFECTION

Headache often occurs with systemic infection, in particular with influenza or with fever. Generally it is not helpful in the diagnosis or management of the systemic infection. The ICHD specifies headaches due to viral, bacterial, and "other systemic infections." Table 8–25 lists the diagnostic criteria for headache attributed to systemic infection.

Table 8–23 Headache Attributed to Brain Abscess

Diagnostic criteria:

A. Headache with at least one of the following characteristics and fulfilling criteria C and D:
1. Bilateral
2. Constant pain
3. Intensity gradually increasing to moderate or severe
4. Aggravated by straining
5. Accompanied by nausea

B. Neuroimaging and/or laboratory evidence of brain abscess

C. Headache develops during active infection

D. Headache resolves within 3 months after successful treatment of the abscess

Table 8–24 Headache Attributed to Subdural Empyema

Diagnostic criteria:

A. Headache with at least one of the following characteristics and fulfilling criteria C and D:
   1. Unilateral or much more intense on one side
   2. Associated with tenderness of the skull
   3. Accompanied by fever
   4. Accompanied by stiffness of the neck
B. Neuroimaging and/or laboratory evidence of subdural empyema
C. Headache develops during active infection and is localised to or maximal at the site of the empyema
D. Headache resolves within 3 months after successful treatment of the empyema

HEADACHE ATTRIBUTED TO HIV/AIDS

Headache in the setting of HIV is common and important. The criteria do not allow for a separation from other forms of headache, such as primary headache. In clinical practice headache is often a presenting symptom of intracranial infection such as toxoplasmosis, a common infection, where brain imaging generally reveals single or multiple ring-enhancing lesions. The basal ganglia is a favored site for toxoplasmosis. Such lesions can also be caused by neoplasia (for example, lymphoma, which occurs commonly in the HIV population). Headache may the presentation of HIV-related meningitis or other meningeal infection such as cryptococcus, which is often associated with raised intracranial pressure, and a dull continuous headache. Many HIV patients have a few extra white blood cells in their CSF chronically. Central nervous system infections in the HIV population are much more likely to occur when the CD4 count is less than 200. Table 8–26 lists the diagnostic criteria for headache attributed to HIV/AIDS (Figs. 8–19, 8–20, 8–21, 8–22, and 8–23).

CHRONIC POST–BACTERIAL MENINGITIS HEADACHE

Many patients develop long-term headache problems after CNS bacterial infections and less so after viral infection. Table 8–27 lists the diagnostic criteria for chronic post–bacterial meningitis headache.

Table 8–25 Headache Attributed to Systemic Infection

Diagnostic criteria:

A. Headache with at least one of the following characteristics and fulfilling criteria C and D:
   1. Diffuse pain
   2. Intensity increasing to moderate or severe
   3. Associated with fever, general malaise or other symptoms of systemic infection
B. Evidence of systemic infection
C. Headache develops during the systemic infection
D. Headache resolves within 72 hours after effective treatment of the infection

Table 8–26 Headache Attributed to HIV/AIDS

Diagnostic criteria:
A. Headache with variable mode of onset, site and intensity fulfilling criteria C and D
B. Confirmation of HIV infection and/or of the diagnosis of AIDS, and of the presence of HIV/AIDS-related pathophysiology likely to cause headache, by neuroimaging, CSF examination, EEG and laboratory investigations
C. Headache develops in close temporal relation to the HIV/AIDS-related pathophysiology
D. Headache resolves within 3 months after the infection subsides

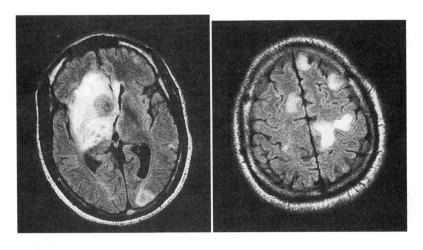

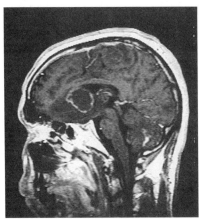

Figures 8–19, 8–20 and 8–21 Two FLAIR MR images and a T1 post-gadolinium MR image from a man immunocompromised with HIV and toxoplasmosis infection. The large contrast-enhancing right basal ganglia lesion is typical, and other lesions are noted. The main differential is a neoplasm like lymphoma. Toxoplasmosis infection like this responds well to treatment.

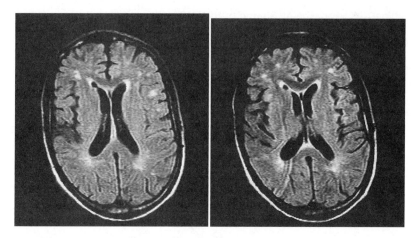

Figures 8–22 and 8–23 These images are axial FLAIR MR studies in an immunocompromised patient with HIV and cryptococcal meningoencephalitis. Scattered hyperintensities are seen in the subcortical white matter. It is unknown how many of these lesions are old and related to HIV and how many are new and related to the meningoencephalitis.

SUMMARY

This chapter covered the secondary headaches in Sections 7 and 9 of ICHD-II to facilitate a comprehensive review of secondary headache.

Alterations in intracranial pressure are a common cause of headache, and as imaging is often normal, it is particularly important to keep this group of secondary headaches under diagnostic consideration. Inflammatory disorders involving the meninges are destined to cause headache and commonly include bacterial and viral meningitis. Other inflammatory disorders may need more careful diagnostic consideration, especially in patients who are immunocompromised.

Table 8–27 Chronic Post–Bacterial Meningitis Headache

Diagnostic criteria:
A. Headache with at least one of the following characteristics and fulfilling criteria C and D:
   1. Diffuse continuous pain
   2. Associated with dizziness
   3. Associated with difficulty in concentrating and/or loss of memory
B. Evidence of previous intracranial bacterial infection from CSF examination or neuroimaging
C. Headache is a direct continuation of *Headache attributed to bacterial meningitis*
D. Headache persists for >3 months after resolution of infection

Neoplasms causing headache typically do this by direct invasion of pain-sensitive structures or raised intracranial pressure. Referred pain to the face from intrathoracic cancer has been described, possibly from involvement of the vagus nerve.

Review Questions

1. Of the following medications, which one is least likely to result in aseptic meningitis?
   a. Trimethoprim
   b. Ibuprofen
   c. Immunoglobulins
   d. Aspirin
2. A 25-year-old overweight woman is reviewed by you for neck pain. On direct questioning she has had no recent headache history and her only medication is the estrogen ring for contraception. You are concerned that she has papilledema. A brain CT is normal and a lumbar puncture demonstrates a pressure of 260 mm. Cerebrospinal fluid studies are normal. An ophthalmology consult states that her disks are consistent with papilledema. The most likely diagnosis is:
   a. Secondary cause for intracranial hypertension
   b. Idiopathic intracranial hypertension
   c. CSF leak
   d. Venous sinus thrombosis
3. A slim man has a lumbar puncture and 48 hours later develops a postural unilateral headache, worse when upright, quickly relieved with recumbency. The headache persists until an epidural blood patch a week later. Which of these statements is most appropriate?
   a. This is a post-LP headache but does not fulfill ICHD criteria due to its unilateral nature.
   b. This is a post-LP headache but does not fulfill ICHD criteria due to the time needed to develop the headache (less than 48 hours).
   c. This is a post-LP headache but does not fulfill ICHD criteria due to the time delay and the unilateral nature.
   d. This is a post-LP headache and fulfills ICHD criteria for same.
4. A 37-year-old man develops a clinical episode characterized by a holocephalic throbbing headache, right arm weakness, and no visual symptoms and was evaluated at a local emergency department. There was no meningismus or fever and he was well up until the time of the headache. Lumbar puncture demonstrated an opening pressure of 260mm, 130 white cells, 95% lymphocytes, protein 86 mg/dL, culture negative. This had happened twice before in the past 6 weeks, with similar clinical syndrome and workup. He has no other background

headache history. Symptoms resolved completely within 24 hours. What diagnosis is most appropriate?

a. Hemiplegic migraine
b. Mollaret's meningits
c. HaNDL syndrome
d. Viral meningitis

5. A 40-year-old woman is reviewed for daily headache. She states that 10 years ago she had an episode of bacterial meningitis, for which she was treated and recovered well. Since then she has had daily headache. There is no headache history before that. What diagnosis is most appropriate?

a. New-onset persistent daily headache
b. Chronic post–bacterial meningitis headache
c. Headache attributed to intracranial hypertension secondary to hydrocephalus
d. Headache attributed to non-infectious inflammatory disease

6. A 25-year-old obese woman is followed for idiopathic intracranial hypertension. Topiramate is used to help the chronic headache after she did not tolerate acetazolamide. She is admitted to the hospital with a severe exacerbation in headache, without fever or meningismus. A non-contrast brain CT is unremarkable. Opening pressure on LP is 230 mm, much improved from her historical pressure of 400 mm on initial diagnosis of idiopathic intracranial hypertension. What is the most appropriate step to take next?

a. Repeat the LP
b. Trial of a triptan or DHE
c. Morphine
d. MRI of the brain
e. MR venography

7. A 22-year-old college student is brought to the emergency department with headache. The headache started that day, and he has been forgetting things and complaining of smells that are not there. He has a fever of 101° F. A CT of the brain was normal. A lumbar puncture demonstrated clear CSF, 18 white cells, 50% neutrophils, 7 red cells, protein 60 mg%, with normal glucose. A roommate recalls that he had had some bad headaches in the past but no confusion. The most appropriate step to take next would be:

a. Acyclovir and antibiotics
b. Acyclovir
c. Urgent EEG
d. Antibiotics
e. Steroids

8. A 28-year-old woman develops a headache disorder characterized by unilateral sharp attacks lasting an hour or so. An MRI demonstrated

a 7-mm pituitary microadenoma without suprasellar extension or compression of surrounding structures. The prolactin level was 60 ng/mL, over twice normal limits. Treatment with bromocriptine markedly exacerbated the pain and had to be discontinued. Numerous other medical therapies were poorly effective at treating her headaches, and she had a transsphenoidal resection of the pituitary lesion. Afterwards the headache attacks resolved. Which statements are most appropriate?

 a. The headaches are attributed to pituitary hypersecretion.
 b. The headache diagnosis is likely cluster headache incidental to the pituitary lesion.
 c. The headache is attributed to the pituitary hypersecretion but does not fulfill
    ICHD criteria for pituitary-related headache due to the small size of the lesion.
 d. A tumor that small could never cause headache.

9. Imaging findings in low-pressure headache include all but which one of the following?

 a. Enlargement of the ventricles
 b. Descent of the cerebellar tonsils
 c. Subdural fluid collections
 d. Enlargement of the pituitary

10. The following are all associated with idiopathic intracranial hypertension except which one?

 a. Cis-retinoic acid
 b. Lithium
 c. Growth hormone
 d. Carbamazepine

10. d
9. a
8. a
7. a
6. b
5. b
4. c
3. d
2. b
1. a

SUGGESTED READING

Graham, C.B., & Wippold, F.J. Headache in the HIV patient: A review with special attention to the role of imaging. *Cephalalgia* 21 (2001): 169–174.

Marchioni, E., Tavazzi, E., Bono, G., et al. Headache attributed to infection: Observations on the IHS classification (ICHD-II). *Cephalalgia* 26 (2006): 1427–1433.

Mokri, B. Low cerebrospinal fluid pressure syndromes. *Neurology Clinics* 22, no. 1 (Feb. 2004): 55–57.

Moris, G., & Garcia-Monco, J.C. The challenge of drug-induced aseptic meningitis. *Archives of Internal Medicine* 159 (1999): 1185–1194.

Purdy, R.A., & Kirby, S. Headaches and brain tumors. *Neurology Clinics* 22, no. 1 (2004): 39–53.

9

Classification and Diagnosis of Secondary Headaches: Substances, Metabolic Disorders, EENT Causes, and Neuralgias

Lawrence C. Newman, MD

This chapter is divided into four separate sections incorporating many seemingly disparate disorders, some which may be commonly seen in clinical practice and others that are quite obscure. Nonetheless, knowledge of these disorders is essential in that they are all secondary and misdiagnosis may have dire consequences. This chapter encompasses Chapters 8, 10, 11, and 13 in the ICHD-II.

HEADACHE ATTRIBUTED TO A SUBSTANCE OR ITS WITHDRAWAL

In the ICHD-II, substance-related headaches are divided into four subtopics: headache induced by use of or exposure to acute substances, medication overuse headache, headache as an adverse event attributed to chronic medication, and headache attributed to substance withdrawal.

The definitive diagnosis of headache attributed to a substance can be made only after the headache resolves or greatly improves after 3 months has passed after termination of the exposure; if the headache does not resolve or significantly improve after 3 months the diagnosis "chronic post-substance exposure headache" (included in the ICHD-II appendix) is considered.

Although 3 months is the time point required for improvement for headache due to acute use or exposure, a period of 2 months is mandated for medication overuse headache; prior to 2 months, the diagnosis "probable medication overdose headache" is indicated. In cases of medication overuse headache, if the headache does not resolve or revert to the original pattern within 2 months of discontinuation, the diagnosis must be discarded.

Headache Induced by Acute Substance or Exposure

According to the ICHD-II description, headache disorders can be induced in three manners: as an unwanted effect of the toxic substance, as an unwanted effect of the substance in normal therapeutic use, or in experimental studies. In double-blind, placebo-controlled trials, headache can be regarded as a true side effect only if it occurs more often with the active agent. Under this group of disorders are headaches from nitric oxide (NO), phosphodiesterase (PDE), carbon monoxide, alcohol, components and additives such as MSG, cocaine, cannabis, histamine, and CGRP. Also included in this chapter are headaches that occur as an acute adverse event better attributed to medications used for other indications, headaches induced by acute substance use or exposure, medication overuse headaches, headaches as an adverse event attributed to chronic medication, and headaches attributed to substance withdrawal. This chapter will review several of these more important disorders.

NO Donor–Induced Headache

Nitric oxide may cause either an immediate or delayed headache. These headaches are typically bilateral, pulsating, and frontotemporal. They may worsen with routine activity. In the immediate subtype, the headache develops within 10 minutes after absorption of an NO donor and resolves within 1 hour after release of NO has ended; in the delayed subtype, headache develops after NO is cleared from the blood and resolves within 72 hours after a single exposure. The delayed subtype occurs in patients with pre-existing primary headaches.

PDE Headache

These headaches are bilateral, frontotemporal, and throbbing and worsen with activity. They develop within 5 hours of exposure and resolve within 72 hours. These headaches follow the use of sildenafil and dipyridamole. Unlike NO headaches, these headaches have only a monophasic form.

Alcohol-Induced Headache

Alcohol-induced headaches may be either immediate or delayed; in the immediate subtype headache develops within 3 hours and resolves within 72 hours of exposure. The delayed subtype occurs as a result of different degrees of ingestion; a modest amount of alcoholic beverage is required by migraineurs, an intoxicating amount by non-migraine sufferers. These headaches may be bilateral, frontotemporal, pulsating, and aggravated by routine physical activity.

Histamine-Induced and CGRP-Induced Headache

Histamine causes an immediate headache in non-headache sufferers and an immediate and delayed headache in migraineurs. Migraine and tension-type headaches develop after 5 to 6 hours, whereas cluster headaches develop after only 1 to 2 hours.

CGRP may also induce an immediate or delayed type of headache. The ICHD-II criteria are similar for both of these headache disorders.

Medication Overuse Headache

Patients with a pre-existing primary headache who develop a new type of headache or whose migraine or tension-type headache is made markedly worse during medication overuse should be given both the diagnosis of the preexisting headache and the diagnosis of medication overuse headache. If the offending medication has not yet been withdrawn or if the overuse has ceased within the last 2 months but the headache has not yet resolved or reverted to its previous pattern, the "probable" designation should be used. In the ICHD-II classification there exist subtypes for ergotamine, triptan, analgesic, opioid, combination medications, and combinations of the above, as well as a subcategory for other medications.

For analgesic overuse headaches, the intake of simple analgesics must occur on 15 or more days per month for more than 3 months; however, for all the other forms of medication overuse headaches, intake has to occur only 10 or more days monthly. The actual descriptions of the headaches have been eliminated in revisions to the criteria.

Headaches Attributed to Substance Withdrawal

The ICHD-II criteria discuss caffeine withdrawal, opioid withdrawal, estrogen withdrawal, and withdrawal from chronic use of other substances in this section.

Caffeine withdrawal headaches are bilateral and/or pulsating. These headaches occur when there is interruption of caffeine consumption in patients who have been ingesting 200 mg or more of caffeine per day for more than 2 weeks. These headaches develop within 24 hours of cessation of caffeine and are relieved within 1 hour of ingestion of 100 mg of caffeine, or the headache resolves within 7 days after total withdrawal.

Estrogen withdrawal results in a headache or migraine that occurs after an interruption in the daily usage of exogenous estrogen for 3 or more weeks. These headaches develop within 5 days after the last use of estrogen and resolve within 3 days.

Headache Attributed to Withdrawal from Chronic Use of Other Substances

Although significant evidence does not exist, it has been postulated that the withdrawal of corticosteroids, tricyclic antidepressants, selective serotonin reuptake inhibitors, and nonsteroidal anti-inflammatory agents may produce headache (Table 9–1). The ICHD-II criteria state that if these medications have been used for more than 3 months and then discontinued, a headache will develop in close temporal relationship. These headaches should resolve within 3 months after complete withdrawal.

HEADACHE ATTRIBUTED TO DISORDERS OF HOMEOSTASIS

Chapter 10 of the ICHD-II contains disorders that were previously referred to as "headaches associated with metabolic or systemic disease." In this section headaches due to hypoxia or hypercapnia, dialysis, arterial hypertension, hypothyroidism, fasting, and cardiac cephalalgia are discussed.

Table 9–1 Medications that May Induce Headaches

Medication class	Medications
Nonsteroidal antiinflamatory	Indomethacin, diclofenac
Beta-blocker	Atenolol
Calcium channel blocker	Nifedipine
Histamine receptor blocker	Cimetidine, ranitidine
Antibiotics	Tetracyclines, trimethaprim-sulfamethoxazole
Vasodilators	Isosorbide dinitrate, glyceryl trinitrate
Hormones	Danazol, ethinylestradiol, oral contraceptives
Others	Angiotensin-converting enzyme inhibitors, monoamine oxidase inhibitors, selective serotonin receptor inhibitors

High-Altitude Headache

Headache commonly occurs when climbing to altitudes greater than 2,500 meters. The disorder affects women more often than men and affects younger people more often, possibly because of the lack of brain atrophy

High-altitude headaches are bilateral and frontal or frontotemporal in location and are usually dull or pressing in nature. High-altitude headaches are usually mild to moderate in severity and may be aggravated by movement, exertion, straining, coughing, or bending. These headaches develop within 24 hours of ascent and will resolve within 8 hours of descent. The headache may awaken the sufferer from sleep or be present upon awakening in the morning. High-altitude headache appears to be independent of an individual's previous headache history, although patients with migraine may describe a more severe headache that resembles their typical migraine attacks.

Diving Headache

These headaches occur following dives below 10 meters. The headache has no typical characteristics and is associated with one or more features of CO_2 intoxication. The headache may be associated with lightheadedness, confusion, dyspnea, flushing, or a feeling of incoordination. Diving headaches resolve within 1 hour of 100% oxygen therapy. These headaches usually intensify during the decompression phase of a dive or upon resurfacing.

Sleep Apnea Headache

These recurrent headaches occur on more than 15 days per month and are bilateral, pressing, and not accompanied by nausea, photophobia, or photophobia. Individual headaches are present upon awakening and resolve within 30 minutes. According to the ICHD-II criteria sleep apnea must be demonstrated by overnight polysomnography. The criteria also mandate that headache resolves within 72 hours and does not recur after effective treatment of the sleep apnea.

Dialysis Headache

A majority of patients receiving dialysis complain of headaches. The characteristics of these headaches are not described in the ICHD-II. They commonly occur in association with hypotension and the dialysis disequilibrium syndrome. The disequilibrium syndrome may begin as a headache, progressing to obtundation and coma with or without seizures. According to the criteria, these headaches develop during at least half of the hemodialysis sessions. Additionally, the criteria state that headaches resolve within 72 hours after each session and/or cease altogether after successful kidney transplantation. Because caffeine is rapidly removed by dialysis, the ICHD-II criteria also note that the diagnosis "caffeine withdrawal headache" should be considered in patients who consume large quantities of caffeine.

HEADACHE RELATED TO ARTERIAL HYPERTENSION

Mild or moderate hypertension does not cause headache; a variety of disorders that lead to paroxysmal, abrupt, or severe elevations in blood pressure, however, are associated with headaches.

Pheochromocytoma

Pheochromocytomas are catecholamine-producing tumors arising from chromaffin cells. The disorder should be considered in patients who suffer from headaches that are associated with hypertension, autonomic disturbances, and panic attacks. Although these tumors are usually found within the adrenal medulla, they may also occur elsewhere in the body.

Patients with pheochromocytomas often report sudden-onset, severe headaches. The headaches may localize to the frontal or occipital regions and are pulsatile or steady in quality. These headaches are notable for their short duration, typically lasting 1 hour or less. Although the ICHD-II states that headache develops concomitantly with the abrupt rise in blood pressure and that the headache resolves or markedly improves within 1 hour of normalization of blood pressure, approximately 13% of sufferers have normal blood pressure and 8% are asymptomatic. Nonetheless, the vast majority of patients with pheochromocytoma are hypertensive, and approximately half of all sufferers have paroxysmal hypertension.

Associated with the headache, patients may experience sweating, palpitations, anxiety, and facial pallor or flushing. The paroxysms of pain can occur spontaneously or be provoked by exertion, stress, pressor medications, or postural changes.

Increased 24-hour urinary excretion of catecholamines or catecholamine metabolites is needed for the diagnosis. A CT or MRI of the neck, chest, abdomen, and pelvis may demonstrate the tumor.

Headache Attributed to Hypertensive Crises Without Hypertensive Encephalopathy

Paroxysmal hypertension may occur in a number of important clinical situations. It may follow carotid endarterectomy or irradiation of the neck, or occur in patients with pheochromocytomas. Headaches develop during the hypertensive crises (a rise in blood pressure to above 160/120). These headaches are bilateral, pulsating, and precipitated by exertion. The headache should resolve within 1 hour after normalization of the blood pressure.

Headache Attributed to Hypertensive Encephalopathy

Sudden and severe increases in blood pressure may produce an acute encephalopathy. In normotensive patients this syndrome may develop when the blood pressure reaches 160/100; in patients with chronic hypertension, encephalopathy usually does not develop until the systolic blood pressure rises above 250 and diastolic blood pressure rises above 120. The ICHD-II criteria state that this blood pressure elevation is associated with at least two of the following: confusion, reduced level of consciousness, visual disturbances, and seizures. The headache should develop in close temporal relationship to the blood pressure elevation, and it should be bilateral, pulsating, or aggravated by routine physical activity. Furthermore, the criteria state that the headache should resolve within 3 months following the control of the elevated blood pressure.

Abnormalities on brain MRI include posterior white matter edema, especially in the parietal occipital regions with spread to the basal ganglia, brain stem, and cerebellum.

Headache Attributed to Pre-eclampsia and Eclampsia

Pre-eclampsia consists of hypertension, edema, and proteinuria (>0.3 g/2 hours). Eclampsia is characterized by all of the above plus the presence of seizures. The ICHD-II states that both disorders can occur up to 4 weeks postpartum. The risk of developing these disorders is increased if the patient has a prior history of hypertension, or if there is a prior or family history of pre-eclampsia and chronic hypertension. Additional risk factors include nulliparity or multiple pregnancies.

The headache may be bilateral, pulsatile, or worse with exertion. The headache should develop during periods of high blood pressure and resolve within 7 days after effective treatment of the hypertension. Thunderclap headache has been reported to occur with these disorders, but it is not mentioned in the ICHD-II criteria.

Headache Attributed to Fasting

Headaches as a result of fasting are more common in people with a prior history of headache; in migraine sufferers, the headache attributed to fasting may resemble migraine. These headaches do not appear to be related to hypoglycemia, nor are they related to the duration of sleep, or caffeine withdrawal. These headaches are more likely to develop as the duration of the fast increases.

Fasting headaches are usually frontal, diffuse, nonpulsatile, and of mild or moderate intensity. They are precipitated by a fast of greater than 16 hours and resolve within 72 hours after resumption of food intake.

Headache Attributed to Hypothyroidism

Approximately 30% of patients with hypothyroidism complain of headache. These headaches have a female preponderance, and sufferers often have a childhood history of migraine. These headaches are bilateral, nonpulsatile, or continuous and are not associated with nausea or vomiting. These headaches develop within 2 months after other symptoms of hypothyroidism become clinically evident and resolve within 2 months after effective therapy.

Cardiac Cephalalgia

Cardiac cephalalgia is a headache that develops concomitantly with acute myocardial ischemia. The disorder begins in close proximity to the onset of vigorous exercise and subsides with the rest or anti-anginal treatments. The headache may be associated with nausea. Although not contained in the ICHD-II criteria, reports of cardiac cephalalgia have occurred in patients while at rest. Additionally, headaches may be unilateral (not ICHD-II) and are not precipitated by a Valsalva maneuver (not ICHD-II).

The diagnosis of cardiac cephalalgia is made by documenting the relationship between headache onset and simultaneous cardiac ischemia during either treadmill or nuclear cardiac stress testing. It is of paramount importance to distinguish this disorder from primary headache disorders because the use of vasoconstrictors such as ergots or triptans is contraindicated in patients with ischemic heart disease.

HEADACHE OR FACIAL PAIN ATTRIBUTED TO DISORDERS OF CRANIUM, NECK, EYES, EARS, NOSE, SINUSES, TEETH, MOUTH, OR OTHER FACIAL OR CRANIAL STRUCTURES

Disorders of the cervical spine and other structures of the head and neck are commonly implicated as causing headache. However, in many disorders, a true causative effect has not been delineated. Chapter 11 of the ICHD-II contains a variety of headache disorders that are attributed to disorders of cranial bones, neck, eyes, ears, teeth, jaws, and temporomandibular joint. That chapter also covers headache attributed to rhinosinusitis.

Headache Attributed to Disorder of Cranial Bone

Most disorders of the skull are not associated with headache, but important exceptions to this rule include osteomyelitis, Paget's disease, and multiple myeloma. Lesions of the mastoid and petrositis may also cause headaches.

Cervicogenic Headache

The headache of cervical origin is nonspecific. The headache may be unilateral or bilateral.

The pain may be triggered by flexion, coughing, or straining. Occasionally cervicogenic headaches may mimic low-cerebrospinal-fluid-pressure headache in that the headaches have a positional component. These headaches may be associated with vertigo, facial numbness, limb weakness, or ataxia (Table 9–2).

The diagnosis of cervicogenic headache may be made using an ipsilateral blockade of the C2 root or greater occipital nerve, which allows differentiation between cervicogenic headache due to irritation of the C2 root and another primary headache disorder, in which only a short-lived benefit would be observed.

Headache Attributed to Retropharyngeal Tendinitis

Retropharyngeal tendinitis is a rare condition of unknown etiology. The disorder is characterized by the acute onset of unilateral or bilateral upper cervical and occipital pain. The pain is nonpulsatile and is aggravated by bending the head backwards. Patients may develop a mild to moderate fever and an increased sedimentation rate. X-rays may demonstrate an increased thickness of the C1–C4 paravertebral soft tissues. The pain is alleviated within 2 weeks of treatment with nonsteroidal anti-inflammatory drugs. It is important to rule out upper carotid dissection prior to making the diagnosis.

Headache Attributed to Craniocervical Dystonia

A number of local dystonias of the head and neck are accompanied by pain. These include pharyngeal dystonia, spasmodic torticollis, mandibular dystonia, lingual dystonia, and a combination of the cranial and cervical dystonias. The pain from these dystonias arises as the result of continuous muscle contraction. Headaches are common in this condition and may be unilateral but most commonly are occipital. The typical sensation is that of a cramp, tension, or pain in the neck that radiates to the back of the head or into the entire head.

Table 9–2 Accepted Cervical Causes of Headache

Developmental anomalies of craniovertebral junction and upper cervical spine
Paget's disease of skull with secondary invagination
Osteomyelitis of upper cervical vertebrae
Rheumatoid arthritis /Ankylosing spondylitis of upper cervical spine
Traumatic subluxation
Retropharyngeal tendinitis
Craniocervical dystonias

Modified from *The headaches*, 3rd ed., ed. Olesen, J., et al. Philadelphia: Lippincott Williams & Wilkins, 2006, p. 1005.

Headache Attributed to Disorder of Eyes

The ICHD-II lists the following disorders under this subsection: acute glaucoma, refractive errors, heterophoria or heterotropia, and ocular inflammatory disorder. Headaches are often assumed to be the result of an ocular disorder and many patients not surprisingly first consult optometrists and ophthalmologists for their recurring headaches. In general, however, ocular causes of headache are not common.

Acute angle-closure glaucoma results from an increase in intraocular pressure and causes severe ocular, retro-orbital and periorbital pain that is associated with conjunctival injection, corneal clouding, and blurring of the vision. The diagnosis is made by documenting increased intraocular pressure. Acute angle-closure glaucoma is an ophthalmic emergency; failure to recognize and treat the disorder rapidly may lead to permanent blindness.

Although eyestrain is frequently misattributed as the cause of headache, in fact errors of refraction are rarely associated with headache. Patients with eyestrain are more likely to report a mild ache or dull pain in the eyes, although patients with pre-existing migraine or tension-type headaches may develop pains in the head as a manifestation of refraction errors. The ICHD-II criteria for these headaches suggest that the pain is typically mild, located frontally and in the eyes. These headaches are not present upon awakening; they result from prolonged visual tasks at the distance or angle where the vision is impaired. The refractive problems associated with these headaches include hyperopia (farsightedness), astigmatism, presbyopia, and wearing incorrect glasses.

Headache Attributed to Rhinosinusitis

Sinus infections are overdiagnosed; in fact, migraine and tension-type headache are often confused with sinus headache. Paradoxically, sinus disease is also underdiagnosed since sphenoid sinusitis is frequently missed.

The ICHD-II criteria for rhinosinusitis state that a frontal headache, accompanied by pain in one or more regions of the face, ears, or teeth, should develop simultaneously with the onset or acute exacerbation of rhinosinusitis, and that the headache or facial pain should resolve within 1 week after remission or following successful treatment. Chronic sinusitis is not a validated cause of headache. Rhinosinusitis, therefore, represents either an acute infection or an acute exacerbation of a chronic condition.

In general, acute sinus infections are usually manifested by facial pain and tenderness, congestion, and a purulent nasal discharge. Other signs include anosomia, pain on chewing, halitosis, and fever.

Sphenoid sinusitis accounts for only 3% of all acute rhinosinusitis cases and is frequently overlooked. The pain associated with sphenoid sinusitis is usually localized to the occipital, frontal, or temporal regions but may also be peri-orbital. The headache is worsened by standing, walking, or bending. Sphenoid sinusitis has been reported to have a thunderclap onset. The headache may be associated with nausea and vomiting but is not usually accompanied by nasal discharge or congestion. At times the headache may be associated with pain or paresthesia in the face, photophobia, and tearing. Clinically this disorder is notable because it interferes with sleep and may be resistant to treatment with opioids.

Diagnosis is made by neuroimaging the sinus, either with MRI or CT (Fig. 9–1). Complications of sphenoid sinusitis include bacterial meningitis, cavernous sinus and cortical vein thromboses, subdural abscess, and pituitary insufficiency.

CRANIAL NEURALGIAS AND CENTRAL CAUSES OF FACIAL PAIN

The ICHD-II states that pain in the head and neck is mediated by afferents in the trigeminal nerve, nervus intermedius, glossopharyngeal and vagus nerves and upper cervical nerves via the occipital nerves. Stimulation of these nerves by compression, distortion, exposure to cold, or a lesion in central pathways may cause stabbing or constant pain in the innervated region.

Difficulties within the classification are seen with trigeminal and glossopharyngeal neuralgias, because if the pain is due to compression of the nerve from a vascular loop found at operation, the neuralgia is designated as "secondary." Because many patients do not undergo surgery it is impossible to determine if the cause is primary or secondary. Therefore, the ICHD-II uses the terms

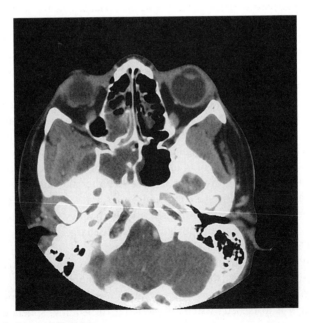

Figure 9–1 Spenoid Sinusitis.

"classical" and "symptomatic"; "secondary" is reserved for patients who have a vascular loop revealed at surgery.

Table 9–3 lists clinical features of the cranial neuralgias.

Trigeminal Neuralgia

Trigeminal neuralgia (TN) is the most common neuralgic syndrome of the elderly, with a female-to-male ratio of 3:2. The majority of cases are caused by compression of the nerve root by an aberrant vascular loop. Other causes include tumors (posterior fossa meningiomas or neuromas) that distend or infiltrate the nerve root or ganglion. Approximately 2% to 4% of patients with TN have multiple sclerosis, and multiple sclerosis should be considered in all patients who develop TN prior to age 50 years. Other causes of TN in young patients include myeloma or metastasis of the sphenoid, meningiomas, acoustic neuromas, cholesteatomas, and basilar artery aneurysms.

Clinically, TN is characterized by paroxysms of very brief, electric-like, lancinating pains usually affecting the regions of the face supplied by the second and third divisions of the trigeminal nerve; the first division is involved less than 5% of the time. Paroxysms begin and end abruptly and last from a fraction of a second to 2 minutes each. In some sufferers, a dull ache may be present between painful exacerbations. These painful episodes may be evoked by touching trigger zones on the face, typically around the ipsilateral orbit, nares, and chin, but they may also occur spontaneously. Attacks may be precipitated by washing the face, shaving, brushing the teeth, eating, or exposure to a breeze. At times, the pain may be triggered by somatosensory stimuli outside the distribution of the trigeminal nerve. The pain often evokes a muscle spasm of the ipsilateral face mimicking a facial tic (hence the name tic douloureux). Following the painful exacerbations there is usually a refractory period during which time pain is not induced by the above precipitants.

On neurologic examination, no deficits should be present. Impairment of sensation suggests a structural, demyelinating, or compressive cause for the neuralgia. In symptomatic TN, the ICHD-II criteria state that in addition to the above features, there may or may not be a persistent ache between paroxysms, and a causative lesion other than vascular compression has been found.

Glossopharyngeal Neuralgia

Glossopharyngeal neuralgia is a rare syndrome with an onset usually in the sixth decade of life. In this condition pain occurs in the areas supplied by the somatosensory branches of the glossopharyngeal and vagus nerves. Like TN, glossopharyngeal neuralgia may be caused by vascular cross-compression. Symptomatic causes include cerebellopontine angle tumors, nasopharyngeal carcinoma, carotid aneurysms, and peritonsillar abscesses. Ten percent of sufferers have both TN and glossopharyngeal neuralgia.

Clinically, glossopharyngeal neuralgia is characterized by severe paroxysms of stabbing pain, lasting a fraction of a second to 2 minutes. The pain is felt

Table 9–3 Clinical Features of Cranial Neuralgias

	Trigeminal	Glossopharyngeal	Nervus Intermedius	Superior Laryngeal
Gender Predominance	Female	Female	Female	Male
Age of Onset	>50	>50	Middle age	Middle age
Pain Quality	Electric/lancinating	Stabbing	Sharp/lancinating	Severe
Pain Location	V2-V3	Tonsil, tongue, larynx to oropharynx and ear	Auditory canal	Submandible to ipsilateral ear, eye, shoulder
Pain Duration	Seconds – 2 minutes	Seconds – 2 minutes	Seconds – minutes	Seconds – minutes
Triggers	Touching/washing/shaving face, brushing teeth, breeze striking face	Swallowing, coughing, talking, yawning	Touching posterior wall of auditory canal	Swallowing, straining voice, turning head, coughing, sneezing, yawning, blowing nose. Also trigger point on lateral aspect of throat over hypothyroid membrane
Associated Features	Facial tic	Coughing, hoarseness, syncope, seizures	Salivation, rhinorrhea, tinnitus, bitter taste	Irresistable urge to swallow, inability to speak

predominantly in the tonsil, tongue, and larynx and radiates back from the oropharynx into the ipsilateral ear. Unlike TN, the pain has an abrupt onset, persists for approximately 1 minute, and abruptly ends ("square-wave" pain). Attacks recur 5 to 30 times daily and may occur throughout the night as well. Some patients experience a dull, deep pain between exacerbations.

Glossopharyngeal neuralgia may be triggered by swallowing, coughing, talking, or yawning. The pain is associated with coughing, hoarseness, syncope, and seizures. Bouts may occur in clusters lasting weeks to months, followed by remission periods lasting months to years.

Nervus Intermedius Neuralgia

Nervus intermedius neuralgia is a rare disorder that affects middle-aged adults. It affects women more often than men. It arises from a disturbance of the sensory portion of cranial nerve VII, which innervates part of the external auditory canal and tympanic membrane, the skin between the angle of the ear and mastoid, and the tonsillar region.

The disorder is characterized by very brief paroxysms of severe sharp or lancinating pains in the auditory canal. There is often local tenderness of the pinna or external auditory canal; stimulation of these regions will precipitate an attack. Associated with the pain, patients experience excessive salivation, rhinorrhea, tinnitus, vertigo, or a bitter taste.

Superior Laryngeal Neuralgia

The superior laryngeal nerve is a branch of the vagus nerve and innervates the cricothyroid muscle of the thyroid. The nerve is sometimes injured during carotid endarterectomies. The disorder affects middle-aged men and is characterized by pain paroxysms lasting seconds to minutes. The pain arises in the submandibular region and radiates into the ipsilateral ear, eye, or shoulder and is often precipitated by swallowing, straining the voice, head turning, coughing, sneezing, yawning, or blowing the nose. The painful exacerbations are accompanied by an irresistible urge to swallow (which exacerbates the pain) and the inability to speak.

Neck–Tongue Syndrome

This syndrome is characterized by acute onset of pain in the occiput or upper neck that lasts seconds to minutes. It may occur with or without dysesthesia of the ipsilateral tongue and is precipitated by sudden neck turning, which compromises the C2 root.

Tolosa-Hunt Syndrome

This rare syndrome is due to granulomatous inflammation of the cavernous sinus, superior orbital fissure, or orbit. It is characterized by one or more episodes of unilateral orbital pain with paralysis of cranial nerves III, IV, and VI.

Untreated, the disorder lasts 8 weeks; if treated with steroids, relief occurs within 72 hours. The disorder may be mimicked by aneurysm, diabetes, paranasal mucocele, parasellar tumor, carotid-cavernous fistula, and sphenoid sinusitis.

Persistent Idiopathic Facial Pain

"Persistent idiopathic facial pain" is the new ICHD-II term replacing what had been previously called "atypical facial pain." This disorder is manifested by persistent pain in the face that does not have the characteristics of the cranial neuralgias and is not associated with physical signs or a demonstrable organic cause. Sufferers are usually middle-aged, and women are affected significantly more often than men.

Clinically, patients describe daily unremitting pain that is characterized as deep and poorly localized. Initially the pain is limited to one side of face, but over time it may spread to involve the upper or lower jaws or a wider area of the face and neck. No associated sensory loss or other physical findings accompany the syndrome. Laboratory testing and radiographic examinations of the face and jaw are normal.

It is of paramount importance to realize that facial pain may be a manifestation of a more serious disorder, and that "atypical" facial pain is a descriptive term, not a diagnosis. Constant, severe, aching pain in the face with radiation into the ear may be the result of carcinoma of the lung.

SUMMARY

The disorders reviewed in this chapter highlight the need to be cognizant of the many causes of head, neck, and facial pain. Headache and facial pain syndromes can arise as the result of perturbations of normal structures, homeostatic mechanisms, or exposure to myriad substances. Familiarity with these disorders is essential for all clinicians, for failure to recognize these conditions can lead to significant disability and in some instances mortality.

Review Questions

1. Delayed headaches in migraine sufferers occur with all of the following except:
   a. Alcohol
   b. Histamine
   c. Nitric oxide
   d. CGRP
   e. Carbon monoxide
2. Intake on more than 15 days/month for more than 3 months causes medication overuse headache from:
   a. Ergots
   b. Triptans
   c. Simple analgesics

    d. Combination analgesics

    e. Opioids

3. A 35-year-old woman presents with an increased frequency of her migraine headaches without aura since beginning oral contraception. Headaches worsen with menses and are more frequent at other times of the month as well. Diagnoses include which of the following?

    a. Menstrually related migraine without aura

    b. Estrogen withdrawal headache

    c. Exogenous hormone-induced headache

    d. Idiopathic intracranial hypertension

    e. A and C only

4. Headaches attributed to a disorder of homeostasis include all except:

    a. Cardiac cephalgia

    b. Hypertensive crises without encephalopathy

    c. Hypertensive encephalopathy

    d. Hyperthyroidism

    e. Diving

5. Cardiac cephalgia:

    a. Is associated with vomiting

    b. Occurs during acute myocardial infarction

    c. Is worsened by nitroglycerin

    d. Is precipitated by the Valsalva maneuver

    e. Is often unilateral

6. A 65-year-old man presents with a 3-month history of facial pain. The pain is short-lived and stabbing and begins abruptly. The pain starts in the back of his throat and radiates into his ear. Attacks may be triggered by swallowing and coughing. What is the diagnosis?

    a. Glossopharyngeal neuralgia

    b. Persistent idiopathic facial pain

    c. Nervus intermedius neuralgia

    d. Cluster headache

    e. Superior laryngeal neuralgia

7. The cranial neuralgia associated with the inability to speak is:

    a. Symptomatic trigeminal

    b. Glossopharyngeal

    c. Nervus intermedius

    d. Superior laryngeal

    e. Classical trigeminal

8. A 57-year-old women presents with a 9-month history of facial pain. The pain is aching, deep, and poorly localized. She reports stabbing pains in her ear as well. There are no trigger zones and no refractory period. The most appropriate test to establish the diagnosis is:

    a. CT without contrast of the brain

    b. CT with contrast of the brain

   c. Chest x-ray

   d. MRA of brain

   e. MRI of brain

9. Headaches associated with sleep apnea:

   a. Occur on a nightly basis

   b. Last 1 to 2 hours each

   c. Resolve within 1 week of correction of apnea

   d. Are bilateral

   e. May be associated with nausea but not vomiting

10. A 25-year-old woman with a 10-year history of migraine without aura presents to your practice for the first time. Over the past 4 months she has been suffering from daily low-level headaches as well as episodic migraine headaches. She has been treating her daily headaches with an OTC product containing aspirin, acetaminophen, and caffeine, four tablets daily, for the past 4 months. According to ICHD-II guidelines, her current diagnosis for her most recent headache is:

   a. Transformed migraine

   b. Chronic migraine

   c. New daily persistent headache

   d. Probable chronic migraine

   e. Probable medication overuse headache

10. e

9. d

8. c

7. d

6. a

5. e

3. d

2. c

1. e

SUGGESTED READING

Headache in clinical practice, 2nd ed., eds. Silberstein, S.D., Lipton, R.B., & Goadsby, P.J. London: Martin Dunitz Ltd., 2002, pp. 335–344.

The headaches, 3rd ed., eds. Olesen, J., Goadsby, P.J., Ramadan, N.M., et al. Philadelphia: Lippincott Williams & Wilkins, 2006, pp. 989–1027.

La Mantia, L., Curone, M., Rapoport, A.M., & Bussone, G. Tolosa-Hunt syndrome: Critical literature review based on IHS 2004 criteria. *Cephalalgia* 26 (2006): 772–781.

Wolff's headache and other head pain, 7th ed., eds. Silberstein, S.D., Lipton, R.B., & Dalessio, D.J. New York: Oxford University Press, 2001, pp. 434–535.

10

Psychiatric Comorbidity and Causes of Headache

Steven M. Baskin, PhD

It is widely acknowledged that psychological factors can have a significant influence on headache. There are numerous hypotheses in the literature about psychological interactions with headache. Some include personality traits that may predispose to headache; psychological and stress factors that may be associated with the onset, exacerbation, and maintenance of headache; psychiatric comorbidity where both headache and psychiatric disorders coexist; and headache as purely symptomatic of psychiatric illness.

The headache and psychiatric literature reveal significant correlations between daily stress levels and attacks of migraine. Stress may also exacerbate chronic daily headache, and levels of daily minor stress have been associated with migraine. In this case, as in many medical disorders, headache is influenced by psychological factors. This chapter will be concerned with psychiatric comorbidity and headache as well as headache attributed to psychiatric illness.

Comorbidity is the presence of any additional coexisting illness in a patient with a particular index disease. When one disorder occurs with greater-than-chance frequency with another disorder, they are said to be comorbid, a more-than-coincidental association between two conditions. Comorbidities may complicate the differential diagnosis, contribute to disease burden, affect adherence to treatment, lead to therapeutic opportunities and limitations, give insight into mechanisms, and alter the course of the index disease, in some cases leading to a poorer prognosis, including chronification.

There are methodologic issues that may confound comorbidity data. Selection bias has to do with the deviation of results from a true value because of differences in characteristics between those selected to be investigated and those that are not studied. Selection biases can lead to misleadingly high rates of comorbidity in treatment-seeking samples. Berkson's bias or paradox is the non-random co-occurrence of two conditions attributed to artifacts of the methodology employed—for example, a sample that was selected from a clinical setting that was not representative of the general population of individuals with the particular index disease. Berkson's bias arises because individuals with more than one disorder can seek treatment for any or all disorders and thus tend to be treated more often than those with only one disorder. Hence, individuals with two or more conditions may be overrepresented in a clinical sample. As a result, disproportionately more individuals with comorbid disorders are included in clinical samples than in community studies. Comorbidity studies are most valid when they are population studies. Measurement or assessment bias occurs when there is a systematic error arising from inaccurate measurement or classification of subjects. For example, the co-occurrence of two disorders may be due to overlapping diagnostic criteria, coding biases, or assessment methods used to gauge the criteria. Comorbidity studies must use operational definitions and systematic methods for diagnosing all index diseases. An operational definition is a clear and specific description of what is to be observed and measured, such that different people collecting, using, and interpreting data will do so consistently. Studies on comorbidity must apply systematic diagnostic methods for identifying migraine and the other conditions under study. Finally, studies may be either cross-sectional or longitudinal. Only longitudinal studies can indicate directionality to see if one condition predisposes one to another condition (unidirectional) or if the relationship is bidirectional, where there exists a "two-way street" with each disorder increasing the subject's susceptibility to the other condition.

The mechanisms of comorbidity include chance, one disorder causing another (for example, diabetes and neuropathic pain), or shared genetic or environmental risk factors (such as post-traumatic headache and post-traumatic seizure disorder), or genetic and environmental factors may predispose to a brain state that may lead to both conditions (most likely the case in psychiatric comorbidity and migraine).

Numerous clinic-based studies as well as more recent community samples using International Headache Society and *Diagnostic and Statistical Manual* (DSM) criteria have shown a relationship between migraine and a number of psychiatric disorders.

"Headache attributed to psychiatric illness" is a new diagnostic category of secondary headache in the *International Classification of Headache Disorders*, 2nd edition (ICHD-II). In the earlier diagnostic schema, this category did not exist, and psychiatrically caused headaches were considered a variant of tension-type headache.

MIGRAINE AND MOOD DISORDERS

The studies examining the relationship between migraine and major depression have odds ratios (OR) varying from 2.2 to 4.0 (Table 10–1). Early studies established a cross-sectional relationship between the disorders, whereas later researchers examined the temporal relationships from depression to migraine and from migraine to depression.

The Zurich Cohort Study used an epidemiologic cohort of 27- and 28-year-olds in Zurich and was one of the first population-based studies of psychiatric comorbidity associated with migraine. Diagnoses did not strictly adhere to IHS

Table 10–1 Association Between Migraine and Depression: IHS-Based Community Studies

Reference	Association	Odds Ratio
Breslau (1998)	Yes	
Migraine with aura		4.0
Migraine without aura		2.2
Swartz et al. (2000)	Yes	2.3
Breslau et al. (2000)	Yes	3.5

Modified with permission from Low and Merikangas, 2003.

criteria. Migraine was strongly associated with major depression (OR 2.2) and bipolar spectrum disorders (OR 2.9). There were also associations, in this early cross-sectional study, between migraine and numerous anxiety disorders. There was an added increased risk of migraine among subjects with both major depression and an anxiety disorder. For most diagnoses, migraine with aura was more strongly associated with psychiatric disorders. In this study, migraineurs with comorbid depression met the criteria for atypical depression, with weight gain and hypersomnolence predominating. Merikangas and colleagues reported that in most cases, anxiety first appeared in childhood, followed by the occurrence of migraine, and then by episodes of depression. Moreover, persons with migraine with or without major depression are at higher risk for suicide attempts than those without any history of migraine.

Breslau and colleagues have done numerous studies examining the relationship between migraine and major depression. They initially showed a bidirectional relationship between major depression and migraine in a research study in 1994. One study in 2000 reported that the lifetime prevalence of major depression was approximately three times higher in persons with migraine and persons with non-migrainous severe headaches but not with a non-headache control group. The association was greater in migraine with aura than in subjects with migraine without aura. Significant bidirectional relationships were found between migraine and major depression, with migraine increasing the risk for the first onset of depression and major depression increasing the risk for the first onset of migraine. Persons with non-migrainous severe headaches had a higher incidence of first-onset depression, but major depression did not predict an increase in the incidence of other severe headaches.

Breslau and colleagues reported similar results in a 2-year longitudinal population-based study in 2003. In this study, migraine at baseline increased the risk of first-onset major depression (OR 5.8) and major depression at baseline increased the risk of incident migraine (OR 3.4). With respect to other severe headaches, there was no increased risk associated with baseline major depression (OR 0.6) and a questionable risk in the reverse direction (OR 2.7, 95% confidence interval [CI] 0.9 to 8.1).

The combination of these studies suggests that the bidirectional relationship is specific to migraine and not to all severe headaches. There was one study by Swartz and associates that did not support a bidirectional relationship, but methodologic limitations may account for this negative study.

In Breslau's 2003 study, subjects with comorbid major depression did not have a greater frequency or persistence of attacks and did not differ in progression of migraine-related disability over time compared to migraine sufferers without depression. Migraine with aura was a risk factor for suicide attempts. In a recent research study by Fasmer and Oedegaard, the frequency of suicide attempts was higher among the patients having migraine with aura than in the patients having migraine aura without headache. In another study by the same group, the authors compared patients having migraine with aura with those having aura without headache in a large sample of patients with major depression. The group who had aura without headache had a significantly lower rate of "affective temperaments" and suicide attempts. Oedegaard and colleagues recently examined, in a multiple logistic regression analysis, the association between anxiety disorder/depression and migraine with and without aura. They reported that depression and depression with comorbid anxiety disorder were more likely in women having migraine with aura compared to those having migraine without aura. There was no difference in "pure" anxiety disorders, across all anxiety diagnoses, between migraine with and without aura in women. The authors reported no difference in the prevalence of depression and anxiety disorders between migraine with and without aura in men.

Zwart and colleagues investigated the relationship between migraine, non-migrainous headache, and headache frequency in a large cross-sectional population-based study. The ORs for depression and anxiety disorders among both migraine and non-migraine sufferers were higher with increasing headache frequency. These relationships seemed more dependent on higher-frequency headache rather than diagnosis.

A population-based study by McWilliams and associates examined associations between three pain conditions (migraine, back pain, arthritis) and three frequently diagnosed psychiatric conditions (depression, generalized anxiety disorder, panic disorder). They reported that 28.5% of subjects with migraine were determined to be clinically depressed; only 12.3% of subjects without migraine were classified as depressed.

Patel and colleagues studied the prevalence of major depression in subjects with migraine, those with probable migraine, and controls in a health maintenance organization using telephone interviews. They found an overall prevalence of major depressive disorder of 28.1% for the migraine group, 19.5% for the probable migraine group, and 10.3% for the controls.

Current major depression is also significantly more frequent in migraineurs than in non-migraineurs, as shown in two different studies. It also appears that migraine and depression exert a significant but independent impact on quality of life. Lipton and colleagues, in a recent population-based case–control study, confirmed that there was a higher risk of current depression in those suffering from migraine and that migraine and depression are independently associated with decreases in quality of life. Wang and colleagues studied a geriatric sample in a population-based study and found that the risk of current depression was much greater in migraine sufferers than in non-migraine patients.

The relationship between migraine and bipolar spectrum disorders is less studied than the relationship between migraine and major depression; however, it has been studied in clinical as well as population-based studies (Table 10–2). The Zurich Cohort Study showed that migraine was associated with bipolar spectrum disorders: 8.8% of the 61 migraine subjects and only 3.3% of the controls met their criteria for bipolar spectrum disorder. Breslau reported similar results in a study with young adults, with an OR for bipolar I of 7.3 and bipolar II of 5.2. Migraine with aura had a stronger relationship than migraine without aura.

Oedegaard and Fasmer in a recent study reported that a comorbid migraine and depression group resembled bipolar II patients more than unipolar depressives, and the authors concluded that migraine in depressed patients might be a bipolar spectrum trait. To avoid misdiagnosis it can be helpful to use a screening instrument for bipolar disorder such as the Mood Disorder Questionnaire, which exhibits adequate sensitivity and very good specificity.

MIGRAINE AND ANXIETY DISORDERS

Anxiety disorders are also associated with migraine (Table 10–3). Merikangas and coworkers in 1990 reported a stronger relationship between migraine and anxiety disorders than between migraine and the affective disorders. Migraineurs are three to ten times more likely to suffer from panic disorder, with the highest OR in migraine with aura. One study by Breslau and colleagues

Table 10–2 Association Between Migraine and Bipolar Disorder: Community Studies

Reference	Odds Ratio
IHS-Based	
Breslau (1998)	
Bipolar I Migraine with aura	7.3
Migraine without aura	2.4
Bipolar II Migraine with aura	5.2
Migraine without aura	2.5
Non-IHS-Based	
Merikangas et al. (1990)	
Bipolar spectrum	2.9

Modified with permission from Low and Merikangas, 2003.

Table 10–3 Association Between Migraine and Anxiety: Community Studies

Reference	Panic	GAD	OCD	Phobia
	Odds Ratio			
Breslau et al. (1998)				
Migraine with aura	10.4	4.1	5.0	2.9
Migraine without aura	3.0	5.5	4.8	1.8
Swartz et al. (2000)	3.4		1.3	1.4
Breslau et al. (2001)	3.7			
Merikangas et al.	3.3	5.3		2.4 (simple)
(1990; 1993)				3.4 (social)
McWilliams (2004)		3.9		

Modified with permission from Low and Merikangas, 2003.
GAD, generalized anxiety disorder; OCD, obsessive–compulsive distorder.

found that migraineurs were four to five times more likely to suffer from generalized anxiety disorder and five times more likely to suffer from obsessive–compulsive disorder. Swartz and colleagues did not replicate these associations in a later study with an older sample. McWilliams and associates, in their recent large-scale prospective community study, reported that 9.1% of subjects with migraine, compared with only 2.5% of people without migraine, had comorbid generalized anxiety disorder.

Breslau and colleagues explored the temporal relationship between migraine and panic disorder and between non-migrainous severe headache and panic disorder. The results showed that the comorbidity of panic disorder was not specific to migraine but included non-migrainous severe headache types as well. There was a bidirectional relationship between headache and panic, but the headache-to-panic direction appears to have greater influence than the reverse direction. Swartz and colleagues did a 13-year prospective study on psychiatric disorders as risk factors for migraine onset and found that only antecedent phobic disorders were predictive of future migraine.

Most patients with a mood disorder also have an accompanying anxiety disorder, whereas many people with anxiety disorders do not suffer from mood disorders. The combined effects of anxiety disorder and migraine, however, dramatically increase the odds for major depression. Therefore, it is important to screen for both mood and anxiety disorders in migraine patients.

Guidetti and colleagues found that those with headache who had two or more comorbid psychiatric disorders in childhood or adolescence had a significantly lower rate of improvement than patients with no or one psychiatric comorbidity after an 8-year follow-up. Anxiety disorders were found to be a negative prognostic factor related to the persistence of migraine and tension-type headache as well as to the future onset of depression.

CHRONIC DAILY HEADACHE

The previously mentioned Zwart study showed increasing ORs for mood and anxiety disorders as headache frequency increased. Chronic daily headache was associated with higher levels of anxiety and mood disorders than was episodic migraine in three studies. This risk seems to be particularly high in "transformed" migraine. There is a high comorbidity between anxiety and depression in this population, and in a study by Verri and associates 90% of the 88 chronic daily headache patients studied had at least one comorbid psychiatric disorder and 45% had comorbid mood and anxiety disorders. There was a trend for mood disorders to be more frequent in individuals who had suffered from chronic daily headache for more than 5 years. The Verri study compared headache patients with low back pain patients and found that headache patients suffered more frequently from all psychiatric disorders except for somatoform disorders. Thus, these comorbidities appear to be specific to a headache population rather than the result of any form of chronic pain.

A study by Juang and colleagues showed that 78% of patients with transformed migraine had psychiatric comorbidity, including major depression (57%), dysthymia (11%), panic disorder (30%), and generalized anxiety disorder (8%), and also had a higher rate of psychiatric issues than patients with chronic tension-type headache. A large-scale study of 245 chronic tension-type headache sufferers by Holroyd and coworkers showed that they were 3 to 15 times more likely to have a comorbid mood or anxiety disorder than matched controls with less than 10 minor headaches per year. They reported that "affective distress" was an important aspect of patient impairment.

Two studies compared episodic migraine patients with chronic daily headache patients with analgesic overuse. Mitsikostas and Thomas found major depression to be associated with all types of headaches studied, but the association was twice as strong in patients with daily headache and chronic substance use. Another study by Radat and colleagues, comparing migraine alone to transformed migraine with chronic substance use, reported a higher prevalence for major depression, panic disorder, and social phobia in transformed migraine patients with chronic substance use.

Recent studies by Atasoy and Radat and their colleagues have shown that comorbid psychiatric disorders are prevalent in medication overuse headache, and the Radat study reported that the psychiatric condition was likely to precede the onset of the medication overuse. Rothrock and colleagues reported that migraine patients with coexisting borderline personality disorder were more likely to have more pervasive headache, more headache-related disability, and less likelihood of responding to standard pharmacologic therapies and were more prone to medication overuse.

Two retrospective studies investigated abuse issues and migraine. Tietjen and colleagues did a cluster analysis of clinic patients and identified three different migraine comorbidity constellations. One subgroup of migraine sufferers was determined by the diagnoses of depression, anxiety, and fibromyalgia. This subgroup had the greatest disability and the lowest quality of life; they more commonly reported physical, emotional, and sexual abuse than the other defined migraine subgroups. Peterlin and colleagues showed that the relative frequency of physical and sexual abuse was higher in the chronic daily headache group compared to an episodic migraine group.

HEADACHE ATTRIBUTED TO PSYCHIATRIC DISORDER

The presence of comorbid psychiatric illness may contribute to treatment refractoriness but is not considered etiologic. "Headache attributed to psychiatric illness" is a new diagnostic category of secondary headache. In this latest classification revision, ICHD-II, somatization disorder and psychotic disorder are specifically delineated as extremely rare secondary causes of headache. To attribute headache to a psychiatric disorder, the headache must occur exclusively during the course of the psychiatric illness. The headache disorder must resolve or show marked improvement after effective treatment or spontaneous remission of the psychiatric condition.

Somatoform disorders are characterized by the presence of physical symptoms that suggest a medical condition but cannot be fully explained by a known medical disorder, another psychiatric condition, or the effects of a substance. These physical symptoms are not the result of conscious malingering or the result of a factitious disorder, where a symptom is intentionally produced to assume a sick role. Somatization disorder is one of the somatoform disorders and has been historically called "hysteria" or Briquet's syndrome. It is characterized by numerous significant somatic complaints beginning before age 30, including at least four pain symptoms from different sites, two non-pain

Table 10–4 Criteria for Headache Attributed to Somatization Disorder

12.1 Headache attributed to somatization disorder
Diagnostic criteria:
A. Headache, no typical characteristics known, fulfilling criterion C
B. Presence of somatization disorder fulfilling DSM-IV criteria:
  1. History of many physical complaints beginning before age 30 that occur over a period of several years and result in treatment being sought and/or in significant impairment in social, occupational or other important areas of functioning
  2. At least four pain symptoms, two non-pain gastrointestinal symptoms, one sexual or reproductive symptom and one pseudoneurological symptom
  3. After appropriate investigation, each of these symptoms cannot be fully explained by a known general medical condition or the direct effects of a substance or medication; or, if there is a related medical condition, the complaints or impairment are in excess of what would be expected from the history, examination or laboratory findings
C. Headache is not atttributed to another cause

Source: ICHD-II, 12.1 Headache attributed to somatisation disorder. Cephalalgia 24 (2004): 122.

Table 10–5 Criteria for Headache Attributed to Psychotic Disorder

12.2 Headache attributed to psychotic disorder
Diagnostic criteria:
A. Headache, no typical characteristics known, fulfilling criteria C–E
B. Delusional belief about the presence and/or etiology of headache occurring in the
    context of delusional disorder, schizophrenia, major depressive episode with psychotic
    features, manic episode with psychotic features or other psychotic disorder fulfilling
    DSM-IV criteria
C. Headache occurs only when delusional
D. Headache resolves when delusions remit
E. Headache is not attributed to another cause

Source: ICHD-II, 12.2 Headache attributed to psychotic disorder. *Cephalalgia* 24(2004): 122.

gastrointestinal symptoms, one sexual or reproductive symptom, and one pseudoneurologic symptom (Table 10–4). Recognition that a patient has a somatization disorder is extremely important. Accurate diagnosis allows for coordination of care between different practitioners, which can help avoid iatrogenic harm from unnecessary or aggressive testing or interventions.

Headache attributed to psychotic disorder is diagnosed when headache is a somatic delusion or part of a different type of delusion (i.e., persecutory) in the context of any DSM-IV psychiatric disorder (Table 10–5). The most common diagnoses include schizophrenia and schizophreniform disorder, delusional disorder, major depressive episode with psychotic features, and manic episode with psychotic features. The delusions are often bizarre in schizophrenia, and headache may be part of a false belief that may include loss of control over mind or body, alien thought (headache) insertion, and delusions of control where outside forces may be manipulating the body.

The ICHD-II appendix contains "candidate criteria" for seven other psychiatric disorders as causes of headache to facilitate research: headache occurring exclusively during episodes of major depression, panic disorder, generalized anxiety disorder, undifferentiated somatoform disorder, social phobia, separation anxiety disorder, and post-traumatic stress disorder. Factitious disorders and malingering are not included in either the main ICHD-II classification or the appendix.

SUMMARY

Mood and anxiety disorders are often comorbid with migraine. These include major depressive disorder, bipolar spectrum disorders, generalized anxiety disorder, panic disorder, obsessive–compulsive disorder, and phobias. Comorbid psychiatric disorders may heighten "affective distress" and increase impairment and may contribute to headache chronification. There appears to be a bidirectional relationship between migraine and depression and most likely between severe headache and panic disorder. There is an increased risk of psychiatric comorbidity with chronic daily headache compared to episodic migraine. Psychiatric comorbidities may be involved in medication overuse headache, and the onset of the psychiatric condition may precede the overuse of medication. A history of physical or emotional abuse and the presence of a personality disorder may further complicate the clinical picture. In rare cases, headache may be directly attributed to a psychiatric disorder.

Review Questions

1. Which of the following statements is true?
   a. Bipolar disorder has a greater comorbidity with migraine without aura than migraine with aura.
   b. Generalized anxiety disorder has a greater comorbidity with migraine with aura than migraine without aura.
   c. Most depression studies show a greater comorbidity with migraine with aura than migraine without aura.
   d. Depression and migraine have only a unidirectional relationship as per Breslau's research, with severe migraine increasing the risk for depression.
2. A researcher is looking at associations between migraine and asthma. Patients are recruited from the neurology outpatient clinic. Which of the following is a possible bias?
   a. Patients with asthma may be referred at a higher frequency because they are unable to take beta blockers.
   b. IHS diagnostic criteria are complex.
   c. These type of population studies often have selection bias.
   d. Headache diaries and asthma diaries have low compliance.
3. Individuals with two or more conditions may be overrepresented in a clinical study. This is referred to as:
   a. Assessment bias
   b. Measurement bias
   c. Berkson's bias
   d. Breslau's paradox
4. An example of a study that may have a selection bias is:
   a. A longitudinal community study
   b. A cross-sectional population study
   c. A study of patients seeking treatment for tension-type headache
   d. An epidemiologic cohort study of all 30-year-olds in a community
5. What type of study allows for directionality of a relationship between two index disorders?
   a. Cross-sectional
   b. Population-based

      c. Double-blind

      d. Longitudinal

6. Epidemiologic research in psychiatric comorbidity suggests which one of the following developmental sequences in migraine patients?

      a. Migraine in childhood followed by depression and then anxiety in adulthood

      b. Phobias in childhood followed by the occurrence of migraine and then by episodes of depression in adulthood

      c. Severe childhood depression followed by migraine at menarche and obsessive–compulsive disorder in adolescence

      d. Migraine in early childhood followed by child abuse and then a personality disorder in adulthood

7. A patient has migraine with aura. Which of the following statements is true?

      a. Frequency of suicide attempts is higher in patients having migraine with aura than in patients having migraine aura without headache.

      b. In a study of patients with major depression, patients having migraine aura without headache had a higher rate of "affective temperaments."

      c. In chronic daily headache, only patients with a history of migraine with aura have a high comorbidity of depression.

      d. Obsessive–compulsive disorder is significantly more prevalent in patients with migraine with aura.

8. What is the best statement concerning the data on bidirectionality between severe headache and major depression and panic disorder?

      a. Persons with non-migrainous severe headaches had a higher incidence of first-onset depression, but major depression did not predict an increase in the incidence of non-migrainous severe headaches.

      b. Significant bidirectional relationships were found between migraine and major depression but not between major depression and first-onset migraine.

      c. The comorbidity of panic disorder was only specific to migraine and not to non-migrainous severe headache.

      d. The longitudinal depression–headache studies suggests that the bidirectional relationship is not specific to migraine but applies to all severe headaches.

9. A patient has a long history of borderline personality disorder, chronic daily headache, and medication overuse. Which one of the following is likely to be false?

      a. She has a high probability of having a comorbid Axis I psychiatric disorder.

      b. Her psychiatric conditions most likely are a result of medication overuse.

    c. She is less likely to respond to standard pharmacologic therapies.

    d. She most likely has a significant amount of headache-related disability.

10. A 35-year-old woman presents for treatment with a 20-year history of new daily persistent headache. It began with a severe migraine, and she reports constant head pain at varying intensities since that episode. At the time of initial evaluation she was overusing narcotics and barbiturate-containing medications. The patient reported a history of multiple, recurring, significant somatic complaints that resulted in some form of medical treatment. She reported a history of daily nausea, bloating, and undiagnosed abdominal pain for months at a time, which would suddenly remit; low back pain resulting in two hospitalizations for "traction" and one failed surgery; severe menstrual pain and irregularities; severe pain during intercourse; intermittent severe facial pain with one failed "TMJ" surgery; and sleep disorder "since infancy." She denied any abuse history. She also reported an episode in her 20s of coordination problems associated with paresthesias, localized weakness, and sleepwalking. She had a negative neurologic workup at that time, with a diagnosis of multiple sclerosis considered. Laboratory, MRI, lumbar puncture, and sleep evaluations have been normal. What psychiatric diagnosis should be considered?

    a. Generalized anxiety disorder

    b. Factitious disorder

    c. Somatic depression

    d. Somatization disorder

10. d

9. b

8. a

7. a

6. b

5. d

4. c

3. c

2. a

1. c

SUGGESTED READING

Baskin, S.M., Lipchik, G.L., & Smitherman, T.A. Mood and anxiety disorders in chronic headache. *Headache* 46, suppl. 3 (2006): S76–S87.

Bigal, M.E., & Lipton, R.B. Modifiable risk factors for migraine progression. *Headache* 46 (2006): 1334–1343.

Breslau, N. Psychiatric comorbidity in migraine. *Cephalalgia* suppl. 22 (1998): 56–61.

Breslau, N., Davis, G.C., Schultz, L.R., & Peterson, E.L. Migraine and major depression: A longitudinal study. *Headache* 34 (1994): 387–393.

Breslau, N., Lipton, R.B., Stewart, W.F., Schultz, L.R., & Welch, K.M. Comorbidity of migraine and depression. *Neurology* 60 (2003): 1308–1312.

Breslau, N., Schultz, L.R., Stewart, W.F., Lipton, R.B., Lucia, V.C., & Welch, K.M. Headache and major depression: Is the association specific to migraine? *Neurology* 54 (2000): 308–313.

Breslau, N., Schultz, L.R., Stewart, W.F., Lipton, R., & Welch, K.M. Headache types and panic disorder: Directionality and specificity. *Neurology* 56 (2001): 350–354.

Frediani, F., & Villani, V. Migraine and depression. *Neurologic Science* 28 (2007): S161–S165.

Guidetti, V., Galli, F., Fabrizi, P., Giannantoni, A.S., Napoli, L., Bruni, O., & Trillo, S. Headache and psychiatric comorbidity: Clinical aspects and outcome in an 8-year follow-up study. *Cephalalgia* 18 (1998): 455–462.

Hamelsky, S.W., & Lipton, R.B. Psychiatric comorbidity of migraine. *Headache* 46 (2006): 1327–1333.

Lake, A.E. Medication overuse headache: Biobehavioral issues and solutions. *Headache* 46, Suppl. 3 (2006): S88–S97.

Lipchik, G.L., & Penzien, D.B. Psychiatric comorbidities in patients with headaches. *Seminars in Pain Medicine* 2 (2004): 93–105.

Low, N.C.P., & Merikangas, K.R. The comorbidity of migraine. *CNS Spectrums* 8, no. 6, (2003): 433–444.

McWilliams, L.A., Goodwin, R.D., & Cox, B.J. Depression and anxiety associated with three pain conditions: Results from a nationally representative sample. *Pain* 111 (2004): 77–83.

Merikangas, K.R., Angst, J., & Isler, H. Migraine and psychopathology. *Archives of General Psychiatry* 47 (1990): 849–853.

Merikangas, K.R., Merikangas, J.R., & Angst, J. Headache syndromes and psychiatric disorders: Association and familial transmission. *Journal of Psychiatric Research* 27 (1993): 197–210.

Oedegaard, K.J., & Fasmer, O.B. Is migraine in unipolar depressed patients a bipolar spectrum trait? *Journal of Affective Disorders* 84 (2005): 233–242.

Oedegaard, K.J., Neckelmann, D., Mykletun, A., et al. Migraine with and without aura: Associations with depression and anxiety disorder in a population-based study. The Hunt Study. *Cephalalgia* 26 (2006): 1–6.

Radat, F., Creac'h, C., Swendsen, J.D., et al. Psychiatric comorbidity in the evolution from migraine to medication overuse headache. *Cephalalgia* 25 (2005): 519–522.

Radat, F., & Swendsen, J. Psychiatric comorbidity in migraine: a review. *Cephalalgia* 25 (2004): 165–178.

Sheftell, F.D., & Atlas, S.J. Migraine and psychiatric comorbidity: From theory and hypotheses to clinical application. *Headache* 42 (2002): 934–944.

Swartz, K.L., Pratt, L.A., Armenian, H.K., Lee, L.C., & Eaton, W.W. Mental disorders and the incidence of migraine headaches in a community sample: Results from the Baltimore Epidemiologic Catchment area follow-up study. *Archives of General Psychiatry* 57 (2000): 945–950.

Tietjen, G.E., Herial, N.A., Hardgrove, J., Utley, C., & White, L. Migraine comorbidity constellations. *Headache* 47 (2007): 857–865.

Verri, A.P., Proietti Cecchini, A., Galli, C., Granella, F., Sandrini, G., & Nappi, G.
    Psychiatric comorbidity in chronic daily headache. *Cephalalgia* 18, Suppl. 21 (1998):
    45–49.
Zwart, J.A., Dyb, G., Hagen, K., et al. Depression and anxiety disorders associated with
    headache frequency. The Nord-Trondelag Health Study. *European Journal of
    Neurology* 10 (2003): 147–152.

IV
Headache Treatment

11

Pharmacologic Treatment of Acute Migraine

Alan M. Rapoport, MD

The pharmacologic treatment of headache is only one part of the entire regimen of optimal management principles for headache patients. Prior to prescribing medication, it is critical for the physician to make an accurate set of diagnoses, to establish a good doctor–patient relationship, to review the details of previous treatment regimens, to go over the various therapeutic options with the patient (including the non-pharmacologic ones), and to reassure the patient that on the basis of the history, examination, and appropriate testing, no other significant neurologic problems exist. Educating patients about how to identify and avoid headache triggers and teaching them to understand how medications work (including avoidance of adverse reactions or drug–drug interactions) are also essential parts of successful headache management.

Acute treatment (also called abortive treatment) is intended to reverse attacks once they begin, limit disability, and reduce and stop the pain and associated symptoms, such as nausea, vomiting, photophobia, phonophobia, and increased pain with movement. Some patients use only occasional acute treatments and obtain fairly rapid and complete relief when needed. For example, evidence exists that when a migraine headache attack is treated shortly after the pain has begun and is still of mild intensity, the medication is more effective, often leading to a pain-free state. This treatment approach is also more likely to cause fewer adverse reactions and reduce the chance of a recurrent headache developing within the next 24 hours.

PRINCIPLES OF PHARMACOLOGICAL TREATMENT

Once an accurate set of diagnoses is made, the next task is to develop a successful treatment plan. The goals in designing and initiating a treatment plan are to:

- Reduce headache attack frequency, severity, and duration
- Avoid headache escalation
- Prevent headaches completely, if possible
- Reduce disability
- Rapidly return the patient to normal functioning

- Improve the patient's quality of life
- Avoid medication overuse
- Educate the patient about self-management of the illness (e.g., trigger avoidance, careful use of acute care medication, and lifestyle changes such as sleeping and eating on time and exercising regularly)
- Use the right treatment the first time (stratified care), which usually means treating significant cases of migraine with the appropriate dose and form of a triptan, not a nonspecific medication

In designing the most appropriate treatment plan for each patient, discussion regarding potential adverse events, preferences as to frequency of dosing, routes of administration, lifestyle considerations (e.g., alcohol consumption, sleeping and eating patterns, use of OTC products, use of herbal or vitamin supplements, among others) will help ensure the patient receives treatment modalities and medications he or she will take as prescribed. Women of childbearing age should be asked if there is any chance they are pregnant, or if they are planning to become pregnant in the near future, or could possibly become pregnant, as this will significantly affect treatment choices.

ACUTE MIGRAINE THERAPY

Management of patients with migraine requires individualized acute care therapies that follow several basic principles:

1. Engage the patient in the treatment plan and management of his or her own illness so there will be a true patient–physician partnership.
2. Tailor treatment to meet the patient's individual headache needs based on severity of illness (disability), prior response to specific medications (including efficacy and presence of adverse events), and presence of comorbid and coexisting medical conditions.
3. Educate headache sufferers about their specific condition and current theories of pathophysiology so they will understand the rationale for the therapy that you present.
4. Use migraine-specific agents (not analgesics) as first-line treatment when possible, especially for more significant headaches.
5. Select a route of administration appropriate for the attack characteristics and patient preferences. Be aware that injections and nasal sprays, by bypassing the gastrointestinal tract, usually work faster than tablets and are optimal for nauseated and vomiting patients and those whose poorly functioning gastrointestinal tracts preclude rapid absorption of oral medication.
6. Follow the patient closely and frequently to help improve efficacy by giving useful tips about taking medication early and repeating it when needed, manage medication side effects, and avoid overuse syndromes.

7. Give the patient a headache calendar (diary) and ask him or her to fill it in daily and bring it to each office visit for review. This will help to track headache frequency, intensity, and duration, use of preventive and acute care medications, menstrual cycle and its relevance to headache causation, and so forth. It may also help to track disability by having the patient take a MIDAS or HIT 6 test.

There are over 40 different medications (Table 11–1) currently prescribed for acute treatment of migraine, of which only 25% have approved indications by

Table 11–1 Acute Therapies for Migraine

Generic Treatment	Dose Range
Aspirin tablets	325 – 1000 mg
Acetaminophen tablets	325 – 1000 mg

Combination Analgesics	Available Doses
Aspirin plus acetaminophen plus caffeine tablets	250 mg plus 250 mg plus 65 mg
Isometheptene mucate plus acetaminophen plus dichloralphenazone tablets (off the market)	65 mg plus 325 mg plus 100 mg
Butalbital plus aspirin plus caffeine tablets	50 mg plus 325 plus 40 mg
Butalbital plus acetaminophen plus caffeine tablets	50 mg plus 325 plus 40 mg

Ergot Alkaloids	Available Doses
Erogotamine tartrate plus caffeine tablet	1 mg plus 100 mg
Ergotamine tartrate plus caffeine suppository	2 mg plus 100 mg
DHE nasal spray	0.5 mg/nostril (repeat in 15 min 1x for 2 mg total dose)
DHE IM or SC	1 mg

NSAIDs	Dose Range
Diclofenac tablets	50 – 100 mg
Flurbiprofen tablets	100 – 300 mg
Ibuprofen tablets	200 – 1,200 mg
Naproxen tablets	250 – 500 mg
Naproxen sodium tablets	550 – 1,100 mg
Piroxicam tablets	40 mg
Tolfenamic acid tablets	200 – 400 mg
Diclofenac sodium IM	50 mg

Cox 2 Inhibitors	
Rofecoxib (off the market)	12.5 – 50 mg
Celecoxib	100 – 200 mg
Valdecoxib (off the market)	10 – 40 mg
Opiate Analgesics	
Butorphanol nasal spray (+ many others)	1 – 2 mg

Continued

Table 11–1 *(Continued)*

Triptans	Available Doses
Almotriptan tablets	12.5 mg
Naratriptan tablets	1 mg or 2.5 mg
Rizatriptan tablets	5 mg or 10 mg
Rizatriptan orally disintegrating tablets	5 mg or 10 mg
Sumatriptan tablets	25 mg, 50 mg, or 100 mg
Sumatriptan nasal spray	5 mg or 20 mg
Sumatriptan SC self-injection	4 or 6 mg
Zolmitriptan tablets	2.5 mg or 5 mg
Zolmitriptan orally disintegrating tablets	2.5 mg or 5 mg
Zolmitriptan NS	5 mg
Frovatriptan tablets	2.5 mg
Eletriptan tablets	20 mg or 40 mg

regulatory authorities. Some are scientifically proven to be clinically useful in migraine, and others are known to be empirically useful but either may lack evidence-based, published supporting data or have it but no indication approved by the FDA. Consequently, choosing a medication for acute therapy is a complex, multistep process that requires a good understanding of the patient's overall health, the range of appropriate treatment options, patient-specific migraine characteristics, and patient preferences.

Simple Analgesics

Some patients can successfully treat a migraine attack by taking simple analgesics, especially if treatment is taken early in the course of the attack when the pain is of mild intensity and not associated with severe nausea. Studies suggest that aspirin monotherapy in selected patients, at a dose of 650 mg, may be helpful in alleviating headache. Conflicting evidence in the literature suggests acetaminophen as monotherapy may not be an ideal first-line treatment choice; however, for selected patients with contraindications to other therapies (e.g., pregnancy, easy bruisability, or aspirin hypersensitivity), a trial of acetaminophen 1,000 mg with a repeat in 2 hours if necessary may be justified. Sometimes the efficacy of simple analgesics has been supplemented by the co-administration of metoclopramide (5 mg or 10 mg orally, given prior to or concomitantly with oral analgesics); this addition may improve absorption of the aspirin, decrease nausea, and improve the therapeutic response. Aspirin can cause gastrointestinal problems and bleeding, acetaminophen can cause liver toxicity, and metoclopramide can cause anxiety and dyskinesia.

Combination Analgesics

Caffeine acts as an analgesic adjuvant, an adenosine antagonist acutely, an adenosine agonist chronically, and a vasoconstrictor in the treatment of headache and other pain disorders. Off-the-shelf combination medications that contain caffeine (e.g., 250 mg aspirin, 250 mg acetaminophen, and 65 mg caffeine in one preparation, or 325 mg aspirin and 32 mg caffeine in another) are sometimes helpful, but there is an increased risk of overuse in patients who have frequent headaches. At doses of 300 to 500 mg/day (the approximate equivalent of drinking three to five cups of coffee), taken several days per week, caffeine can exacerbate the headache syndrome, causing caffeine rebound and withdrawal headaches. We usually take our patients off all caffeine gradually at the start of their treatment. Too much caffeine also causes insomnia, tachycardia, and jitteriness. Other combination medications contain opiates such as codeine or stronger substances. Often these combinations are tried if migraine-specific medications are ineffective or contraindicated. Care must be taken to avoid overuse with resultant dependency and increase in headache (medication overuse headache or rebound). I rarely prescribe opiates for migraine, but would limit their use to two to four times per month if they were necessary. The main side effects are dependency and sleepiness, with decreased ability to function due to drowsiness.

An alternative combination analgesic contains isometheptene mucate 65 mg, acetaminophen 325 mg, and dichloralphenazone 100 mg (Midrin®). It was taken off the market in 2007. Isometheptene mucate is a sympathomimetic amine that constricts blood vessels and also may work centrally. Dichloralphenazone is a mild tranquilizer and chemically related to a sleeping medication. Metamizol, an analgesic (not approved by the FDA but used in several countries outside the United States), can also be combined with isometheptene and caffeine, thereby replacing dichloralphenazone, which makes certain patients very sleepy. Such combinations are most helpful in treating episodic tension-type headache and could help in mild migraine when taken early in the attack. Isometheptene combination agents are good medications given off label for children and can be tried before going to stronger medications. The adult dosage is two capsules at the onset of mild migraine and another one or two capsules in 1 hour if the headache is not substantially improved (totaling four capsules per 24 hours). Combination agents with isometheptene, or any others, should not be used more than 2 days per week. Although isometheptene combination agents are well tolerated, dizziness, drowsiness, and gastrointestinal symptoms have been reported. Importantly, isometheptene-containing medications cannot be used when a patient is on a monoamine oxidase inhibitor (MAOI) or has stopped one within the last 2 weeks. Also remember that isometheptene combinations in the United States contain acetaminophen, so other preparations containing acetaminophen should be avoided.

Another analgesic, tramadol, is found as a combination of this centrally acting opioid-like analgesic with serotonin and norepinephrine reuptake blocking properties and acetaminophen (Ultracet®) and may help when used sparingly. It should not be used on a regular basis as it can cause medication overuse headache or rebound.

Nonsteroidal Anti-inflammatory Agents

Nonsteroidal anti-inflammatory agents (NSAIDs) have been proven clinically effective for acute treatment of migraine. They appear to work peripherally by blocking prostaglandins. Some are long-acting, such as naproxen sodium with a half life of 12 to 16 hours. Most NSAIDs are well tolerated, but they can cause dyspepsia and gastrointestinal bleeding in sensitive patients or when used too frequently. When we keep patients on them over a period of time we prescribe a proton pump inhibitor. This is especially true with indomethacin. Lack of response to one agent does not preclude response to another. Clinical evidence has shown that diclofenac (50 to 100 mg), flurbiprofen (100 to 300 mg), ibuprofen (200 to 800 mg), naproxen sodium (550 to 1,100 mg), piroxicam SL (40 mg), and tolfenamic acid (200 to 400 mg) are effective in migraine treatment. Ketorolac 30 mg given intravenously or 60 mg given intramuscularly can be very effective in an office or emergency department situation. Diclofenac sodium given intramuscularly also was reported to be clinically useful in migraine. Most of the other NSAIDs have been shown empirically to work on certain patients with migraine.

Indomethacin, which works especially well in several specific headache syndromes (e.g. chronic paroxysmal hemicrania, episodic paroxysmal hemicrania, exertional headache, and hemicrania continua), can be given by mouth or compounded by a pharmacy into a 50-mg rectal suppository, which can also be very helpful in the acute care of migraine.

Rofecoxib, celecoxib, and valdecoxib, the COX-2-inhibiting (COX-1-sparing) NSAIDs, are also options. There is some evidence that they are less toxic to the gastrointestinal tract, but that is controversial. Despite studies showing that rofecoxib 25 mg is less effective than a triptan, other studies show that a combination of both can be used to reduce recurrence and enhance effectiveness, achieving a better sustained response. Rofecoxib and valdecoxib have been removed from the market as long-term use in older individuals seems to cause an increase in cardiac deaths, leaving only celecoxib on the market. Recently Arcoxia, another COX-2 inhibitor, was not approved by the FDA, possibly because studies show it to be no better than the others in the class.

If a patient is taking a triptan and has an incomplete response or a good response but a rapid or frequent recurrence of headache, an NSAID is sometimes given along with a triptan. This strategy has been studied in double-blind trials and appears to work significantly better than a triptan alone.

Butalbital-Containing Medications

Butalbital is a short-acting barbiturate that has been used for many years in the United States and Canada to treat headache. Its half-life is much shorter than a long-acting NSAID, but it is usually a combination medication composed of three substances. The original preparation, which is still very much in use, is composed of 325 mg aspirin, 40 mg caffeine, and 50 mg butalbital (Fiorinal®).

Another form of the medication substitutes acetaminophen for aspirin, and both also are available with codeine, 30 mg. Its main adverse events are either drowsiness or hyperactive state. Although not specifically tested in placebo-controlled, randomized studies in migraine patients, clinical experience clearly supports the efficacy of butalbital-containing compounds for the early treatment of mild migraine, and even more so the milder episodic tension-type headache.

Although the combination of butalbital, caffeine, simple analgesics, and opiates (codeine) may confer additional clinical benefits compared to using the individual components separately, these combination agents may lead to increased risks of sedation, dependency, and toxicities from aspirin, acetaminophen, and caffeine. Of greatest concern is the tendency to overuse these medications, which often leads to mediction overuse headache or rebound headache, dependency, and great difficulty detoxifying the patient. Patients on birth control pills should not take large amount of barbiturates because they can decrease levels of estrogen and impair the effectiveness of the birth control pill.

Most headache specialists feel these medications should either be banned from the market or used very sparingly and prescribed in small amounts with no refills. A typical dose is one or two tablets stat, which may be repeated in 1 to 4 hours one time. Most headache specialists who prescribe these medications would limit them to 1 or 2 days per week. The common brand names are Fiorinal®, Fioricet®, and Esgic®.

Opiate Analgesics

Opiate analgesics have been used for centuries to control pain. Efficacy studies in migraine are limited, but the results do support a therapeutic role in moderate to severe pain, even when benign. Butorphanol, which is available as an injectable but is most commonly used as a nasal spray in a 1-mg dose, was used more widely a few years ago. However, given the risk of dependency from frequent use, butorphanol should be reserved for occasional rescue therapy when first-line migraine medications fail. It should not be used more than 2 days per week except in special circumstances; care must be taken when prescribing butorphanol as it comes in a multidose vial with up to 14 available doses. Prescriptions should be limited to no more than one vial per month except in unusual circumstances. Patients have to be warned to use the medication only when in bed as it can cause dizziness, sleepiness, and dysphoria. Its benefits include rapid onset of action (15 to 20 minutes), sleep induction, and pain relief. Most headache specialists no longer prescribe it.

Similarly, codeine-containing medication and all other opioids and opiates may be used to reduce the pain of migraine. They are not usually as effective at getting rid of headache as triptans. Opiates or opioids do not usually reduce the disability from migraine as well as triptans do, and they often cause drowsiness and decreased cognitive sharpness. However, opiates maybe useful as rescue medications when used on an occasional basis, especially when other medications have failed.

Other opiate medications used mostly for rescue and in emergency room settings include fentanyl by injection, dermal patch, or transmucosal "lollipop," hydrocodone, hydromorphone, levorphanol, meperidine, methadone, morphine, oxycodone, pentazocine, and propoxyphene. If a patient comes to an emergent care setting and a vasoactive medication has either failed or is contraindicated, then an opiate may be used either alone or in combination with promethazine or other antiemetic. Although meperidine is commonly used, it should be avoided as it may cause a paradoxical reaction due to its metabolite normeperidine. Sometime it can cause a hyperactivity state, and its beneficial effect is inadequate and short in duration.

Some patients claim that no other category of medication works on their migraine, and they deny becoming drowsy or disabled from opiate use. Although this may be true, it also suggests that the patient is tolerant and using too much of the drug or may be drug-seeking. Opiates should not be given to patients who must drive home. Patients should also be advised of the risk of sedation associated with opiate analgesics when working or operating heavy equipment. Use is contraindicated if a patient is taking an MAOI antidepressant (especially the use of meperidine).

A far better choice in an emergent setting is an intravenous treatment as described below rather than an opiate. An oral or parenteral steroid could eventuate in a more complete, although slower, improvement. These intravenous and steroid treatments are off label.

Ergot Alkaloids

Ergotamine Tartrate

Ergotamine tartrate is recognized as a migraine-specific medication as it has pharmacologic actions at the serotonergic receptor, which is involved in the pathophysiology of migraine. It stimulates serotonin 1B and 1D receptors like the triptans, but it also stimulates other receptors, which might cause adverse events like nausea. It has a longer half-life than some of the triptans and causes a lot more long-lasting vasoconstriction. Ergotamine was discovered and first used over 50 years ago and has been available in oral, sublingual, injectable, inhaled, nasal, and rectal preparations. Prior to the availability of the triptans in the early 1990s, it was the only vasoactive medication in widespread use for migraine and cluster headache. Oral ergotamine tartrate is erratically and poorly absorbed, and its bioavailability is less than 5% of the ingested dose. Rectal administration of ergotamine leads to slightly better absorption and better treatment efficacy.

Currently the most commonly used ergotamine tartrate preparations are tablets and suppositories. Selected combination tablets contain 1 mg ergotamine tartrate and 100 mg caffeine. The rectal suppositories contain 2 mg ergotamine tartrate and 100 mg caffeine. Because ergotamine is better absorbed rectally, a smaller dose should be given. It is not uncommon to start with only one quarter of a suppository, which can be repeated in 1 hour if needed. The maximum dose of ergotamine is 4 mg/day, and it should be used only 1 or 2 days per week to prevent ergotamine-induced medication oversue or rebound headache.

The side effect profile of ergotamine tartrate limits its use as a regular acute care migraine treatment. The potential adverse events include exacerbation of nausea or vomiting associated with a migraine attack, abdominal pain, distal paresthesias, and muscle cramps. If used more than two times per week, even in low doses, ergotamine tartrate dependency and medication overuse or rebound headaches may develop. Ergotamine is contraindicated in pregnancy, uncontrolled hypertension, coronary artery disease, peripheral vascular disease including venous stasis, sepsis, and liver and kidney disease. It should not be given to a patient on erythromycin or other macrolide antibiotics (which decrease metabolism and raise blood levels). Today in the United States there are few patients who are started on ergotamine tartrate preparations for migraine treatment unless they have failed to respond to triptans. The triptans work more quickly and completely and also can reduce nausea instead of exacerbating it. Ergotamine tartrate is still used extensively in certain countries in South and Central America.

Dihydroergotamine

Dihydroergotamine (DHE) is a hydrogenated ergot preparation that has been available since the early 1940s. Although it is considered a weaker arterial constrictor and a stronger venoconstrictor than ergotamine tartrate, it carries the same contraindications (should not be used in pregnancy, uncontrolled hypertension, coronary artery disease, peripheral vascular disease, sepsis, and liver and kidney disease, or in conjunction with erythromycin or other macrolide antibiotics). DHE has been tested clinically and proven useful when administered intravenously, intramuscularly, subcutaneously, and intranasally for acute treatment of migraine. Pretreatment with an antinausea medication such as metoclopramide, promethazine, prochlorperazine, or ondansetron is not usually needed unless it is given intravenously. Because DHE is most effective by parenteral administration, it is less convenient than an oral triptan, but it is often quite effective. Although there is no published scientific evidence, it appears clinically to work well into the migraine attack, even if the patient has developed central sensitization and allodynia. The half-life of DHE is 10 hours, which may contribute to its long-lasting effect and low recurrence rate— although vasoconstriction lasts longer also. There are rare cases of patients becoming pulseless after receiving intravenous DHE and even oral ergotamine tartrate.

The use of DHE for acute treatment of migraine outside the clinic setting is limited to the nasal spray formulation (Migranal), which is administered as a 0.5-mg dose in each nostril, repeated 15 minutes later for a total of four sprays (2 mg total dose). The nasal spray is well tolerated, with some patients developing nasal stuffiness. DHE given by injection in an emergent care or clinic setting is very effective in reducing migraine pain. The starting dose is often 0.25 to 0.5 mg given by slow intravenous push over 5 minutes through a heparin lock, following administration of an antiemetic. Another 0.5 mg can be given in 60 minutes if there are no significant side effects. If the patient is hospitalized for repetitive intravenous DHE, the usual dose is between 0.5 and 1 mg given slowly through a heparin lock every 8 hours over a period of 3 to 5 days. An effective way to use DHE is 1 mg given intramuscularly or subcutaneously with or without an antiemetic such as oral or intramuscular promethazine or prochlorperazine. A 4-mg dose of dexamethasone also can be given orally, intramuscularly, or intra-venously concomitantly, although there is no good evidence in the literature for its effectiveness acutely. It has been shown to be beneficial during detoxification for medication overuse syndromes. Empirically it has been used acutely with good efficacy for years.

Triptans

Triptans are the most highly selective, migraine-specific acute care treatment currently used in the outpatient setting. There are seven triptans available by tablet. In order of their clinical development and approval by the FDA, the tablets are sumatriptan, zolmitriptan, naratriptan, rizatriptan, almotriptan, frovatriptan, and eletriptan. Different triptans are available in various strengths and formulations, including oral tablets, orally dissolving tablets (ODT), nasal sprays, and subcutaneous injection (Table 11–2). In Europe, sumatriptan is available as a suppository, and some countries do not have all the tablets and melt tablets that are available in the United States. Specific differences among the triptans appear to exist as evidenced by different pharmacokinetic profiles,

Table 11–2 Triptan Medications

Generic	Brand	Formulations	Doses	Maximum Daily Dose
Sumatriptan	Imitrex	Tablets	25 mg, 50 mg, 100 mg	200 mg
		Nasal spray	5 mg, 20 mg	40 mg
		Subcutaneous injection	4 mg, 6 mg	12 mg
Zolmitriptan	Zomig	Tablets	2.5 mg, 5 mg	10 mg
	Zomig-ZMT	Orally disintegrating	2.5 mg, 5 mg	10 mg
	Zomig NS	Nasal spray	5 mg	10 mg
Rizatriptan	Maxalt	Tablets	5 mg, 10 mg	30 mg
	Maxalt- MLT	Orally disintegrating	5 mg, 10 mg	30 mg
Naratriptan	Amerge	Tablets	1 mg, 2.5 mg	5 mg
Almotriptan	Axert	Tablets	12.5 mg	25 mg
Frovatriptan	Frova	Tablets	2.5 mg	7.5 mg
Eletriptan	Relpax	Tablets	20 mg, 40 mg	80 mg

including half-life, T_{max} (time to maximal concentration), C_{max} (maximal concentration after a dose), AUC (the sum of the concentrations over time), metabolism, and drug–drug interaction profiles, among others (Table 11–3). How these differences translate to clinical efficacy and tolerability differences is not well understood. Consequently, clinical distinctions among these agents are subtle and require attention to the specific characteristics of the patient as well as the individual features of the drug and its tolerability profile. In certain patients, such as those with nausea and vomiting, delivery systems and route of administration may be more critical than which triptan is used.

The delivery system plays an important role in the onset of action of triptans. Subcutaneous delivery of sumatriptan offers the most rapid and complete pain relief of the triptans, beginning as early as 10 to 15 minutes and with a high percentage of attacks improved by 2 hours; however, it also is associated with a higher incidence of adverse events and a high recurrence rate. The second most rapid onset of action of the triptans is achieved through nasal spray deliveries of sumatriptan and zolmitriptan nasal spray. Sumatriptan nasal spray has been shown to begin to work in 15 minutes in three of five double-blind, placebo-controlled studies, but many patients do not like the taste. Zolmitriptan nasal spray has been shown to work in 10 minutes in one study and 15 minutes in another. Two recent multicenter studies using zolmitriptan nasal spray for treatment of cluster headache show statistical efficacy beginning as early as 10 minutes versus placebo when a 10-mg dose is used (higher than the 5 mg approved for migraine). All seven of the triptans are available as conventional tablets, and two (rizatriptan and zolmitriptan) are also available in an orally disintegrating formulation. These formulations are more convenient to use and can be taken when the patient is nauseated, but they do not work faster than tablets in studies.

Besides delivery options, other clinical distinctions to consider among the triptans are pharmacokinetic differences, the duration of action, the percentage of patient attacks attaining either headache relief or a pain-free state at 2 hours, and frequency of headache recurrence or persistence (Table 11–4). Sumatriptan has been available for the longest time (since 1993 as an injection in the United States) and has been given successfully to the largest number of patients when all three forms are considered. Zolmitriptan is the only triptan proven effective when repeated for a persistent headache, and the nasal spray seems to be rapidly effective, with a long-lasting effect and well tolerated. Naratriptan has a slower onset of action but a longer half-life and possibly a longer duration of action, which may help address the clinical challenges of treating migraine associated with menses, or migraine in patients who have a history of long-duration attacks. Rizatriptan has the highest 2-hour pain-free rates and the fastest response rate for an oral tablet. Almotriptan has a slightly better side effect profile than sumatriptan, with fewer side effects of chest pain, with the same efficacy in a head to head study. Frovatriptan is a slower-acting triptan with the longest half-life (26 hours) in the class and may also be especially useful in menstrual migraine and other long-lasting headaches (the company that markets frovatriptan has recently

Table 11–3 Pharmacokinetics of the Triptans

Drug	t_{max} (h)[a]	Lipophilicity	$t_{1/2}$ (h)[a]	Bioavailability(%)[a]	Elimination route/metabolism
Sumatriptan		Low			Hepatic (MAO-A); renal (60% excreted unchanged)
50mg tablet	2.5		2	14	
20mg nasal spray	1		2	17	
6mg subcutaneous injection	0.166–0.2		2	97	
25mg suppository	2.5		2	Not published	
Zolmitriptan		Moderate			Hepatic (one active and two inactive metabolites; CYP/MAO-A)
2.5mg tablet	2		3	40–48	
5mg tablet	2		2.71	40–48	
2.5mg orally disintegrating tablet	3.3		2.5–3.0	40–48	
5mg nasal spray	4		2.82	42	
Rizatriptan		Moderate			Hepatic (MAO-A); renal (30% excreted unchanged)
10mg tablet	1.2		2	45	
10mg orally disintegrating tablet	1.6–2.5		2	45	
Naratriptan[b]	2.0–3.0	High	5.0–6.3	63 (men), 74 women)	Hepatic (CYP not MAO-A); renal (70% excreted unchanged)
Almotriptan[b]	1.4–3.8	Unknown	3.2–3.7	80	Hepatic (CYP/MAO-A; 15% active N-desmethyl metabolite); renal (26–35% excreted unchanged)
Eletriptan[b]	1.0–2.0	High	3.6–5.5	50	Hepatic (CYP3A4; 15% active N-desmethyl metabolite: not MAO-A)
Frovatriptan[b]	2.0–4.0	Low	26	24–30	Hepatic (CYP); renal (26–35% excreted unchanged)

[a] When a single value is given, it represents the mean.
[b] Available as conventional oral tablets only.
CYP = cytochrome P450; MAO-A = monoamine oxidase. A: t_{max}=time to peak plasma concentration; $t_{1/2}$ = half-life.

Table 11–4 Clinical End-Points for the Triptans From Selected Clinical Trials

Drug	Dose (mg) and route	Therapeutic gain at 2h (%)[ab]	Recurrence rate (%)[a]
Sumatriptan	6; subcutaneous injection	51	34–38
	50; oral	29–36	32
	20; nasal spray	28–55	32–34
	25; suppository	31–43	35
Zolmitriptan	2.5; oral	34	22–37
	5.0; oral	37	32
	2.5; orally disintegrating tablet	41	ND
	5.0; nasal spray	40	26
Naratriptan	2.5; oral	22	17–28
Rizatriptan	10; oral	27–40	30–47
	10; orally disintegrating tablet	19–46	ND
Almotriptan	12.5; oral	26–32	18–29
Eletriptan	40; oral	22–41	19–23
Frovatriptan	2.5; oral	16–19	7–25

[a] When a single value is given, it represents the mean.
[b] Defined as the difference in headache response at 2-hours post-administration between placebo- and drug-treated patients.
ND = no data.

applied to and been turned down by the FDA for a mini-prophylaxis indication for menstrually related migraine). One third of the patients studied who were taking frovatriptan had an early response and remained early responders in subsequent dosing. Eletriptan is the most recent triptan tablet to enter the market and it works rapidly, with a low recurrence rate.

Despite these distinctions, the triptans are more similar than different. However, one cannot predict which triptan will work best for any given patient. If the first triptan tried is not ideal in all clinical respects, a second or third should be tried. The patient should be questioned carefully to determine if the triptan he or she is taking is the right one in terms of rapid onset of action, complete response, lack of recurrence, long time to recurrence, and minimal side effects. If it is not but has been given in the maximum dose at an early time point in the attack for two or three headache attacks, then another triptan should be tried.

Adverse event profiles of triptans may be helpful in determining which triptan is best for a particular patient. Sumatriptan, rizatriptan, and zolmitriptan should not be used with MAOI antidepressants. Rizatriptan requires a dose reduction to 5 mg in patients taking propranolol, but not other beta blockers. Clearance of naratriptan is reduced with concomitant administration of oral contraceptives so it should be avoided in patients on birth control pills or other forms of estrogen, as well as smokers. Eletriptan should not be used with seven contraindicated CYP3A4 inhibitors (ketoconazole, itraconazole, nefazodone, troleandomycin, clarithromycin, ritonavir, and nelfinavir). Zolmitriptan should be avoided if a patient is on birth control pills or other forms of estrogen, and the dose should be decreased if the patient is on cimetidine.

As a class, triptans are all vasoconstrictive agents causing peripheral and central arterial wall narrowing. Each one stimulates serotonin 1B receptors on blood vessels to cause constriction and 1D receptors on peripheral and brain stem nerves to decrease inflammation and prevent central transmission of nerve signals. In vitro studies report that the vasoconstriction associated with coronary arteries is minimal with therapeutic doses. However, as a safety precaution, patients with specific vascular risk factors or on other vasoconstrictive medications should not take triptans. Triptan contraindications include coronary artery disease and risk factors for coronary artery disease that have not been carefully evaluated (e.g., smoking, obesity, family history of early or severe coronary disease, diabetes, lack of exercise, high cholesterol, peripheral vascular or cerebrovascular disease, uncontrolled hypertension, and cardiac conduction pathway disorders). Triptans should be used cautiously in patients with Raynaud's disease. They should not be used in patients with unusual or prolonged auras, basilar migraine, or hemiplegic migraine. Patients who have migraine with aura, as long as there is no weakness, can take a triptan (that includes symptoms of aphasia, numbness, and visual field defects).

If given to patients with migraine who have no contraindications or cardiac risk factors, triptans are very safe drugs. No single triptan has been reported as being any safer than another, even though some (e.g., almotriptan, frovatriptan, and naratriptan) appear to have caused fewer side effects in clinical trials. There is a warning about giving a triptan when a patient is taking a selective serotonin reuptake inhibitor for fear of causing serotonin syndrome, with irritability, increased temperature, and many other symptoms. This is a very rare condition but must be considered. Sumatriptan has a sulfa moiety but does not appear to cause allergic reactions in patients with a "sulfa" allergy.

Corticosteroids

The mechanism of action of steroids in migraine is not clearly understood but may relate to their effect on the perivascular neurogenic inflammation in the meninges, thought to be one of the neuropathologic mechanisms causing the pain of migraine. Although scientific evidence is limited supporting the use of corticosteroids for acute migraine treatment, several headache specialists and headache centers use it as an oral rescue medication when a triptan is not effective in controlling a migraine attack. Use of oral corticosteroids may decrease the chance of recurrence within 24 hours and often for several days more. When corticosteroids work, they gradually decrease both the headache and the associated symptoms. The literature contains a few studies suggesting possible efficacy when steroids are given intravenously as a rescue medication in status migrainosus. Steroids also have been shown to be helpful in treating medication overuse headache. Specifically, studies using dexamethasone (with or without an antiemetic) and hydrocortisone suggest a possible clinical response to treatment.

Physicians should always consider the large number of side effects from long-term use of corticosteroids when choosing this option. Although there is no consensus, it appears clinically that steroid use for 2 days a month or a 1-week burst given every 2 to 3 months is safe in patients who have no risk factors for corticosteroid use, such as diabetics. Steroids may also be among the safest medications to use to terminate a migraine attack in a pregnant woman after the first trimester, although there is no evidence for this in the literature. There are few adverse events from short-term use of high-dose steroids, the most common being inability to sleep, hyperactivity, and unmasking of psychological conditions.

CGRP Antagonists

Olcegepant was studied as an intravenous preparation in a controlled trial and published as an effective CGRP antagonist that effectively treated migraine with few adverse events, no typical triptan adverse events, and no significant vasoconstriction. It has not yet been developed into a more usable form of medication. MK-0974 is an oral tablet that has undergone phase 3 trials in the United States and Europe. A phase 2B dose-range-finding trial suggests that is has similar properties to olcegepant with few triptan adverse events and may have good 24-hour sustained pain-free results. If the phase 3 trials are significantly positive and demonstrate good tolerability and safety, the company that manufactures the drug might apply for FDA approval for this new class of acute migraine treatment in 2009.

Antiemetics

If triptans do not sufficiently relieve nausea, consider oral medications such as 2 or 4 mg ondansetron, 50 mg promethazine, 10 mg prochlorperazine, 50 mg hydroxyzine, 10 mg metoclompramide, and others. Consider also the orally disintegrating form of ondansetron and the injectable or suppository forms of the above medications. Many of these neuroleptics are dopamine antagonists and work well to decrease migraine acutely when given intravenously, as explained in the next paragraph.

HEADACHE IN THE EMERGENCY ROOM

In an emergency department or headache clinic, a patient might be given intravenous medication for a severe, acute headache. If it is a thunderclap headache or the first or worst headache a patient has ever had, or if there are neurologic symptoms or signs, a non-contrast CT scan should be performed urgently to rule out hemorrhage and other incracranial pathology. It may be necessary to follow up with an MRI scan of the head. If the headache is diagnosed as a migraine attack and triptans and ergots have not been taken within 24 hours, then the patient can receive injectable or intranasal DHE or triptans. Other options, especially if vasoactive drugs have already been tried within the preceding 24 hours, are intravenous prochlorperazine, metoclopramide, chlorpromazine, promethaz-ine, diphenhydramine, valproate, magnesium sulfate, ketorolac, and steroids.

PREVENTING REBOUND HEADACHE (MEDICATION OVERUSE HEADACHE)

Migraine is a chronic disease, and for those with frequent, disabling headaches, daily preventive therapies, behavioral medicine techniques, as well as acute care medications taken properly are usually required. Without proper education, these patients are at great risk of overusing acute care medications, and this may lead to rebound syndromes, now termed medication overuse headache. Overuse of medications used to treat acute headaches not only increases the frequency and intensity of headaches, but it also may prevent the usually effective triptans and preventive medications from working. The regular overuse of selected acute care therapies (and even some preventive therapies) may be complicated by analgesic rebound headache and even long-term dependency concerns (e.g., with opiates, barbiturates, benzodiazepines, ergots, triptans, various nasal sprays, and all types of off-the-shelf or prescription simple and combination analgesics). When patients take acute care medication more than 2 days per week, they may need to be tapered off them completely to see if their headaches improve. The same may be true of patients averaging 6 ounces of regular coffee or more per day.

TREATMENT OF EPISODIC TENSION-TYPE HEADACHE

There are no medications properly studied for treating the occasional tension-type headache. Most patients treat these headaches with over-the-counter med-ications containing aspirin, acetaminophen, caffeine, and NSAIDs. Doctors also prescribe the butalbital-containing medications, prescription-strength NSAIDs, and occasionally opiates. Tension-type headaches are usually easy to self-treat unless they are too frequent and lead to medication overuse headache.

TREATMENT OF MIGRAINE IN CHILDREN

Triptans are not approved for use in patients younger than age 18, although double-blind studies show them to be safe in children with migraine. The best initial treatment in children is either a small dose of acetaminophen, or if that is not effective, a small dose of an over-the-counter NSAID. Aspirin should not be given to children to avoid Reye's syndrome.

SUMMARY

Acute pharmacotherapy of migraine should be designed to stop the migraine process completely as quickly and as consistently as possible. You should use stratified care, selecting a triptan in an optimal dose and formulation for your patient from the first visit. If you can make your patient pain-free in 2 hours or less, there is a better chance the patient will achieve sustained pain-free status for 24 hours and have no recurrence or the need for rescue medication or redosing.

Choose your favorite one of the five fast-acting triptans (sumatriptan, zolmitriptan, rizatriptan, almotriptan, or eletriptan), at maximal recommended dose for your desired route of administration. Then instruct the patient to take the full dose within 30 minutes of the start of migraine symptoms. If there is not almost complete relief at 2 hours, that dose should be repeated once more at 2 hours. If that does not work, the choices are usually a steroid (4 mg dexamethasone), an opiate of your choice, a sedative or sleeping pill, or a visit to the emergency department, where parenteral medications including neuroleptics might be appropriate. Some intravenous options are prochlorperazine, metoclopramide, chlorpromazine, promethazine, diphenhydramine, valproate, magnesium sulfate, ketorolac, steroids, as well as others.

If the triptan does not work taken properly for two or three migraine attacks, or if it causes adverse events, switch to a second or even a third triptan. Consider adding a large dose of an NSAID to the triptan to increase effectiveness or decrease recurrence. Do not give sumatriptan, zolmitriptan, or rizatriptan to patients on an MAOI. If the patient is on propranolol (not other beta blockers), cut the dose of rizatriptan in half. If the patient is on macrolide antibiotics, do not use DHE, ergotamine tartrate, or eletriptan. If the patient is on a selective serotonin reuptake inhibitor, use triptans with caution. Theoretically the patient could develop a serotonin syndrome. Most headache specialists have not found problems using these two types of medication together, but they should warn their patients. If the patient is a smoker or on birth control pills, avoid naratriptan. If the patient is on birth control pills or cimetedine, avoid zolmitriptan or reduce the dose. Patients on any of these potent CYP3A4 inhibitors should not take eletriptan: ketoconazole, itraconazole, nefazodone, troleandomycin, clarithromycin, ritonavir, and nelfinavir.

Carefully and regularly using a headache calendar to record clinical and medication information will help both the patient and physician to accurately track headaches, triggers, menstrual patterns, and medication usage. The regular assessment of disability and the impact of migraine on daily life (using such disability tools as MIDAS or HIT-6) will help document the severity of the disability and track the response to the patient's treatment plan. Using a headache calendar over the long term will also help identify improvement in illness severity parameters and regression of the patient's headaches.

Review Questions

1. A 37-year-old male construction worker noticed the gradual onset of mild headache in both temples once per week, in the afternoon. It was

steady, holocephalic, and not associated with nausea, vomiting, photophobia, or phonophobia. He had no history of migraine. His examination, lumbar puncture, and MRI were normal. Which medication should he take for a headache?

a. Frovatriptan 2.5 mg
b. DHE nasal spray 2.5 mg, 4 sprays
c. Rizatriptan 10 mg
d. Dexamethasone 12 mg
e. Naproxen sodium OTC 220 mg

2. A 46-year-old woman with frequent attacks of migraine without aura was on methysergide intermittently for 10 years. When it became unavailable, her doctor switched her to methylergonovine 0.2 mg tid. Which of the following medications can she take for an acute migraine attack?

a. Zolmitriptan 5 mg
b. Frovatriptan 2.5 mg
c. Dexamethasone 4 mg
d. Almotriptan 12.5 mg
e. Ergotamine tartrate 1 mg

3. A 50-year-old woman has migraine without aura and is on a 10-day course of ampicillin. Which, if any, of the following triptans are contraindicated?

a. Sumatriptan
b. Naratriptan
c. Almotriptan
d. Eletriptan
e. None of the above

4. A 35-year-old male engineer is on a 10-day course of erythromycin for a minor illness. He develops a severe migraine and goes to his physician. Which acute care medication, if any, is contraindicated?

a. Dihydroergotamine 1 mg IM
b. Zolmitriptan 5 mg
c. Rizatriptan 10 mg
d. Frovatriptan 2.5 mg
e. None of the above

5. A 41-year-old woman with 4 days per week of migraine without aura and tension-type headache takes four tablets of aspirin 325 mg per day, 4 days per week. Her headaches are increasing in frequency, without much nausea or photophobia. Which treatment modality is appropriate?

a. Oxycodone 10 mg 4 times per week
b. Decrease and stop her aspirin
c. Ondansetron 2 mg 4 times per week
d. Almotriptan 12.5 mg 4 times per week
e. Frovatriptan 2.5 mg bid for 6 days as mini-prophylaxis

6. A 6-year-old boy has four severe headaches per year followed by vomiting and he then falls asleep for an hour. What treatment should be tried first?
   a. Ibuprofen 200 mg
   b. Aspirin 1,000 mg
   c. Ergotamine tartrate 1 mg with caffeine 100 mg
   d. Oxycodone 5 mg
   e. Sumatriptan 100 mg

7. A 43-year-old male computer programmer with migraine without aura has a thunderclap headache. What should he receive first in the emergency department?
   a. Dexamethasone 12 mg IV
   b. Sumatriptan 6 mg by SC injection
   c. Morphine 10 mg IV
   d. Emergency CT scan without contrast
   e. MRI scan with gadolinium and MRV

8. A 29-year-old female high school teacher with migraine without aura is given DHE nasal spray for migraine and gets no relief and goes to the emergency department. Which medicine should be given for rescue?
   a. Demerol 75 mg IM plus phenergan 50 mg IM
   b. Sumatriptan 6 mg SC injection
   c. Ergotamine tartrate 1 mg plus caffeine 100 mg
   d. Zolmitriptan 5 mg nasal spray
   e. Eletriptan 40 mg

9. A 20-year-old female college student has migraine with aura and occasional episodes of hemiplegia on the right side. During one of these severe episodes she comes to the emergency department. Which treatment should she get?
   a. Sumatriptan 25 mg
   b. Prochlorperazine 10 mg IV
   c. Frovatriptan 2.5 mg
   d. DHE 1 mg IV
   e. Almotriptan 12.5 mg

10. A 35-year-old male bartender who has both migraine with and without aura develops severe numbness on the right side with some dysphasia. Which, if any, of these treatments, is contraindicated?
    a. DHE 1 mg IV
    b. Zolmitriptan 5 mg nasal spray
    c. Sumatriptan 6 mg SC injection
    d. All of the above
    e. None of the above

1. e
2. c
3. e
4. a
5. b
6. a
7. d
8. a
9. b
10. e

SUGGESTED READING

Altura, B.M., & Altura, B.T. Magnesium and vascular tone and reactivity. *Blood Vessels* 15 (1978): 5–16.

Cady, R.K. Treatment strategies for migraine headache. *JAMA* 285 (2001): 1014–1015.

Goadsby, P.J., Lipton, R.B., & Ferrari, M.D. Migraine—Current understanding and treatment. *New England Journal of Medicine* 346 (2002): 257–270.

Hawkey, C.J. COX-2 inhibitors. *Lancet* 353 (1999): 307–314.

Klapper, J., & Stanton, J. The emergency treatment of acute migraine headache; a comparison of intravenous dihydroergotamine, dexamethasone, and placebo. *Cephalalgia* 11, suppl. 11 (1991): 159–160.

Krymchantowski, A.V., & Barbosa, J.S. Rizatriptan combined with rofecoxib vs. rizatriptan for the acute treatment of migraine: An open-label pilot study. *Cephalalgia* 22, no. 4 (2002): 309–312.

Kuzybski, W. Metamizole and hydrocortisone for the interruption of a migraine attack—preliminary study. *Headache Quarterly* 3, no. 3 (1992): 326–328.

Longmore, J., Razzaque, Z., Shaw, D., et al. Comparison of the vasoconstrictor effects of rizatriptan and sumatriptan in human isolated cranial arteries: Immunohistological demonstration of the involvement of 5-HT1B-receptors. *British Journal of Clinical Pharmacology* 46, no. 6 (1998): 577–582.

Matchar, D.B., Young, W.B., Rosenberg, J.H., Peitrzak, M.P., Silberstein, S.D., Lipton, R.B., Mathew, N.T., Kailasam, J., & Fischer, A. Early intervention using rofecoxib alone, rizatriptan alone and combination of rizatriptan and rofecoxib in acute migraine. (Abstract presented at the 10th Congress of the International Headache Society). *Cephalalgia* 21 (2001): 405–432.

Peatfield, R. Drugs acting by modification of serotonin function. *Headache* 26 (1986): 129–131.

Ramadan, N.M. Evidence-based guidelines for migraine headache in the primary care setting: Pharmacological management of acute attacks. Available at: www.neurology.org, April 2000.

Ramadan, N.M., Silberstein, S.D., Freitag, F.G., Gilbert, T.T., & Frishberg, B.M. Evidence-based guidelines for migraine headache in the primary care setting: Pharmacological management for prevention of migraine. Available at: www.neurology.org, April 2000.

Rapoport, A.M., Sheftell, F.D., & Purdy, A. *Advanced therapy of headache.* Hamilton: BC Decker Inc., 2002.

Rapoport, A.M., & Tepper, S.J. Triptans are all different. *Archives of Neurology* 58 (2001): 1479–1480.

Rapoport, A.M., Tepper, S.J., Bigal, M.E., & Sheftell, F.D. The triptan formulations: How to match patients and products. *CNS Drugs* 17, no. 6 (2003): 431–447.

Welch, K.M., & Ramadan, N.M. Mitochondria, magnesium and migraine. *Journal of Neurologic Science* 134 (1995): 9–14.

12

Preventive Pharmacologic Treatment of Migraine and Tension-Type Headache

Stewart J. Tepper, MD

Daily migraine-prevention medication should be prescribed when migraine frequency and disability are high. Medications should be selected based on comorbidity to treat multiple disorders at the same time, using the highest level of evidence possible. Treatment is initiated at a low dose, with gradual escalation to the effective dose range, and maintained for at least 2 to 3 months, with headache calendars maintained to evaluate outcomes. Headache treatment fails when medication overuse headache or chronic daily headache is present, the wrong drug is selected, too high an initial dose is used, too low a final dose is maintained, too short a duration of treatment is completed, or the patient or doctor has unrealistic expectations. The highest level of evidence for preventive medications in migraine exists for amitriptyline, propranolol, timolol, valproate, and topiramate. Few randomized controlled trials (RCTs) have been performed on frequent or chronic tension-type headache, with the best evidence for amitriptyline.

MIGRAINE

Pathophysiology and Mechanisms of Action for Preventive Medications in Migraine

The genesis of migraine remains controversial. Migraine is most frequently an inherited disorder of neuronal hyperexcitability, and the initiation of an attack is linked to neuronal activation. Debate exists as to whether the onset of migraine is the same for both migraine with aura and without aura, or different for each. The question is whether the start of all migraine is due to cortical spreading depression (CSD), or whether CSD occurs just in those with aura, while those without aura have the onset of migraine in a central brain stem generator in the midbrain or pons region.

The "depression" term in CSD is a misnomer, as the events of CSD are actually characterized by an *activation* of neurons and glia with associated hyperemia suggesting spreading activation, and the events can be started by trauma, embolus, or electrical or chemical (e.g., potassium ion) stimulation. Following initial activation there is a wave of decreased brain activity, the actual depression, with oligemia. "Cortical" is not fully accurate, as the waves of activation and depression can occur not only in cortex but also in the cerebellum and hippocampus. Cortical spreading depression is the basis for human aura, but as noted above its relationship to the beginning of migraine without aura is controversial. Cortical spreading depression opens the blood–brain barrier through activation of brain matrix metalloproteinases (MMP), such as MMP-9, and this alteration of the blood–brain barrier may be necessary for access to the brain central compartments for preventive medications.

Cortical spreading depression is associated with increased transmission at excitatory cortical glutamatergic synapses, and this increased glutamatergic tone is best exemplified by the three forms of familial hemiplegic migraine (FHM), which also shed light on preventive medication mechanisms.

FHM3 mutations occur on chromosome 2q24 in the SCN1A gene. SCN1A codes for channels necessary for propagation of action potentials along axons, the neuronal voltage-gated sodium (Na) channels located on axonal membranes. *Gain of function* occurs when FHM3 mutations lead to faster recovery of the Na channels after axonal depolarization. This allows an increase in action potentials propagated per unit time, thereby releasing more glutamate into synapses.

FHM1 mutations are on chromosome 19p13 in the CACNA1A gene. CACNA1A codes for the alpha-1A subunit of the cav2.1 P/Q calcium channel located on presynaptic neuronal membranes. Action potentials provoke calcium influx at presynaptic membranes, and this triggers synaptic vesicle fusion and glutamate release into the synapse via these P/Q calcium channels. FHM1 mutation *gain of function* leads to more presynaptic calcium transport at glutamatergic synapses and increased glutamate release. This elevated glutamate release lowers thresholds for CSD with faster propagation of CSD, all of the results excitatory.

FHM2 mutations are on chromosome 1q21 in the ATP1A2 gene. ATP1A2 codes for the alpha-2 subunit of the sodium/potassium (Na/K) ATPase pump located on astrocyte membranes. This pump helps to maintain ionic gradient across astrocytic plasma membranes and provides energy for passive astrocyte membrane transporters. After glutamate is released into the synapse from neuronal presynaptic membranes, the glutamate transporter EAAT1 or GLAST, a passive transporter, removes the excess glutamate. In FHM2, a *loss of function* of the Na/K ATPase pump results in the failure of passive astrocyte membrane transporters such as EAAT1/GLAST, and this in turn results in more glutamate becoming available for postsynaptic glutamate receptors. Increased excitatory tone facilitates CSD because glutamate is not removed and continues to stimulate postsynaptic receptors.

Returning to the issue of CSD in migraine without aura, for CSD to occur without aura, it must occur in silent areas of the brain, or at subclinical intensity. In one classic case report, a patient at UCLA was undergoing positron emission tomography (PET) for cognitive testing when she developed a migraine without aura attack. The PET showed unequivocal bilateral CSD, so it is possible that CSD does in fact occur in non-aura migraineurs as an initiating event.

The midbrain/periaqueductal gray/dorsal raphe/locus ceruleus area was first proposed as a unilateral generator for contralateral migraine without aura after the observation that stimulation of this region produces headaches with characteristics of migraine, and that this area showed regional cerebral blood flow (rCBF) increases contralateral to the migraine pain in men with migraine without aura in a PET study.

Following the activation of the central generator (either CSD or brainstem), trigeminovascular efferents initiate meningeal migraine pain mechanisms in the form of neurogenic inflammation, vasodilation, and plasma protein extravasation. These pain mechanisms include release of neuroinflammatory peptides such as substance P, inflammatory cytokines, and calcitonin-gene related peptide (CGRP), the latter of which causes vasodilation, plasma extravasation, and mast cell degranulation with further release of the same chemicals, and repetitive pathology. Neurogenic inflammation and vasodilation, in turn, sensitize trigeminovascular nociceptive sensory afferents that carry pain signals back to the brain stem via the trigeminal ganglion to the trigeminal nucleus caudalis (TNC) in the caudal brain stem. Activation of these peripheral nociceptors is referred to as peripheral sensitization, while activation of the TNC and rostral brain structures is associated with central sensitization.

Migraine can be conceptualized as occurring in three steps: central generator activation, peripheral meningeal pain mechanisms, and central integration. Mechanisms of action of preventive medications in migraine include inhibition of CSD through blocking Na and Ca channels, inhibition of MMPs, and inhibition of CSD through blocking gap junctions used in conveying the CSD signals themselves. Dr. Michael Welch has pointed out that most migraine preventive agents lower central neuronal excitatory tone. Thus, in addition to inhibiting CSD, other preventive medications work by reducing the likelihood or magnitude of central generator firing, which may be the same thing as inhibiting CSD if the generator is always CSD, or may be brainstem inhibition in migraine without aura.

No medications have been designed specifically for migraine prevention since the synthesis of methysergide. Thus, preventive medications have been found by serendipity, and their preventive mechanisms have been investigated only after the empiric discovery of limited efficacy common to them all. Different preventive medications also likely have multiple mechanisms of action in prophylaxis of migraine.

Mechanisms of Action of Specific Classes of Medication

Tricyclic Antidepressants

Tricyclic antidepressants (TCAs) vary by type and class but all inhibit, to a lesser or greater extent, norepinephrine (Nor) and serotonin (5-HT) high-affinity uptake. Tricyclic antidepressants downregulate beta-adrenergic receptors and reduce excitatory tone. Whether these actions are the actual mechanisms preventing migraine is uncertain, because in migraine excitatory influences mediated by 5-HT2 receptors may be in excess of inhibitory influences mediated by 5-HT1 receptors. Some TCAs, such as amitriptyline, do block 5-HT2 receptors or downregulate 5-HT2 receptor binding over time, and blocking 5-HT2, in addition to being inhibitory, may also prevent the initiation of arachidonic acid metabolism at the onset of a migraine attack, preventing neurogenic inflammation.

Tricyclic antidepressants also upregulate gamma-amino butyric acid (GABA)-B receptors. GABA, a major inhibitory neurotransmitter, increases inhibitory tone in the excitatory migrainous state and can thus reduce neuronal firing.

Finally, TCAs inhibit neuronal reuptake of adenosine, resulting in agonist effect at adenosine A1 receptors, which appears to work against pain mechanisms.

Beta-Blockers

Beta-blockers decrease adrenergic tone and may thereby reduce excitatory central tone in the hyperexcitable state of migraine via a variety of mechanisms. Blockade of presynaptic noradrenergic receptors and, as a result, decrease in Nor release, blockade of tyrosine hydroxylase with resultant reduced Nor synthesis, inhibition of central beta-adrenergic receptors, and decreased firing of the adrenergic locus ceruleus all contribute to decreased excitatory tone. Returning to blockade of CSD, beta-blockers may prevent CSD by blocking both kainate and N-methyl-D-aspartic acid (NMDA) glutamate receptors.

Calcium Channel Blockers

As described above, the mutation of FHM1 is a calcium (Ca) channelopathy, resulting in a gain of function, and increased glutamate availability, leading to increased CSD. The inevitable next step is to try calcium channel blockers (CCBs) for migraine. There is indirect evidence for Ca channelopathies in other more common forms of migraine, with descriptions of jitter on single-fiber electromyography (EMG) and subclinical cerebellar dysmetria in migraineurs, both suggesting dysfunctional Ca channels. Thus, the blocking of Ca influx and reduction of glutamate release would be the probable modes of action for CCBs for those migraineurs with inherited Ca channelopathies, which appear to be more frequent in those with aura. Finally, CCBs inhibit 5-HT release, which may alter central migraine tone.

Angiotensin-Converting Enzyme Inhibitors and Angiotensin Receptor Blockers

There are two small, positive RCTs for lisinopril and candesartan in the prevention of migraine. Tronvik and colleagues point out that angiotensin II modulates both potassium channels and Ca activity in cells and increases the level of the main 5-HT metabolite, 5- hydroxyindoleacetic acid (5HIAA). The actual sequence whereby this would prevent migraine is not worked out at this time.

Anti-epilepsy Drugs

Three anti-epilepsy drugs (AEDs) have RCT data proving effectiveness in preventing migraine, but their mechanisms of action differ (valproate, topiramate, gabapentin).

Valproate increases brain GABA and is an inhibitory AED. Valproate enhances GABA synthesis, inhibits GABA degradation, and increases responsiveness to GABA by hyperpolarizing postsynaptic membranes through increased potassium conductance. Thus, by increasing GABAergic tone, it has an overall inhibitory *central* effect. The GABAergic central effects may also modulate 5-HT, as valproate helps suppress the rostral brain stem generator or modulator. Valproate inhibits NMDA depolarization and thus also reduces glutamate responses, suppressing CSD.

Valproate also decreases *peripheral* meningeal neurogenic inflammation via GABA-A receptors and directly attenuates nociceptive neurotransmission. Therefore, valproate's multiple preventive mechanisms include both central and peripheral inhibition.

Topiramate, a derivative of the naturally occurring monosaccharide D-fructose, also has multiple actions, all of which appear to be inhibitory and help prevent migraine. Topiramate blocks both voltage-gated Na and Ca channels, enhances GABAergic inhibitory activity through GABA-A receptors similar to valproate, and inhibits excitatory glutamatergic receptors such as α-amino-3-hydroxy-5-methylisoxazole-4-propionic acid (AMPA)/kainate receptors. Each of these mechanisms can reduce CSD.

In the medulla and spinal cord, topiramate inhibits central activation of the TNC and cervical cord. Finally, topiramate is a carbonic anhydrase inhibitor, although the significance of this action for antimigraine effect has not been explained.

Gabapentin blocks voltage-gated Ca but not Na channels. Gabapentin, as with valproate, raises brain GABA concentrations and probably increases GABA synthesis. Gabapentin increases 5-HT concentrations in human whole blood, which may have inhibitory effects on migraine. Finally, gabapentin may inhibit glutamate synthesis. Once again, the overall impact of gabapentin appears inhibitory.

Anti-serotonin Drugs

Anti-serotonin medications include the ergots methysergide and methylergonovine, as well as cyproheptadine and pizotifen. All of these medications

block 5-HT-2B and -2C excitatory receptors, implicated in migrainous vasodilation via CGRP/nitric oxide mechanism. The ergots also have agonist effects
at 5-HT1B and 1D receptors, which antagonize migraine via presynaptic inhibition of the release of neuroinflammatory peptides, postsynaptic vasoconstriction, and inhibition of the transduction of peripheral nociceptive signals
to the brainstem. The ergots have mixed agonist/antagonist effects at 5-HT2
receptors and thus may depend on other mechanisms of action for benefit,
while cyproheptadine and pizotifen are more pure 5-HT2 blockers. However,
simply blocking 5-HT2 is not sufficient for antimigraine effects, as buspirone
and ketanserin, both 5-HT2 blockers, failed as preventive agents.

Herb, Minerals, Vitamins, and Supplements

Magnesium blocks NMDA glutamate receptors, and low magnesium levels are
associated with increased NMDA glutamate activation and CSD. Magnesium
supplementation and intravenous acute administration has been found to be
helpful in patients with low brain ionized magnesium and in migraine with aura.

Mitochondriopathy is implicated in some forms of migraine, as a low
phosphorylation ratio of ADP/ATP has been reported in migraine brain.
Flavinoids are a cofactor in the Krebs cycle, and **riboflavin** is a precursor for
flavin mononucleotides in the electron transport chain in mitochondria.
Coenzyme Q10 is not a cofactor, but it transfers electrons in the electron transport chain in mitochondrial function. Both supplements have been reported to
prevent migraine in RCTs, and the proposed mechanism of action is a suggested treatment of mitochondriopathy.

An extract of the butterbur root, *Petasites hybridus*, has anti-inflammatory
properties and blocks leukotriene synthesis. Leukotrienes are released in
migrainous neurogenic inflammation. Two RCTs have reported efficacy for
petasites in migraine prevention.

Evidence of Effectiveness

The U.S. Headache Consortium published guidelines and technical reports on
preventive medications in 2000. These reports evaluated preventive agents
based on strength of evidence, scientific effect measures, and clinical impression of effect. Also, the medications were placed in groups (Table 12–1).

Since that time, additional RCTs have been published that change the position and evidence on a number of important preventive agents, and these will
be covered below.

Goals and Guidelines for Clinical Use of the Preventive Agents

The U.S. Headache Consortium lists the following goals for preventive treatment:

1. Decrease attack frequency (by 50%), and decrease intensity and duration
2. Improve responsiveness to acute treatment
3. Improve function and decrease disability

Table 12–1 Preventive Therapies for migraine‡‡

Group 1: Medium to high efficacy, good strength of evidence, and a range of severity (mild to moderate) and frequency (infrequent to frequent) of side effects	Group 2: Lower efficacy than those listed in first column, or limited strength of evidence, and mild to moderate side effects	Group 3: Clinically efficacious based on consensus and clinical experiences, but no scientific evidence of efficacy	Group 4: Medium to high efficacy, good strength of evidence, but with side effect concerns	Group 5: Evidence indicating no efficacy over placebo
Amitriptyline Divalproex sodium Lisuride* Propranolol Timolol	Aspirin‡‡, Atenolol, Cyclandelate*, Fenoprofen, Feverfew, Flurbiprofen, Fluoxetine (racemic), Gabapentin, Guanfacine, Indobufen*, Ketoprofen, Lornoxicam*, Magnesium, Mefenamic acid, Metoprolol, Nadolol, Naproxen, Naproxen sodium, Nimodipine, Tolfenamic acid*, Verapamil, Vitamin B2	**a. mild-to-moderate side effects** Bupropion, Cyproheptadine, Diltiazem, Doxepin, Fluvoxamine, Ibuprofen, Imipramine, Mirazepine, Nortriptyline, Paroxetine, Protriptyline, Sertraline, Tiagabine, Topiramate, Trazodone, Venlafaxine **b. side effect concerns** Methylergonovine (methylergometrine) Phenelzine	Methysergide Flunarizine* Pizotifen* TR-DHE*	Acebutolol, Alprenolol*, Carbamazepine, Clomipramine, Clonazepam, Clonidine DEK*, Femoxetine*, Flumedroxone* Indomethacin, Iprazochrome*, Lamotrigine, Mianserin*, Nabumetone, Nicardipine, Nifedipine, Oxprenolol*, Oxtirptan*, Pindolol, Tropisetron*, Vigabatrin*

‡‡Does not include combination products.
* Currently not available in the US.

4. Intervene to prevent transformation into chronic daily headache, medication overuse headache, or rebound headache

The guidelines consider the following circumstances as warranting daily preventive medications:

1. Recurring migraine that significantly interferes with the patient's daily routine despite acute treatment (e.g., two or more attacks a month that produce disability that lasts at least 3 days or headache attacks that are infrequent but produce profound disability)
2. Failure of, contraindication to, or troublesome side effects from acute medications
3. Overuse of acute medications
4. Special circumstances, such as hemiplegic migraine or attacks with a risk of permanent neurologic injury
5. Very frequent headaches (more than two a week), or a pattern of increasing attacks over time, with the risk of developing medication overuse headache or rebound with acute attack medicines
6. Patient preference (i.e., the desire to have as few acute attacks as possible)

Daily preventive medication should be selected when the circumstances fit those listed by the U.S. Headache Consortium, but several more comments are in order. First, the decision to use prevention is most often based on a balance of patient headache frequency and disability. Thus, the higher the frequency of headache, the greater the need for daily prevention, and the higher the disability from the migraines, the greater the need for daily prevention as well. The balance occurs when frequency is low but disability is high, and then prevention may be indicated even with very few headache days per month.

Overall, the decision based on frequency is linked to the fact that increased frequency of headache days and increased frequency of acute medication treatment days increase the risk of transformation of episodic migraine into chronic daily headache or medication overuse headache. When to intervene is controversial.

The American Migraine Prevalence and Prevention (AMPP) study by Lipton and colleagues convened an expert panel who made the following recommendations, which are not validated:

1. Prevention should be offered to migraine subjects reporting either more than 6 headache days per month, more than 4 headache days with at least some impairment, or more than 3 headache days with severe impairment or requiring bed rest.
2. Prevention should be considered in migraineurs with 4 or 5 migraine days per month with normal functioning, 3 migraine days with some impairment, or 2 migraine days with severe impairment.

3. Prevention is not indicated in migraineurs with less than 4 headache days per month and no impairment, or subjects with less than 1 headache day per month regardless of the impairment.

The AMPP group pointed out:

> The criteria applied for "offer" or "consider" preventive treatment are intended as an operational rule for epidemiologic research and not as a clinical management guideline. They were admittedly somewhat arbitrary … We acknowledge that there are patients in the "offer prevention" group who might be well-managed by modifying acute treatment, and there are patients with infrequent severe attacks, perhaps with persistent neurologic deficits, who may be best treated with a preventive.

In other words, migraineurs who have 6 headache days per month, which are in fact three multiple-day attacks, could be given acute migraine-specific medication at optimal dose early in an attack when the pain is mild and achieve sustained pain-free results, reducing the headache days per month to 3 and at the same time lowering disability. Thus, the suggestions by the AMPP group may be too aggressive for clinical decisions on prescribing daily preventive medications.

On the issue of frequency alone, Katsarava and colleagues offer the following guidance. In following patients with episodic migraine over a year, the German group found an odds ratio of 6.2 for developing chronic daily headache for patients starting off the year with 6 to 9 headache days per month compared to those with 0 to 4 headache days per month. Patients with 10 to 14 days per month were considered to be in a critical state, with an odds ratio of 20.1 compared to the low-frequency group, for developing chronic daily headache. If acute treatment is yielding sustained pain-free results, thus keeping disability down, one could recommend a discussion of prevention with the use of a headache diary if headache days are more than 5 per month, but one should try very hard to get patients who have more than 9 headache days per month to accept daily prevention, based on this evidence.

Silberstein and colleagues state that for optimal prevention, clinicians should do the following:

1. Start the drug at a low dose.
2. Give each treatment an adequate trial.
3. Avoid interfering, overused, and contraindicated drugs.
4. Re-evaluate therapy.
5. Be sure that women of childbearing potential are aware of any potential risks.
6. Involve patients in their care to maximize compliance.
7. Consider comorbidity and choose medications to treat several coexisting disorders where possible.

8. Choose a drug based on its proven efficacy, the patient's preferences and headache profile, the drug's side effects, and the presence or absence of coexisting or comorbid disease.

To summarize, choose prevention based on comorbid illnesses—that is, choose a medication that can treat at least two problems at the same time (e.g., a beta-blocker to treat migraine, hypertension, and anxiety). Data based on RCTs suggest that responder rates are quite similar at the highest level of evidence, so the choice should be individualized given the patient's specific clinical history.

Finally, two admonitions:

1. All patients who are on daily preventive medication merit migraine-specific acute treatment. Their disability and frequency have mandated the prevention; the disability also predicts the need for specific acute treatment such as triptans. No patient should ever be placed on daily preventive medications without prescriptions for as-needed migraine-specific treatment, preferably triptans in those without vascular contraindications.
2. Preventive daily medications, as well as migraine-specific acute medications, do not work well, if they work at all, if a patient is in rebound (i.e., has transformed into medication overuse headache and chronic daily headache). A common reason for failure of prophylaxis is that a patient is in medication overuse headache, and this is often not recognized without a headache diary. Detoxification is necessary to restore the effectiveness of daily preventive medications.

Supportive Evidence and Dosing for the Preventive Medications

Tricyclic Antidepressants

The best evidence for effectiveness in this class is for amitriptyline, a tertiary amine TCA (Table 12–2). The quality of evidence, according to the U.S. Headache Consortium, is A ("multiple well-designed randomized clinical trials, directly relevant to the recommendation, yielded a consistent pattern of findings"). The scientific effect for amitriptyline was 3+ ("the effect is statistically significant and far exceeds the minimally clinically significant benefit"), and the clinical impression of effect was 3+ ("the medication is very effective: most people get clinically significant improvement"). Amitriptyline is listed in Group 1 ("medium to high efficacy, good strength of evidence, and a range of severity [mild to moderate] and frequency [infrequent to frequent] of side effects"). Amitriptyline is approved by government regulatory bodies as a migraine preventive medication in the United Kingdom and other countries, but not the United States.

One other TCA, nortriptyline, has 3+ clinical effect, but the grade of evidence for nortriptyline, protriptyline (tertiary amines), doxepin (a secondary

Table 12–2 Tricyclic Antidepressants in Migraine Prevention

Medication	Quality of Evidence	Clinical Effectiveness	Optimal Dose/Day
Amitriptyline	A	3+	30–150 mg
Nortriptyline	C	3+	25–100 mg
Doxepin, Imipramine	C	+	30–150 mg
Protriptyline	C	2+	10–40 mg

Ratings from Ramadan et al., 2000.

amine), and imipramine is C ("the U.S. Headache Consortium achieved consensus on the recommendation in the absence of relevant RCTs"). All are listed in Group 3a ("clinically efficacious based on consensus and clinical experience, but no scientific evidence of efficacy"—that is, no RCTs).

TCAs work well in the setting of comorbid depression, anxiety, and neck pain.

The side effects of TCAs begin with "the four horsemen of the apocalypse"—dry mouth, constipation, sedation, and weight gain, the latter from antihistaminic effects. The anticholinergic adverse events include the dry mouth and constipation, along with a risk for tachycardia, blurry vision, and urinary retention. The older the patient, the greater the risk for confusion and other adverse central nervous system (CNS) effects, and TCAs can also lower the seizure threshold.

The combination of anticholinergic and alpha-adrenergic effects can lead to cardiac arrhythmias and orthostatic hypotension, and overdose is often fatal. Other adverse effects include the syndrome of inappropriate ADH secretion (SIADH), and the precipitation of mania in bipolar patients.

Serotonin Reuptake Inhibitors

The efficacy of serotonin reuptake inhibitors (SSRIs) in migraine prevention has been disappointing, and the RCT data are conflicting. The U.S. Headache Consortium listed fluoxetine as Grade B for quality of evidence and 1+ for clinical effectiveness and placed it in Group 2 ("lower efficacy than in Group 1, or limited strength of evidence, and mild to moderate side effects"). Fluoxetine doses ranged from 10 to 80 mg/day. The other SSRIs were rated even lower, and none represents first-line treatment for migraine prevention.

Serotonin Norepinephrine Reuptake Inhibitors

There have been two small, positive RCTs on venlafaxine, a serotonin norepinephrine reuptake inhibitor (SNRI), since the U.S. Headache Consortium guidelines were written. Based on these two studies, venlafaxine would have Grade B scientific evidence and at least a 2+ clinical effect and would be placed in Group 2. Effective dose was 150 mg, and one crossover study suggested effectiveness comparable to amitriptyline. No randomized controlled data exist for duloxetine, the other SNRI available, in migraine prevention.

Monoamine Oxidase Inhibitors

The U.S. Headache Consortium lists phenelzine as having Grade C scientific evidence but 3+ clinical effect. It is in Group 3b ("clinically efficacious based on consensus and clinical experience, but no RCTs, and with side effect concerns"). The consortium notes that monoamine oxidase inhibitors (MAOIs) such as phenelzine require "complex management with special dietary restrictions and have high potential for drug–drug interactions."

MAOIs have common side effects, including diaphoresis, hypotension, weight gain, and sexual dysfunction. They are activating and can cause insomnia. The greatest concern is the risk for hypertensive crisis when combined with dietary tyramine or sympathomimetic drugs.

Beta-Blockers

Propranolol, a nonselective beta-blocker, has Grade A scientific evidence and 3+ clinical effect and is in Group 1 (Table 12–3). It is approved for migraine prevention by the U.S. Food and Drug Administration (FDA) and the U.K. regulatory agencies, as well as in other countries. Dosage range is 120 to 240 mg/day.

Timolol, also nonselective, also has Grade A scientific evidence and Group 1 placement but only 2+ clinical effect. It is indicated for migraine prevention in the United States. Dosage range is 20 to 30 mg/day.

Nadolol, a nonselective beta-blocker, and atenolol and metoprolol, beta-1-selective beta-blockers, have Grade B scientific evidence and are in Group 2. Overall, 43% to 80% of patients treated with beta-blockers have a 50% reduction in migraine frequency after 2 to 3 months on a therapeutic dose (responder rate; Fig. 12–1).

All beta-blockers are best used in patients with comorbid hypertension or anxiety. They are relatively contraindicated in patients with diabetes mellitus, asthma, Raynaud's syndrome, depression, congestive heart failure, and hypotension. They can also cause bradycardia, exercise intolerance, and erectile dysfunction.

Table 12–3 Beta-Blockers in Migraine Prevention

Medication	Scientific Evidence	Clinical Effect	Optimal Dose/Day
Propranolol	A	3+	120–240 mg
Timolol	A	2+	20–30 mg
Atenolol	B	2+	100 mg
Nadolol	B	3+	80–240 mg
Metoprolol	B	3+	200 mg

Ratings from Ramadan et al., 2000.

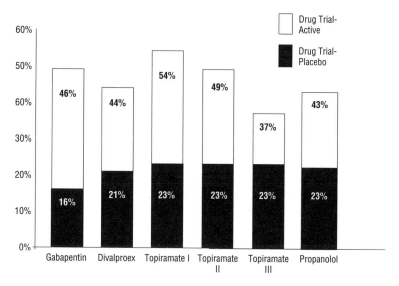

Figure 12–1 50% Responder rates for major preventive drugs in randomized controlled trials.

Calcium Channel Blockers

Flunarazine and verapamil are the two-best studied CCBs in migraine prevention. Flunarazine (not available in the United States) has Grade B scientific evidence, is generally considered to have excellent clinical effectiveness, and is listed in Group 4 ("medium to high efficacy, good strength of evidence, but with side effect concerns, due to the risk of sedation, weight gain, depression, and extrapyramidal signs").

Verapamil has Grade B scientific evidence and 1+ clinical effectiveness and is in Group 2. There are even fewer or no data for all of the other CCBs, although diltiazem has Grade B scientific evidence and is also in Group 2.

As noted in the discussion of mechanisms, because of the discovery of Ca channelopathy in FHM1, and the finding of indirect evidence for Ca channelopathies in other migraine forms, most commonly in migraine with aura, CCBs are frequently used for migraine with aura patients, as well as in the setting of hemiplegic and basilar-type aura.

The adverse events associated with CCBs include constipation, hypotension, and peripheral edema. The drugs can have cardiac effects, including arrhythmia, bradycardia, and atrioventicular block. Flunarazine is also associated with depression, weight gain, and extrapyramidal side effects.

Angiotensin-Converting Enzyme Inhibitors and Angiotensin Receptor Blockers

Since the U.S. Headache Consortium was published, there has been one small positive RCT for lisinopril 20 mg, an angiotensin-converting enzyme inhibitor

(ACE inhibitor) and another for candesartan 16 mg, an angiotensin receptor blocker (ARB).

Anti-epilepsy Drugs

Valproate has Grade A scientific evidence and 3+ clinical effectiveness, is in Group 1, and is approved in its divalproex sodium form by the FDA for prevention of migraine (Table 12–4). Dosage range is 500 to 1,500 mg/day. Overall, 44% of patients obtained at least a 50% reduction in migraine frequency with divalproex (see Fig. 12–1).

The most common adverse events with valproate, in order, are nausea, asthenia, and dyspepsia. Hepatotoxicity is rare but more common in children under 2 years old. This risk increases with co-administration of medications that induce the cytochrome p450 system, such as barbiturates. Other problems in treatment include alopecia, tremor, weight gain, and, rarely, thrombocytopenia and other bone marrow dysfunction, and pancreatitis.

The biggest concern with valproate therapy is its teratogenicity, neural tube defects occurring at a rate of 1% to 2%. In addition, in the Systematic Treatment Enhancement Program for Bipolar Disorder study, polycystic ovarian syndrome occurred in 10.5% of menstruating patients within 1 year. For these reasons, valproate should not be used as a first-line treatment for young, menstruating women, and when used in anyone optimally should be prescribed in monotherapy.

Since the guidelines were published, one large RCT found **gabapentin** effective in migraine prevention (Grade B scientific evidence, 2+ clinical effectiveness, and Group 2). Dosage range was 900 to 2,400 mg/day in divided doses. Forty-six percent of patients achieved at least a 50% reduction in migraine frequency in a modified, completer, intent-to-treat analysis (see Fig. 12–1). Side effects with gabapentin were primarily the two D's, drowsiness and dizziness. Since it is excreted unchanged in the urine, it has no drug–drug interactions.

Also since the guidelines were published, two large regulatory RCTs found **topiramate** effective in migraine prevention (Grade A scientific evidence, 3+ clinical effectiveness, and Group 1). It is approved by the FDA for migraine prevention. Over three RCTs, a mean of 47% of subjects had at least a 50% reduction in migraine frequency at the optimal dose, 100 mg/day (see Fig. 12–1).

Table 12–4 Anti-epilepsy Drugs in Migraine Prevention

Medication	Scientific Evidence	Clinical Effectiveness	Optimal Dose/Day
Valproate	A	3+	500–1,500 mg
Gabapentin	B	2+	900–2,400 mg
Topiramate	A	3+	100 mg

Ratings from Ramadan et al., 2000.

The most common adverse events with topiramate are paresthesias in close to half of patients treated. Fatigue, weight loss, anorexia, and diarrhea can occur. Weight loss occurred in 9% of patients at 100 mg, compared to 1% with placebo, and the mean weight loss in those losing weight over a year was 3%. Of concern are CNS side effects, including aphasia, memory difficulty, and concentration problems. In addition, rare narrow angle-closure glaucoma can occur early in treatment. Hyperchloremic acidosis, usually not clinically significant, can happen in more than 10% of patients. Nephrolithiasis occurs at a rate of 1% as a byproduct of topiramate's carbonic anhydrase inhibition. There is also a rare risk of oligohydrosis, which can result in potentially fatal hyperthermia, more common in younger patients and at higher doses.

There are no RCTs supporting the use of other AEDs in the prevention of migraine. Lamotrigine, ineffective in an RCT for migraine, appeared useful in open-label studies for preventing aura.

Anti-serotonin Drugs

Cyproheptadine (available in the United States) and pizotifen (not available in the United States) are both 5-HT2 antagonists with relatively low clinical effectiveness. The scientific evidence for cyproheptadine is C, for pizotifen A. Cyproheptadine is in Group 3a, pizotifen Group 4 ("medium to high efficacy, good strength of evidence, but with side effect concerns") The dose for cyproheptadine is 4 to 12 mg/day, for pizotifen 1.5 to 6 mg/day. The side effects for both are weight gain and drowsiness.

Methysergide (not available in the United States, but approved by the FDA for migraine prevention) and methyergonovine (methylergometrine) are both ergots. Methysergide, which breaks down to methylergonovine, has 3+ clinical effectiveness. The scientific evidence for methysergide is A, for methylergonovine C. Methysergide is in Group 4, methylergonovine in Group 3b. Doses are up to 6 mg/day for methysergide and up to 0.6 mg/day for methylergonovine. These drugs can produce gastrointestinal side effects of nausea, pain, or diarrhea and occasionally cause drowsiness or leg aches.

The serious side effect of idiosyncratic fibrosis in gut, lung, or heart (including valvular fibrosis and resultant regurgitation and heart failure) can occur in 1/1,500 to 1/5,000 patients after 6 months of steady use of methysergide. Methylergonovine has never been described in the literature as causing fibrotic complications; however, every other ergot used clinically has been associated with fibrotic complications, so absence of evidence for methlyergonovine's potential for fibrosis is not evidence of absence. Indeed, the risk for fibrotic complications may be related to 5-HT2B agonist effects, and methylergonovine is a potent 5-HT2B agonist. Therefore, prudence suggests the use of methylergonovine as methysergide was used, with drug holidays every 6 months based on the hope rather than any evidence that this will prevent fibrotic complications, and regular surveillance of patients who are on the drug chronically with CT scans of the abdomen and lungs, and echocardiography.

Finally, the FDA has contraindicated the simultaneous use of ergots and triptans, so that the use of methylergonovine in prevention precludes the use of triptans for acute therapy.

Herbs, Minerals, Vitamins, and Supplements

Petasites, magnesium, riboflavin, and coenzyme Q10 all have Grade B scientific evidence and 2+ clinical efficacy and are appropriately placed in Group 2. Doses are 150 mg/day of petasites, 400 to 600 mg/day of chelated magnesium, 25 to 400 mg/day of riboflavin, and 300 mg/day of coenzyme Q10. Side effects are burping for petasites, diarrhea for magnesium, and rash for vitamin B2 and coenzyme Q10.

Other Preventive Agents

Aspirin and some NSAIDs such as naproxen and ketoprofen have been studied in migraine prevention. Scientific evidence is Grade B and clinical efficacy 1 to 2+, and all are in Group 2.

Summary of Responder Rates

The responder rate is defined as the proportion of subjects demonstrating at least a 50% reduction in migraine frequency at therapeutic doses for a reasonable therapeutic trial, usually 3 months, in a RCT. There are some small differences in the endpoints in the preventive trials in terms of outcomes, measured as reduction of migraine attacks, days of headaches, or 24-hour "migraine periods," but it is not clear that these methodologic differences prevent some comparison across studies of the responder rates. What is clear is that using this marker, antimigraine drugs with high-level evidence are remarkably similar, with approximately 45% of subjects reporting at least a 50% reduction in their migraines in RCTs (see Fig. 12–1). This underlines the need to select medication with the best evidence based on the comorbidity of the individual patient.

Short-Term Prevention

Menstrual migraine represents a unique opportunity for prevention of migraine, as the patient often has migraine at a fixed time during menses. In patients with predictable migraines, linked to a particular day of flow, short-term prevention can be used rather than daily preventive medication and can reduce the severity and duration of menstrual migraines, sometimes prevent them, and often increase their responsiveness to acute treatment. Figure 12–2 is an algorithm for consideration of short-term prevention.

Very small RCTs described nonspecific treatments in short-term prevention for menstrual migraine: two for magnesium and one for naproxen sodium. All of these studies had patients treat for approximately 14 days, from ovulation to flow for magnesium and from day –7 to +6 of menses for naproxen sodium. All showed modest preventive benefit. Hormonal preventive strategies, treating

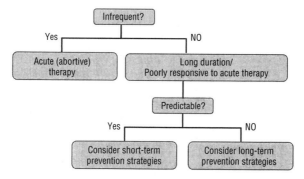

Figure 12–2 Algorithm for short-term prevention. (Tepper, 2006)

with estrogen in various formulations just before menstruation, continue to be used for menstrual migraine prevention. However, in the most definitive and negative of the estrogen short-term prevention RCTs, benefit during treatment was offset by deferred estrogen withdrawal, triggering post-dosing migraine immediately after estrogen gel was stopped.

Triptans have been studied in larger RCTs for menstrual migraine short-term prevention. Sumatriptan administered for 5 days beginning 2 days before the expected first day of menstrual headache was effective in a pioneering open-label study by Newman and associates in 1998. Subsequently, RCTs have been published demonstrating the effectiveness of naratriptan, frovatriptan, and zolmitriptan in short-term prevention. The concept is generally the same, namely beginning a daily scheduled BID dosing of the triptan 2 days before the expected onset of menstrual migraine for a total of 5 or 6 days. No fully peer-reviewed safety extension data have been published on using triptan short-term prevention, but preliminary and favorable data for a year of cycled use from a frovatriptan safety extension trial are available in abstract form. At the time of this writing (July 2007), the FDA is considering an application for the use of frovatriptan in short-term prevention of menstrually related migraine.

Summary of Prevention in Migraine

Daily migraine prevention should be chosen based on the balance of frequency and disability of migraines. Drug selection is predicated on comorbidity (so that multiple disorders can be treated at the same time) and using the highest level of evidence possible. Treatment is initiated at a low dose, working up to an effective dose to be maintained for at least 2 to 3 months, with headache diary monitoring for outcome. Poor outcome is associated with the presence of medication overuse headache/chronic daily headache, picking the wrong drug, an excessive initial dose, an inadequate final dose, too short a duration of treatment, or unrealistic expectations. Also of importance is that prophylaxis is less effective in the setting of medication overuse headache, which requires detoxification. The best evidence for preventive medications exists for amitriptyline, propranolol, timolol, valproate, and topiramate. RCTs for short-term prevention for menstrual migraine exist in limited form for magnesium and naproxen sodium and more extensively for the triptans.

PREVENTION IN TENSION-TYPE HEADACHE

Evidence for prevention in tension-type headache is extremely limited. Many clinicians use tricyclics and SSRIs, but RCTs are small and the results are often equivocal or negative. All trials are for treatment of chronic tension-type headache; sadly, no usable RCTs exist for the prevention of episodic tension-type headache.

Tricyclic Antidepressants

Amitryptiline

Multiple RCTs of amitryptiline have shown mixed results. The first RCT (1964) barely showed statistical significance and preceded ICHD classification diagnostic criteria. Another very early trial (1971) found 25 mg amitriptyline more effective than placebo, but not 150 mg. In a third RCT, 75 mg of a slow-release formulation of amitriptyline was tested on chronic tension-type headache and on headache-associated neurophysiologic parameters (EMG activity, exteroceptive suppression of temporal muscle activity, contingent negative variation, and experimental pain sensitivity). The data showed a statistically relevant reduction of daily headache duration. However, they also showed that amitriptyline only partly alleviated chronic tension-type headaches. In a fourth trial, amitriptyline 50 to 75 mg daily was not significantly more effective in chronic tension-type headache than placebo. In a fifth RCT, amitriptyline did not eliminate chronic tension-type headache but provided a clinically important reduction of headache in the majority of otherwise treatment-resistant patients. In a classic study, Holroyd found that amitriptyline, in combination with nonpharmacologic treatment such as stress management, resulted in significant reduction of headache index scores compared to placebo.

Clomipramine

In one positive RCT, 82 subjects with chronic tension-type headache were treated with placebo, clomipramine, or mianserin in a double-blind parallel group comparison. A decrease in headache for both clomipramine and mianserin was significant compared to placebo.

SSRIs

For citalopram, there are two negative RCTs. For paroxetine, there are two negative RCTs.

For fluoxetine, there is one positive RCT and one negative study. In the positive study, after a 1-month single-blind baseline on placebo, subjects with chronic daily headache (n = 64) were randomly assigned to a 3-month trial of fluoxetine (20 mg) or placebo. The fluoxetine dose was increased to 40 mg in the second month, depending on patient response. For the group of chronic daily headache patients on fluoxetine, overall headache status after 3 months compared to the end of the single-blind placebo baseline improved a mean of 50% versus 11% for those receiving placebo ($P = 0.029$), with 47% versus 23% improving at least 50% ($P = 0.097$, NS). Fluoxetine patients showed significant improvement in monthly mood ratings compared to placebo ($P = 0.001$ by the end of the study) and modest but significant improvement in daily records of headache frequency ($P = 0.019$) but not pain severity.

The negative study was a pediatric study that showed a statistically significant decrease in headache frequency that was independent of the drug. The authors concluded that fluoxetine's efficacy is not higher than that of placebo in the prophylaxis of chronic daily headache in children and adolescents.

In short, despite their clinical use, SSRIs were ineffective in all RCTs in chronic daily headache, which is not necessarily the same precise diagnosis as chronic tension-type headache.

Miscellaneous Agents

Mirtazepine

There is one positive RCT for mirtazepine for chronic tension-type headache. Twenty-four nondepressed patients with chronic tension-type headache took mirtazapine 15 to 30 mg/day or placebo for 8 weeks, separated by a 2-week washout period. Mirtazapine reduced duration × intensity by 34% more than placebo. However, a second study by the same group failed to confirm this finding, and adding ibuprofen to the mirtazapine actually worsened the chronic tension-type headaches.

Gabapentin

There is one positive RCT for gabapentin for chronic daily headache (as noted above, not necessarily chronic tension-type headache). There was a 9.1% difference in headache-free rates favoring gabapentin over placebo ($P = 0.0005$). Benefits for gabapentin were also demonstrated for other secondary endpoints. Gabapentin may represent a therapeutic option for patients with chronic daily headache.

Summary on Prevention of Tension-Type Headache

There is limited positive evidence as to the effectiveness of amitriptyline, and clomipramine has a single positive RCT for chronic tension-type headache, while gabapentin has a single positive RCT for chronic daily headache. Careful review of the SSRI data suggests uniformly negative studies, although some of the RCTs were on nonspecific chronic daily headache and not ICHD-defined chronic tension-type headache.

Review Questions

1. In the history of the United States, what are the five medications approved by the FDA for the prevention of migraine?
   a. Amitriptyline, propranolol, gabapentin, topiramate, verapamil
   b. Propranolol, timolol, divalproex, topiramate, methysergide
   c. Propranolol, nadolol, metoprolol, divalproex, topiramate
   d. Amitiriptyline, propranolol, verapamil, gabapentin, topiramate
2. In what group is nortriptyline listed in the summary table for the U.S. Headache Consortium, and based on how many RCTs?
   a. Group 1, based on two large RCTs
   b. Group 2, based on one large RCT
   c. Group 3, clinically efficacious based on consensus and clinical experience, but no scientific evidence of efficacy—that is, no RCTs
   d. Group 4, not clinically efficacious
3. Name two antiepileptic drugs that affect GABA and glutamate and are proven with randomized controlled trials to prevent migraine.
   a. Divalproex and pregabalin
   b. Gabapentin and pregabalin
   c. Divalproex and topiramate
   d. Topiramate and lamotrigine
4. Name four serotonin-2 antagonists effective in the prevention of migraine.
   a. Buspirone, trazodone, nefazodone, bromocriptine
   b. Buspirone, methysergide, clomipramine, pizotifen
   c. Buspirone, methysergide, ketanserin, pizotifen
   d. Cyproheptadine, methysergide, methylergonovine, pizotifen
5. At a dose of 100 mg, what percentage of topiramate patients had weight loss in the regulatory trials, and what was the mean weight loss at 100 mg over 1 year?
   a. 20%, 10 pounds
   b. 25%, 15 pounds
   c. 9%, 3% body weight
   d. 5%, 25% body weight
6. A diabetic patient who has had a myocardial infarction and has a history of kidney stones wants migraine prevention. Which medication would be optimal?
   a. Amitriptyline
   b. Topiramate
   c. Divalproex
   d. Methylergonovine
7. A young, obese patient with high-frequency headaches desires daily prevention. Which choice is optimal?
   a. Amitriptyline
   b. Topiramate

    c. Divalproex
    d. Propranolol
8. A very anxious patient with no history of depression wants daily prevention for migraine. Name two potential choices that optimally treat both disorders.
    a. Amitriptyline, topiramate
    b. Divalproex, propranolol
    c. Propranolol, venlafaxine
    d. Fluoxetine, venlafaxine
9. A depressed patient with chronic tension-type headache and glaucoma would like prevention. What is the best choice?
    a. Amitriptyline
    b. Clomipramine
    c. Paroxetine
    d. Mirtazepine
10. A healthy young patient has depression, sleep disorder, and both migraine and chronic tension-type headache. What is the best choice?
    a. Amitriptyline
    b. Topiramate
    c. Divalproex
    d. Timolol

10. a
9. d
8. c
7. b
6. c
5. c
4. d
3. c
2. c
1. b

SUGGESTED READING

Ayata, C., Jin, H., Kudo, C., Dalkara, T., & Moskowitz, M.A. Suppression of cortical spreading depression in migraine prophylaxis. *Annals of Neurology* 59 (2006): 652–661.

Bach, F.W., Langemark, M., Ekman, R., Rehfeld, J.F., Schifter, S., & Olesen, J. Effect of sulpiride or paroxetine on cerebrospinal fluid neuropeptide concentrations in patients with chronic tension-type headache. *Neuropeptides* 27 (1994): 129–136.

Bendtsen, L., Buchgreitz, L., Ashina, S., & Jensen R. Combination of low-dose mirtazapine and ibuprofen for prophylaxis of chronic tension-type headache. *European Journal of Neurology* 14 (2007): 187–193.

Bendtsen, L., & Jensen, R. Mirtazapine is effective in the prophylactic treatment of chronic tension-type headache. *Neurology* 62 (2004): 1706–1711.

Bendtsen, L., Jensen, R., & Olesen, J. A non-selective (amitriptyline), but not a selective (citalopram), serotonin reuptake inhibitor is effective in the prophylactic treatment of chronic tension-type headache. *Journal of Neurology, Neurosurgery & Psychiatry* 61 (1996): 285–290.

Bendtsen, L., Jensen, R., & Olesen, J. Amitriptyline, a combined serotonin and noradrenaline re-uptake inhibitor, reduces exteroceptive suppression of temporal muscle activity in patients with chronic tension-type headache. *Electroencephalography Clinics Neurophysiology* 101 (1996): 418–422.

Bendtsen, L., Jensen, R., & Olesen, J. A non-selective (amitriptyline), but not a selective (citalopram), serotonin reuptake inhibitor is effective in the prophylactic treatment of chronic tension-type headache. *Journal of Neurology, Neurosurgery & Psychiatry* 61 (1996): 285–290.

Bigal, M.E., Bordini, C.A., Tepper, S.J., & Speciali, J.G. Intravenous magnesium sulphate in the acute treatment of migraine without aura and migraine with aura. A randomized, double-blind, placebo-controlled study. *Cephalalgia* 22 (2002): 345–353.

Bolay, H., Reuter, U., Dunn, A.K., Huang, Z., Boas, D.A., & Moskowitz, M.A. Intrinsic brain activity triggers trigeminal meningeal afferents in a migraine model. *Nature Medicine* 8 (2002): 136–142.

Brandes, J.L., Saper, J.R., Diamond, M., Couch, J.R., Lewis, D.W., Schmitt, J., Neto, W., Schwabe, S., Jacobs, D., and the MIGR-002 Study Group. Topiramate for migraine prevention: A randomized controlled trial. *JAMA* 291 (2004): 965–973.

Bulut, S., Berilgen, M.S., Baran, A., Tekatas, A., Atmaca, M., & Mungen, B. Venlafaxine versus amitriptyline in the prophylactic treatment of migraine: Randomized, double-blind, crossover study. *Clinical Neurology & Neurosurgery* 107 (2004): 44–48.

Cohen, G.K. Migraine prophylactic drugs work via ion channels. *Medical Hypotheses* 65 (2005): 114–122. Cutrer, F.M., Limmroth, V., & Moskowitz, M.A. Possible mechanisms of valproate in migraine prophylaxis. *Cephalalgia* 17 (1997): 93–100.

Diamond, S., & Bates, B. Chronic tension headache treated with amitriptyline: A double-blind study. *Headache* 11 (1971): 110–116.

Gherpelli, J.L., & Esposito, S.B. A prospective randomized double blind placebo controlled crossover study of fluoxetine efficacy in the prophylaxis of chronic daily headache in children and adolescents. *Arq Neuropsiquiatr* 63 (2005): 559–563.

Gobel, H., Hamouz, V., Hansen, C., Heininger, K., Hirsch, S., Lindner, V., Heuss, D., & Soyka, D. Chronic tension-type headache: Amitriptyline reduces clinical headache-duration and experimental pain sensitivity but does not alter pericranial muscle activity readings. *Pain* 59 (1994): 241–249.

Gursoy-Ozdemir, Y., Chu, J., Matsuoka, N., Bolay, H., Bermpohl, D., Jin, H., Wang, X., Rosenberg, G.A., Lo, E.H., & Moskowitz, M.A. Cortical spreading depression activates and upregulates MMP-9. *Journal of Clinical Investigation* 113 (2004): 1447–1455.

Heninger, G.R., & Charney, D.S. "Mechanism of action of antidepressant treatments: Implications for the etiology and treatment of depressive disorders." In: *Psychopharmacology: the third generation of progress*, ed. H.Y. Meltzer. New York: Raven Press, 1987:535–544.

Holroyd, K.A., O'Donnell, F.J., Stensland, M., Lipchik, G.L., Cordingley, G.E., & Carlson, B.W. Management of chronic tension-type headache with tricyclic antidepressant medication, stress management therapy, and their combination: a randomized controlled trial. *JAMA* 285 (2001): 2208–2215.

Jacquy, J., & Lanaerts, M. Effectiveness of high-dose riboflavin in migraine prophylaxis. *Neurology* 50 (1998): 466–470.

Joffe, H., Cohen, L.S., Suppes, T., McLaughlin, W.L., Lavori, P., Adams, J.M., Hwang, C.H., Hall, J.E., & Sachs, G.S. Valproate is associated with new-onset oligoamenorrhea with hyperandrogenism in women with bipolar disorder. *Biological Psychiatry* 59 (2006): 1078–1086.

Klapper, J. Divalproex sodium in migraine prophylaxis: A dose-controlled study. *Cephalalgia.* 17 (1997): 103–108.

Lance, J.W., & Curran, D.A. Treatment of chronic tension headache. *Lancet* 1 (1964): 1236–1239.

Langemark, M., Loldrup, D., Bech, P., & Olesen, J. Clomipramine and mianserin in the treatment of chronic tension headache. A double-blind, controlled study. *Headache* 30 (1994): 118–121.

Langemark, M., & Olesen, J. Sulpiride and paroxetine in the treatment of chronic tension-type headache. An explanatory double-blind trial. *Headache* 34 (1998): 20–24.

Lipton, R.B., Bigal, M.E., Diamond, M.D., Freitag, F., Reed, M.L., Stewart, W.F., & AMPP Advisory Group. Migraine prevalence, disease burden, and the need for preventive therapy. *Neurology* 68 (2007): 343–349.

Lipton, R.B., Gobel, H., Einhäupl, K.M., Wilks, K., & Mauskop, A. (2004). *Petasites hybridus* root (butterbur) is an effective treatment for migraine. *Neurology* 63 (2004): 2240–2244.

Lipton, R.B., Silberstein, S.D., Saper, J.R., Bigal, M.E., & Goadsby, P.J. Why headache treatment fails. *Neurology* 60 (2003): 1064–1070.

MacGregor, E.A., Frith, A., Ellis, J., Aspinall, L., & Hackshaw, A. Incidence of migraine relative to menstrual cycle phases of rising and falling estrogen. *Neurology* 67 (2006): 2154–2158.

Mathew, N.T., Rapoport, A., Saper, J., Magnus, L., Bernstein, P., Klapper, J., Ramadan, N., Stacey, B., & Tepper, S. Efficacy of gabapentin in migraine prophylaxis. *Headache* 41 (2001): 119–128.

Newman, L.C., Lipton, R.B., Lay, C.L., & Solomon, S. A pilot study of oral sumatriptan as intermittent prophylaxis of menstruation-related migraine. *Neurology* 51 (1998): 307–309.

Ophoff, R.A., Terwindt, G.M., & Vergouwe, M.N. Familial hemiplegic migraine and episodic ataxia type-2 are caused by mutations in the Ca2+ channel gene CACNLA4. *Cell Tissue Research* 87 (1986): 543–552.

Pffafenrath, V., Diener, H.C., Isler, H., Meyer, C., Scholz, E., Taneri, Z., Wessely, P., Zaiser-Kaschel, H., Haase, W., & Fischer, W. Efficacy and tolerability of amitriptylinoxide in the treatment of chronic tension-type headache: A multi-centre controlled study. *Cephalalgia* 14 (1994): 149–155. Pietrobon, D., & Striessnig, J. Neurobiology of migraine. *Nature Reviews Neuroscience* 4 (2003): 386–398.

Ramadan, N.M. Prophylactic migraine therapy: Mechanisms and evidence. *Current Pain Headache Reports* 8 (2004): 91–95.

Ramadan, N.M., Silberstein, S.D., Freitag, F.G., Gilbert, T.T., & Frishberg, B.M. Multispecialty consensus on diagnosis and treatment of headache: Pharmacological management for prevention of migraine. *Neurology* (2000), serial online, at: http://www.aan.com/professionals/practice/pdfs/g10090.pdf

Raskin, N.H., Hosobuchi, Y., & Lamb, S. Headache may arise from perturbation of brain. *Headache* 27 (1987): 416–420.

Roth, B.L. Drugs and valvular heart disease. *New England Journal of Medicine* 356 (2007): 6–9.

Sandor, P.S., DiClemente, L., Coppola, G., Saenger, U., Fumal, A., Magis, D., Seidel, L., Agosti, R.M., & Schenen, J. A randomized controlled trial of coenzyme Q10 in migraine prophylaxis. *Neurology* 64 (2005): 713–715.

Saper, J.R., Silberstein, S.D., Lake, A.E. 3rd, & Winters, M.E. Double-blind trial of fluoxetine: Chronic daily headache and migraine. *Headache* 34 (1994): 497–502.

Schoenen, J., Schrader, H., Stovner, L.J., Helde, G., Sand, T., & Bovim, G. Prophylactic treatment of migraine with angiotensin converting enzyme inhibitor (lisinopril): Randomised, placebo controlled, crossover study. *British Medical Journal* 322 (2001): 19–22.

Silberstein, S.D. Practice parameter: Evidence-based guidelines for migraine headache (an evidence-based review): Report of the Quality Standards Subcommittee of the American Academy of Neurology. *Neurology* 55 (2000): 754–762.

Silberstein, S.D., & Goadsby, P.J. Migraine: Preventive treatment. *Cephalalgia* 22 (2002): 491–512.

Silberstein, S.D., Lipton, R.B., & Goadsby, P.J. *Headache in clinical practice*, 2nd ed. Oxford: Martin Dunitz, 2000, pp. 91–92.

Spira, P.J., Beran, R.G.; Australian Gabapentin Chronic Daily Headache Group. Gabapentin in the prophylaxis of chronic daily headache: A randomized, placebo-controlled study. *Neurology* 61, no. 12 (2003): 1753–1759.

Tepper, S.J. Tailoring management strategies for the patient with menstrual migraine: Focus on prevention and treatment. *Headache* 46 (CME Suppl 2) (2006): S61–S68.

Tronvik, E., Stovner, L.J., Helde, G., Sand, T., & Bovim, G. Prophylactic treatment of migraine with an angiotensin II receptor blocker: A randomized controlled trial. *JAMA* 289 (2003): 65–69.

Weiller, C., May, A., Limmroth, V., Juptner, M., Kaube, H., Schayck, R.V., Coenen, H.H., & Diener, H.C. Brain stem activation in spontaneous human migraine attacks. *Nature Medicine* 1 (1995): 658–660.

Woods, R.P., Iacoboni, M., & Mazziotta, J.C. Brief report: Bilateral spreading cerebral hypoperfusion during spontaneous migraine headache. *New England Journal of Medicine* 331 (1994): 1689–1692.

Ziad el, K., Rahi, A.C., Hamdan, S.A., & Mikati, M.A. Age, dose, and environmental temperature are risk factors for topiramate-related hyperthermia. *Neurology* 65 (2005): 1139–1140.

13

Pharmacologic Treatment of Trigeminal Autonomic Cephalalgias and Other Primary Headaches

Brian E. McGeeney, MD, MPH

The headache disorders in this chapter are considerably less common than migraine and tension-type headache. Because of this, there are few good-quality blinded randomized trials from which to sculpt treatment guidelines, in contrast to therapeutic recommendations for migraine. Consequently, pharmacologic guidelines are based on unblinded or non-randomized trials, case series, reports, and anecdotal experience, which form the entirety of "evidence"; nevertheless, one needs to become familiar with the popular suggested options. The therapies presented presume that any underlying secondary cause such as a structural lesion has been ruled out. All of these syndromes may occur secondary to structural causes, and the literature is replete with examples. This chapter will cover all of the primary headaches recognized by the International Classification of Headache Disorders, 2nd edition, with the exception of migraine and tension-type headache, which have been covered earlier. The therapeutic suggestions are comprehensive but not complete, as there are many medications available. The pharmacologic suggestions made here have some support in the literature and should be given strong consideration.

TRIGEMINAL AUTONOMIC CEPHALALGIAS

The trigeminal autonomic cephalalgias encompass cluster headache, paroxysmal hemicrania, and SUNCT syndrome and share the common features of unilateral short-lived headaches with unilateral autonomic features.

Cluster Headache

The management of cluster headache is nearly always pharmacologic and rarely surgical (Table 13–1). Other interventions are of little benefit, besides avoiding recognizable triggers such as alcohol during vulnerable periods. Treatment can be divided into abortive therapy or prophylactic therapy, and most patients respond well to therapy. The term "transitional prophylaxis" is sometimes used

Table 13–1 Cluster Headache therapy

Most Effective Abortive Treatments	
Treatment	Doses
Sumatriptan	6 mg SC injection
Oxygen	7–10 liters/min non-rebreather mask for 15–30 minutes
Dihydroergotamine IV/IM/SC	1 mg
More Abortive Treatments	
Zolmitriptan nasal spray	5 mg
Sumatriptan nasal spray	20 mg
Dihydroergotamine nasal spray	2 sprays each nostril (0.5 mg per spray). May repeat once.
Lidocaine 4% nasal spray	4 sprays ipsilaterally
Ergotamine (+/− caffeine) tablet	1–2 mg. Max 6 mg/day
Short-Term Prophylaxis to Induce a Remission	
Corticosteroids	Prednisone 60–80 mg/day taper over 1–3 weeks
Ergotamine (+/− caffeine)	1–2 mg PO up to tid
Dihydroergotamine	0.5–1 mg IV q 8h for 3 days or 1 mg IM. 1-2/day for 1 week
Triptans	Naratriptan 2.5 mg bid for 7 days
Prophylaxis	
Verapamil	360–720 mg daily
Lithium	300–1,200 mg daily
Methysergide	2 mg bid–qid
Topiramate	50–200 mg daily
Melatonin	3–10 mg nightly
Valproic acid	1,000–2500 mg daily

to refer to short-term treatment aimed at inducing a remission using agents not suitable for long-term prophylaxis.

Acute Therapy of Cluster Headache

The brief nature of the attacks precludes oral therapies, although sometimes ergotamine and caffeine tablets are used. The best options are subcutaneous suma-triptan, high-flow inhaled oxygen, or intramuscular dihydroergotamine (DHE).

Oxygen therapy Oxygen therapy is a popular choice but has practical limitations due to the bulky nature of the equipment. There are essentially no adverse events associated with the use of oxygen, except in a minority of those with chronic obstructive pulmonary disease who use oxygen saturation as primary respiratory drive, and the flammable hazard with oxygen and fire.

Some patients notice that the use of oxygen only postpones the attack. It is important to administer 7 to 10 liters per minute of 100% oxygen via a face mask for 15 to 25 minutes; the use of a nasal cannula is not as effective. Hyperbaric oxygen has been effective also. The mechanism of action is unknown.

Sumatriptan   Sumatriptan administered by subcutaneous injection at a dose of 4 or 6 mg is arguably the most effective abortive agent for a cluster attack. It is FDA approved for cluster headache and does not appear to be effective for prophylaxis. Sumatriptan 20 mg nasal spray is less effective but still useful. Often there is concern about using ergotamines or triptans in older individuals with cardiac risk factors.

Ergotamine and DHE   Ergotamine is used as an abortive agent using intramuscular, intravenous, subcutaneous, intranasal, oral, rectal, and inhalational routes, but use has generally been superseded by the triptan family. The subcutaneous or intramuscular routes would offer the quickest routes among the options available for home use. A course of DHE can also induce a remission of a cycle. When given parenterally it is often accompanied by an antiemetic due to the frequent occurrence of nausea. The ergotamines have potent actions on the vasculature, which make them unsuitable in many older individuals, and they are contraindicated in those with vascular disease of the heart, cerebral circulation, or periphery.

Other abortive therapy options   Nasal lidocaine 4% spray is a very safe option but it will need to be compounded as it is not commercially available in the United States. Nasal lidocaine is best applied with the head reclined to 45 degrees and rotated to the affected side by 30 to 40 degrees. Zolmitriptan nasal spray 5 mg is also used, and 10 mg has been studied for this purpose. Recently octreotide 100 mcg given subcutaneously (somatostatin analog) has been shown to be effective as an abortive agent.

Direct application of local anesthetics to the nasal mucosa in the region of the sphenopalatine ganglion has resulted in abolition of an attack, as have occipital nerve region blocks with local anesthetic. There does not appear to be a rationale for the use of steroids in occipital blocks, at least when the goal is to break on ongoing cluster attack.

Preventative Therapy of Cluster Headache

Steroids are the quickest way to induce a remission—for example, prednisone 60 to 80 mg daily and tapering over 10 days to 3 weeks. Dexamethasone may also be used. Steroids are usually well tolerated but do carry a very small risk of osteonecrosis. Dihydroergotamine and ergotamine have also been used daily for a short time to induce a remission.

Verapamil   Verapamil is the agent of choice and has demonstrated efficacy, tolerability, and safety in chronic prophylaxis. The starting dose is a 240-mg slow-release tablet daily or 80 mg three times daily. A total of up to 720 mg daily is used. An electrocardiogram is suggested at doses above 240 mg daily due to slowed conduction across the atrioventricular node. Constipation, hypotension, and dizziness are other side effects. Verapamil can result in elevated ethanol blood levels and can reduce lithium levels.

Lithium   Lithium has long been considered a first-line agent for prophylaxis of cluster headache and is reported to be effective in 63% of episodic cluster patients and as many as 78% of chronic cluster patients. Lithium may be used in combination with verapamil. A double-blind crossover trial comparing verapamil to lithium showed similar efficacy. Lithium was not as well tolerated as verapamil. Monitoring of blood levels of lithium is necessary, along with assessment of renal, liver, and thyroid status. Lithium is administered three times daily or as a daily slow-release preparation. The starting dosage is 300 mg twice daily, with a maintenance dosage of 600 to 1,200 mg daily in divided doses. The trough level, measured 12 hours after the last dose, should not exceed 1 mEq/L. Toxicity is manifested by confusion, nausea, vomiting, ataxia, and seizures. Diuretics and nonsteroidal anti-inflammatories can often increase lithium levels by reducing renal excretion. Angiotensin-converting enzyme inhibitors and metronidazole can also increase levels. Lithium has been associated with QT prolongation and even torsades de pointes.

Methysergide   Methysergide is an ergot alkaloid. It is unavailable in the United States but is still available in Canada. Uncommon complications such as retroperitoneal, pleural, and valvular fibrotic changes reduced the use of this agent for migraine and cluster headache prophylaxis. On initiation of therapy some patients experience nausea, cramping, and diarrhea. Short courses of 3 months should avoid these complications, and long-term therapy is coupled with drug-free periods. It is good practice to avoid other ergots and vasoconstrictive agents while on methysergide.

Melatonin   Melatonin is a pineal hormone that is released in a diurnal pattern, with high levels at night and low levels during the day. Reduced serum levels of melatonin have been found in cluster headache patients, particularly during an attack. Melatonin has been shown to have anti-inflammatory and antinociceptive properties. The pattern of cluster headache and abnormal melatonin levels suggests abnormalities in circadian rhythms. Dose recommendations are from 3 to 9 mg nightly.

Other suggested options for cluster prophylaxis include valproic acid, topiramate, and baclofen. Civamide is a capsaicin-like medication that has been studied in cluster prophylaxis. The calcium-channel blockers nifedipine and nimodipine have been used in cluster, albeit rarely.

Surgical Options for Cluster Headache

Surgical options are available, but without evidence, and one must be cautious. Procedures are aimed at lesioning the trigeminal nerve and risk anesthesia dolorosa and secondary trigeminal neuralgia. Deep brain stimulation of the posterior inferior hypothalamus has recently been shown to be effective in a couple of reports using refractory patients.

Paroxysmal Hemicrania

Paroxysmal hemicrania is by definition responsive to indomethacin, if used in a sufficient dose. A suggested regimen would be 25 mg three times daily for 3 days then 50 mg three times daily, although for response 300 mg daily has sometimes been needed. A marked improvement is expected with days. For patents who cannot take indomethacin, a trial of celecoxib should be considered (at least 200 mg daily). Possibly the best alternative to indomethacin when treating paroxysmal hemicrania is verapamil. Some patients with paroxysmal hemicrania have responded to acetylsalicylic acid, naproxen, topiramate, and acetazolamide, but not oxygen or carbamazepine. Prednisone may result in a remission, but this is not suitable for long-term therapy.

Indomethacin, an NSAID, is a potent reversible inhibitor of cyclooxygenase; it also inhibits phosphodiesterase and is an inhibitor of nitrous oxide production. Indomethacin is advocated widely for the headache disorders in this chapter and is administered to headache patients in oral or suppository form. There is currently no commercial form of indomethacin suppository, and compounding pharmacies are used to prepare this product. Indomethacin is highly protein-bound (90%), with a half-life of 3 hours, and it does enter the cerebrospinal fluid. The structure of indomethacin is similar to that of melatonin. Adverse events are common and include gastrointestinal irritation, dizziness, and confusion. The inhibition of cyclooxygenase is thought to be at least partly responsible for the clinical effect, as often these headache disorders will respond to other NSAIDs. Another possible mechanism for the clinical improvement is reduced nitrous oxide production, which has been implicated in many primary headaches. Indomethacin decreases intracranial pressure, likely by multiple mechanisms, and this may be the basis for response with Valsalva-induced headaches.

SUNCT (Short-Lasting Unilateral Neuralgiform Headache Attacks with Conjunctival Injection and Tearing)

These attacks are less responsive to therapy than cluster headaches and the paroxysmal hemincranias. Treatment guidelines are based on anecdotal evidence and refer to prophylaxis as the attacks themselves are of such short duration. Lamotrigine is a suggested first-line agent, followed by gabapentin or topiramate. Intravenous lidocaine or phenytoin has also been used, as have indomethacin, naproxen, valproate, and methysergide. Local anesthetic blocks (occipital or supraorbital) have not been successful. The literature also supports the association between small noncompressive prolactinomas (and other pituitary lesions) and SUNCT (also cluster headache), so the workup should reflect this and it should be treated accordingly. Deep brain stimulation is considered as a very last resort.

OTHER PRIMARY HEADACHE TYPES

Hemicrania Continua

This daily continuous hemicrania differs from the trigeminal autonomic cephalalgias in that it is not short-lived, but they do share unilateral autonomic features. By definition there is a complete response to indomethacin. Other treatments suggested are verapamil, melatonin, and topiramate. Failing these, anticonvulsants such as valproate or beta-blockers may be tried. Occipital nerve stimulation has been performed on some patients with hemicrania continua.

Cough Headache, Exertional Headache, and Headache with Sexual Activity

Sometimes known as the Valsalva-maneuver headaches, reflecting their association with coughing or straining and so forth, these maneuvers cause a transient increase in venous pressure that is transmitted intracranially, resulting in a brief increase in intracranial pressure and a bilateral headache syndrome. All of these headaches are usually responsive to indomethacin, either 25 to 50 mg for occasional use taken 1 hour before activity or on a regular basis in doses of 25 to 150 mg daily. Other NSAIDs such as naproxen may be used. Propranolol is also advocated, as are other beta-blockers such as atenolol. Topiramate or methysergide is an alternative. Cough headache has responded to lumbar puncture, possibly because of the resultant decrease in intracranial pressure. In such cases increased intracranial pressure manifests as cough headache.

Hypnic Headache

Suggested therapies for hypnic headache are caffeine, melatonin, clonazepam, or acetazolamide, taken at night. Lithium is also advocated, and sometimes verapamil.

Primary Stabbing Headache

Indomethacin or other NSAIDs are suggested.

New Daily Persistent Headache

This syndrome is not treated any differently from chronic daily headache, so most clinicians would use the typical array of beta-blockers, antidepressants, anticonvulsants, and other medications.

Primary Thunderclap Headache

There is very limited published experience. If prophylactic treatment is needed, consider an NSAID such as indomethacin. The literature reports on gabapentin and nimodipine also.

SUMMARY

The trigeminal autonomic cephalalgias are distinguished not only by the length and frequency of their attacks but also by their response to therapy. The reader should be completely familiar with the choice of medications for the treatment of cluster, which are effective for most patients. Indomethacin can treat a wide range of primary headache disorders, and by definition paroxysmal hemicrania and hemicrania continua respond to this medication. Interventional therapies such as occipital nerve stimulation and hypothalamic deep brain stimulation are being increasingly investigated for primary headache disorders.

Review Questions

1. The best treatment option for SUNCT is:
   a. Indomethacin
   b. Topiramate
   c. Lamotrigine
   d. Gabapentin
2. Which one of these statements, when applied to melatonin, is false?
   a. It is structurally related to indomethacin.
   b. It is available over-the-counter in the United States.
   c. Cluster patients have low amounts at night compared to the day.
   d. It is generally available in 1-mg and 3-mg pills.
3. A 50-year-old man with cluster headache is treated successfully with methysergide in Canada and on a trip to the United States develops cluster attacks again, ending up in your emergency department. By the time you see him the evening attack is over, and he tells you he usually gets two attacks a day for 3 weeks in a cluster period. There are no cardiovascular risk factors, and he is healthy. Which therapy do you feel would be most suitable?
   a. Componded nasal lidocaine and a short course of prednisone
   b. Sumatriptan 6 mg SC and a short course of prednisone
   c. Dihydroergotamine nasal spray
   d. Sumatriptan 6 mg SC
4. A patient with cough headache is not responding to indomethacin any more. Imaging has been unremarkable. You would next consider:
   a. Lumbar puncture
   b. Verapamil
   c. Ibuprofen
   d. Zonisamide
5. A 70-year-old woman is awakened at night by holocranial headaches that last 30 to 60 minutes, without autonomic features. There is no prior history of headaches, and this has been going on a couple of

times a week for months. She arrives with an unremarkable brain MRI ordered by her primary physician. The first therapy you would consider is:

   a. Caffeine or melatonin at night
   b. Sumatriptan 6 mg SC at onset of attack
   c. Verapamil
   d. Indomethacin 100 mg nightly

6. When patients are taking lithium, which of these statements is false?
   a. Piroxicam and indomethacin can increase lithium levels significantly.
   b. Metronidazole may decrease the lithium level significantly.
   c. Concurrent use of calcium-channel blockers may increase the risk of neurotoxicity.
   d. Diuretic-induced sodium loss may reduce the renal clearance of lithium.

7. When treating a cluster attack, which treatment results in the quickest response?
   a. 5 to 7 liters of oxygen through a nasal cannula
   b. Dihydroergotamine 1 mg intramuscularly
   c. Occipital nerve block with lidocaine
   d. Sumatriptan 6 mg SC

8. The first-line agent for cluster prophylaxis is:
   a. Prednisone
   b. Verapamil
   c. Melatonin
   d. Indomethacin

9. The only FDA-approved medication for cluster headache is:
   a. Verapamil
   b. Sumatriptan
   c. Oxygen
   d. Ergotamine

10. Which of the following statements, when referring to verapamil, is false?
   a. It commonly causes loose stools.
   b. It prolongs the refractory period within the atrioventricular node of the heart.
   c. It can produce significant hypotension.
   d. It significantly inhibits ethanol elimination.

10. a
9. b
8. b
7. d
6. b

5. a
4. a
3. a
2. c
1. c

SUGGESTED READING

Bussone, G., Franzini, A., Proietti Cecchini, A., et al. Deep brain stimulation in craniofacial pain: Seven years' experience. *Neurologic Sciences* 28, Suppl. 2 (May 2007): S146–149.

Matharu, M.S., Cohen, A.S., et al. Short-lasting unilateral neuralgiform headache with conjunctival injection and tearing syndrome: A review. *Current Pain Headache Reports* 7 (2003):308–318.

May, A. Cluster headache: pathogenesis, diagnosis, and management. *Lancet* 366 (2005): 843–855.

May, A., Leone, M., Afra, J., et al. EFNS guidelines on the treatment of cluster headache and other trigeminal-autonomic cephalalgias. *European Journal of Neurology* 13 (2006): 1066–1077.

Rozen, T. Short-lasting headache syndromes and treatment options. *Current Pain Headache Reports* 8 (2004): 268–273.

14

Treatment of Chronic Daily Headache

Fred D. Sheftell, MD

Those who practice by clinical experience alone are bound to repeat their own mistakes .... those who practice by evidence alone are bound to repeat the mistakes of others!

John Edmeads, MD

The above quote by our dear friend and colleague John Edmeads embodies the philosophy of this chapter, in that as David Sackett (the father of evidence-based medicine) stated, the best practice of medicine combines our clinical experience with the best evidence available. These concepts are especially true of the treatment of chronic daily headache of long duration, for there is minimal evidence for the treatment of these disorders, whether we use either the ICHD-II criteria or the Silberstein-Lipton criteria. As you will see, we can count the number of adequate randomized double-blinded placebo-controlled studies on one hand. Those of us who practice in a tertiary care setting or who have specialized in headache medicine truly have had to fly by the seat of our proverbial pants (or skirts) and rely heavily on our clinical experience, given the paucity of evidence in the treatment of very complex disorders and associated comorbidities. Here treatment has truly been more that of the art of medicine than the science. In the years to come, we hope that will change, as clinical research and bench work elucidate mechanisms, but for now, we are left to do the best we can under current circumstances. This chapter will review the "state of the art" of the treatment of chronic daily headache, including chronic migraine, medication overuse headache, chronic tension-type headache, hemicrania continua, and new persistent daily headache. We will review the evidence and include our clinical experience; perhaps together these have become accepted as good clinical practice.

PROBABLE CHRONIC MIGRAINE, PROBABLE MEDICATION OVERUSE HEADACHE, CHRONIC MIGRAINE, AND MEDICATION OVERUSE HEADACHE

In terms of an overview of the treatment of this group of chronic daily headaches, we have to start by assessing risk factors and when present attempting to minimize them. Pharmacologic strategies must include identifying medication overuse headache when present and addressing a variety of "bridge" strategies to transition patients from daily to intermittent medication use (under 10 days per month is the criterion for medication overuse headache). Prophylaxis must be addressed, as well as considering interventional and nonpharmacologic strategies.

Identification of risk factors, including attack frequency, helps determine the need for implementation of preventive strategies while avoiding central sensitization; this also involves the use of successful abortive therapies. Recently Limroth and colleagues, evaluating pooled data from three randomized double-blind placebo-controlled trials, found that topiramate in episodic migraine may reduce the occurrence of chronic migraine and medication overuse headache. In fact, other data suggest that preventive strategies should begin during the period of curtailing medication overuse headache and should not be delayed until after medication overuse headache has been successfully addressed. In fact, introducing these strategies may alone help to decrease medication overuse headache. However, treating medication overuse headache requires decreasing the frequency of acute medication intake with bridge therapies, education, and so forth. If identified, psychiatric comorbidity should be treated aggressively with pharmacotherapy and nonpharmacologic therapy such as cognitive-behavioral therapy, biofeedback, and so forth. Snoring should be evaluated and consideration given to the possibility of sleep apnea.

Treating medication overuse headache generally involves stopping the offending medication, initiating bridge therapies (and treating withdrawal symptoms where appropriate), implementing prophylaxis, and establishing migraine-specific abortive therapies with proper limits. Other key factors are adequate follow-up (at least monthly during the withdrawal period) and educating the patient and family about the mechanisms of medication overuse headache, worsening before improvement, outcome data, and the need to take an active role. The physician must ensure that psychiatric comorbidity will not interfere with treatment.

"Bridge" Therapy Strategies

Strategies may vary from abrupt discontinuation to a gradual process over days to weeks of tapering offending agents, tapering caffeine in diet and medication, and so forth. Generally, abrupt discontinuation is safe for most overused medications, be they over-the-counter or prescription. However, patients generally are very apprehensive about this period of change and a tapering process seems more humane. There is no evidence that one is better than another. However, caution should be observed with butalbital- or benzodiazepine-containing products, given the potential for seizures on abrupt discontinuation. In either event there is evidence that prophylactic medication should be introduced while discontinuing the offending medication.

Pharmacologic bridge therapies include the conversion of short-acting butalbital in Fiorinal/Fioricet/Esgic to long-acting phenobarbital at a ratio of 100 mg butalbital (there is 50 mg butalbital per capsule or tablet) to 30 mg phenobarbital. Benzodiazepines should be tapered slowly as well. In tapering opiates, consider tapering the offending agent by 10% to 15% per day and using clonidine by tablet or patch to ease withdrawal symptoms. In tapering combined butalbital/opiate products consider both tapering strategies just described. Over-the-counter products may be tapered abruptly, but be aware of caffeine-containing products (e.g., ASA 250/APAP 250/caffeine 65 mg). Given the fact that as little as 100 mg of caffeine per day can cause withdrawal symptoms, including headache, we generally calculate combined caffeine content in diet and medication and withdraw 100 mg each day of caffeine-containing tablets.

Ergots and triptans can be tapered by using the product itself, DHE-45 in various formulations such as nasal spray, intramuscular, subcutaneous or intravenous routes, or by changing to a long-acting triptan. Sheftell and associates used naratriptan in one small study and Tepper and Drucker used sumatriptan in another. Other agents that can be used include nonsteroidal anti-inflammatory agents (NSAIDs), steroids, and neuroleptics.

Pharmacologic Prophylaxis

In a review of this topic Saper and coworkers stated, "Unfortunately there is a paucity of controlled trials evaluating the efficacy of preventive drugs for the treatment of TM. The few studies that have been performed have either lacked a control, failed to properly classify patients in the trial, or neglected to account for the overuse of acute medications. Conventional treatments have traditionally included beta-blockers and tricyclic antidepressants, but in the last several years anticonvulsants have emerged as important. Such therapies include valproic acid, topiramate and gabapentin. Tizanidine has also been demonstrated to be potentially useful as an adjunct treatment for patients with TM." More recently topiramate showed a trend toward efficacy in chronic migraine in a randomized double-blind placebo-controlled study by Silberstein and associates that was published in *Headache* in 2007. Other agents with suggested efficacy in chronic daily headache by randomized double-blind placebo-controlled or active comparator trials include gabapentin, amitriptyline, tizanidine, fluoxetine, and botulinum toxin A. Others include citalopram and ritanserin, and open trials include paroxetine, phenelzine, valproate, methylergonovine, naratriptan, and the clonidine patch. However, there are no FDA-approved medications for the treatment of chronic migraine or chronic tension-type headache with or without medication overuse. The choice of agent is largely dependent on its adverse event profile, comorbidities, interactions with current medications, and contraindications.

Interventional strategies include occipital nerve blocks, trigger points, cervical facet blocks, craniosacral manipulation, and acupuncture, none of which has high-grade evidence for use in chronic daily headache. Other interventions currently being evaluated include occipital stimulation and patent foramen ovale closure for refractory populations with daily headache. In a review of emerging therapies, Goadsby states, "Tonaberset (a gap-junction blocker), an inducible nitric oxide synthase inhibitor, and botulinum toxin A are in clinical trials for preventive therapy."

Non-Pharmacologic Prophylaxis

There are reports of stress management, cognitive-behavioral therapy, diet manipulation, exercise, chronobiologic regulation, and individual/family counseling being helpful in chronic daily headache. Given the high percentage of psychiatric comorbidity and the impact these disorders have on sufferers and their families, the author considers these interventions essential in the treatment of these disorders.

In summary:

1. Educate the patient about expectations and mechanisms.
2. Employ non-pharmacologic strategies.
3. Identify and address psychiatric comorbidity.
4. Institute prophylaxis and acute care with limits.
5. Discontinue all offending medications and agents, including caffeine.

CHRONIC TENSION-TYPE HEADACHE

Pharmacologic Approaches

Again, solid evidence is lacking. Difficulties arise in the issue of how chronic tension-type headache is defined. We have seen very few cases of pure chronic tension-type headache: the vast majority of cases are mixed and may even satisfy various definitions of chronic migraine. Fluvoxamine, mianserine, topiramate, 5-hydroxytryptophan, venlafaxine, protriptyline, and amitriptyline have shown possible efficacy in chronic tension-type headache in small studies. Tizanidine, paroxetine, and citalopram had negative outcomes in various studies (some controlled and some uncontrolled, but all small).

To quote Changao and Stillman:

> The first International Headache Society classification defined tension-type headaches (TTHs) by itemising those characteristics of migraines TTHs did not possess ... As a result, TTHs, both episodic and chronic, remain the most nonspecific of all the commonly observed primary headaches. Until recently, there has been little impetus on the part of the pharmaceutical industry to investigate TTHs; many of the potentially useful drugs are now generic and unprofitable. In addition, few investigators have pursued the study of TTHs in lieu of its more glamorous neighbour, migraine. As a result, there are few well-designed studies on the pharmacotherapy of TTHs. The few studies that exist

support the use of age-old standard drug classes, the tricyclic antidepressants and the NSAIDs. New research is now emerging that points to the potential utility of botulinum toxin type A, NMDA-receptor antagonists including Mg(2+) and nitric oxide synthase inhibitors. More scientifically rigorous clinical studies are needed.

I might add that given the high incidence of comorbid depression and anxiety with this disorder, look for the comorbidity and treat it.

In a review by Evers and Olesen in *Cephalalgia* in 2006, outcomes in regard to botulinum toxin in chronic tension-type headache were mixed at best and largely negative.

Two small interventional studies, one involving occipital nerve blocks by Dahlke and associates, was negative with prilocaine and dexamethasone. Another study by Solomon in 1989 suggested that electrocranial stimulation was "potentially effective."

Non-pharmacologic Approaches

A randomized controlled study by Holroyd and coworkers published in *JAMA* demonstrated that combined therapy combining amitriptyline with stress management may be better than monotherapy. Penzien and associates demonstrated that biofeedback therapy, cognitive-behavioral therapy, stress management, nutritional interventions, exercise, and so forth were helpful in this disorder. Other modalities, including physiotherapy, were best for chronic tension-type headache versus frequent or episodic tension-type headache, according to Torelli and colleagues. Complementary/alternative medicine was found to be helpful in 41% of patients with chronic tension-type headache in structured interviews by Rossi and associates.

Goadsby summarized the issues in *American Family Physician*. Amitriptyline is beneficial in the short term. Cognitive-behavioral therapy is likely to be beneficial. The benefits of electromyographic (EMG) feedback, relaxation, acupuncture, selective serotonin reuptake inhibitors (SSRIs), and tricyclic antidepressants (TCAs) other than amitriptyline are "unknown." Benzodiazepines and regular use of acute pain medications are "likely ineffective or harmful."

HEMICRANIA CONTINUA

Hemicrania continua, a syndrome often unrecognized even by experts, is extremely rewarding to treat once recognized because it is almost always responsive to sufficient doses of indomethacin. If one does not inquire about side-lock, this syndrome may be mistaken for chronic migraine, new persistent daily headache, or medication overuse headache. Many patients will find high-dose salicylates or NSAIDs to be somewhat beneficial. Indomethacin treatment may fail at less than 250 to 300 mg per day. Many clinicians often co-administer an H2 blocker or proton pump inhibitor to reduce the risk of gastrointestinal side effects. For patients who require long-term treatment, it is wise to check for occult blood in the stool and monitor BUN, glomerular filtration rate, and creatinine periodically. Starting doses are generally 25 mg TID with meals; the dosage can be doubled every 5 to 7 days to 300 mg if necessary. The biggest problem with maintaining sufficient doses of indomethacin is tolerability. If side effects become intolerable, other therapies have been proposed, as summarized below, especially high dose melatonin whose molecular structure closely resembles indomethacin.

- Trucco and associates in 1992 reported on a case that was responsive to piroxicam-beta cyclodextrin.
- Peres and Silberstein in 2002 tried COX-2 inhibitors (celecoxib and rofecoxib) in 14 patients; 3 in each group had complete response.
- Rozen in 2006 reported on melatonin-responsive hemicrania continua. Doses of up to 24 mg were given at bedtime, titrating by 3 mg every three to five nights.
- Spears in 2006 reported on a case in which a patient experienced complete relief with melatonin (7 mg at bedtime).
- In 2007, Rajabally and Jacob published a case report on hemicrania continua responsive to verapamil (120 mg).
- There have also been scattered anecdotal reports on gabapentin and lamotrigine.

NEW DAILY PERSISTENT HEADACHE

This primary headache, classified under "other primary headaches," is characterized by sudden or at least rapid onset of chronic daily headache in the absence of a prior history of headache. Lance pointed out years ago that a viral infection, even innocuous, often precedes the onset. What is pathognomonic and required to satisfy ICHD-IIR criteria is that the patient can describe the exact time and date of its onset: "I was coming out of Wal-Mart's on February 22 two years ago in the afternoon. I got this headache and it never went away." In a clinic population these patients represent 10% of the population with chronic daily headache of long duration. The first ICHD-II classification stated that these headaches satisfied the criteria for chronic tension-type headache, but the criteria were changed to include migraine as well. In our experience these patients rarely overuse acute medications because "nothing works!"

As rewarding as hemicrania continua is to treat, new daily persistent headache is its polar opposite. Goadsby summarizes the issues well: "It is general experience among those interested in headache management that NDPH of this type is perhaps the most intractable and least therapeutically rewarding forms of headache. In general we classify the dominant phenotype, migraine or tension-type headache, and treat with preventatives according to that subclassification, as for patients with chronic daily headache."

In short, I agree with Peter Goadsby: "Treat the phenotype."

SUMMARY

Though chronic daily headache does not exist as an "official" nosological entity in ICHD-II, it is nonetheless a universally accepted clinical entity among headache specialists. The five subtypes that are official ICHD-II entities are chronic migraine, medication overuse headache, chronic tension-type headache, hemicrania continua, and new daily persistent headache. This chapter focused on evidence-based treatment, and unfortunately there are few well-randomized double-blind placebo-controlled studies to support what headache specialists do to treat this most challenging group of patients. The evidence for prophylactic strategies is largely if not almost exclusively based on study populations with frequent migraine; there is some evidence on chronic tension-type headache but almost none on chronic migraine or chronic daily headache. The existing evidence or lack thereof strongly suggests the need for well-designed prospective studies to give us the proper evidence-based armamentarium we require.

Review Questions

1. A 35-year-old woman presents with a history of intermittent migraine since puberty. Initially her frequency was once per month in association with her menses. Over a period of time her headaches have escalated in frequency to the point where she presents to a tertiary care center with chronic daily headache characterized by daily waxing and waning holocranial pain of mild to moderate intensity with six to eight episodes per month of disabling pain associated with nausea, sensitivity to light and sound, and exacerbation by activity, and requiring bed rest for a portion of the day. She has failed to respond to all preventive medications and her response to migraine-specific medications has diminished over time. Current medications include topiramate at 100 mg, verapamil 240SR, a combination of butalbital/ASA/caffeine at six to eight tablets per day, and "occasional" hydrocodone. She had become more desperate over time, is not sleeping well, and feels hopeless. In terms of treatment your first move would be:
   a. Increase topiramate.
   b. Change verapamil to propranolol.
   c. Add an SSRI.
   d. Educate the patient about medication overuse headache.
2. Pharmacologic treatment for this patient would start with:
   a. Change her preventives and trying something she's never taken
   b. Taper offending medications and simultaneously initiate changes if necessary in her preventives
   c. Taper offending medications and then make changes in her preventives
   d. Stop all acute medications abruptly and tell her to return a month after she is successful

3. The agent with the best evidence for the treatment of chronic migraine is:
   a. Amitriptyline
   b. Valproate
   c. Methergine
   d. Topiramate

4. The recommended method for tapering butalbital is:
   a. Convert to phenobarbital
   b. Treat with clonidine
   c. Stop abruptly
   d. Use steroids

5. Pure chronic tension-type headache without migraine, as observed in the U.S. clinic populations, is reported as:
   a. Nonexistent
   b. Rare
   c. Common
   d. Very common

6. In the patient described above, what is omitted from the history that would lead you to consider another type of primary headache?
   a. Quality of pain
   b. Location of pain
   c. Family history
   d. Marital status

7. Had it been established that the patient's daily background headaches were side-locked, what would you consider?
   a. Chronic paroxysmal hemicrania
   b. Cluster migraine
   c. Hemicrania continua
   d. Unilateral chronic tension-type headache

8. If in fact you consider hemicrania continua, what would be your first consideration?
   a. Gabapentin 300 mg TID
   b. Valproate 500 mg
   c. COX-2 inhibitors with food
   d. Indomethacin 25 mg TID with food

9. If her headaches were as described in the case but had started de novo on a day she could remember, the diagnosis would be:
   a. The same
   b. Conversion disorder
   c. New daily persistent headache
   d. R/O intracranial lesion

10. What would be your initial strategies?
    a. Address medication overuse headache, start prophylaxis, provide migraine-specific therapy with limits

b. Change regimen for one specific for this disorder
c. Oxygen for acute episodes
d. Refer for psychotherapy

10. a
9. c
8. d
7. c
6. b
5. b
4. a
3. d
2. b
1. d

SUGGESTED READING

Bigal, M.E., & Sheftell, F.D. "Chronic daily headache." In *AAN Continuum*, 2006, eds. Saper, J.R., & Rozen, T.D.

Classification Committee of the International Headache Society. International Classification of Headache Disorders II. *Cephalalgia* 24, Suppl. 1 (2004): 1–160.

Goadsby, P.G., Silberstein, P.J., & Dodick, D.W., eds. *Chronic daily headache for clinicians*. Hamilton, Ontario: BC Decker, 2005.

Peres, F.P., & Silberstein, S.D. Hemicrania continua responds to COX-2 inhibitors. *Headache* 42, no. 6 (2002): 530–531.

Rajabally, Y.A., & Jacob, S. Hemicrania continua responsive to verapamil. Case report. *Headache* 45, no. 8 (2007): 1082–1083.

Rozen, T.D. Melatonin-responsive hemicrania continua. *Headache* 46, no. 7 (2006): 1203–1204.

Sheftell, F.D., & Bigal, M.E. "Medication overuse headache." In *AAN Continuum*, 2006, eds. Saper, J.R., & Rozen, T.D.

Silberstein, S.D., Lipton, R.B., & Goadsby, P.J. *Headache in clinical practice*, 2nd ed. Oxford: Isis Medical Media, 2002.

Spears, R. Hemicrania continua: A case in which a patient experienced complete relief on melatonin. *Headache* 46, no. 3 (2006): 524–527.

Trucco, M., Antonaci, F., & Sandrini, G. Headache. A case responsive to piroxicam-beta cyclodextrin. *Headache* 32, no. 1 (1992): 39–40.

V

Treatment of Intractable Headache and Special Populations

15

Headache Treatment in Children, Pregnancy and Lactation, the Elderly, and Renal Disease

Thomas N. Ward, MD

This chapter concerns the treatment of headache in special populations. It serves the practitioner well to be thoroughly familiar with the ICHD-II when approaching patients with headache as the presenting complaint because one must first be able to make correct diagnoses and then understand the underlying pathophysiology and anatomy to move to the next step in choosing treatment options. This is especially true in treating children, pregnant and lactating patients, and patients with other medical illnesses such as renal disease.

HEADACHE TREATMENT IN CHILDREN

Compared to the evidence base for adults, there is much less information available for this age group (under 18 years old). No drug has FDA approval. The AAN Practice Parameter recommends ibuprofen and acetaminophen for acute therapy at appropriate doses; additionally, intranasal sumatriptan is recommended for patients at least 12 years of age. Aspirin should be avoided due to concerns about Reye syndrome. Flunarizine (not available in the United States) is described as probably effective as a prophylactic agent. Non-pharmacologic modalities should be considered especially in this age group.

Antiemetics have practical utility, but children have dystonic reactions at a higher rate than do adults. Some authorities recommend (with little evidence base) propranolol, cyproheptadine, amitriptyline, divalproex, topiramate, and zonisamide.

One should know about ICHD-II 1.3, "Childhood periodic syndromes that are commonly precursors of migraine." 1.3.1, "Cyclical vomiting," consists of recurrent episodes (at least five) of intense nausea and vomiting lasting from 1 hour to 5 days (the vomiting occurs in at least four episodes per hour for at least 1 hour). The child is asymptomatic between episodes and gastrointestinal evaluation excludes other disorders. Appropriate treatment is to stop vomiting, rehydrate the child, and possibly use prokinetic agents (apparently erythromycin has been used for this).

1.3.2, "Abdominal migraine," is also a recurrent disorder in this age group, with episodes of midline abdominal pain lasting 1 to 72 hours (if untreated). The pain is midline or poorly localized and dull and the intensity is moderate to severe. It is accompanied by a least two of the following: nausea, anorexia, vomiting, and pallor. It is "not attributed to another disorder" (as usual for ICHD). Evidence supports the effectiveness of pizotifen (not available in the United States). Propranolol and cyproheptadine (which has some similarities to pizotifen) have also been used.

1.3.3, "Benign paroxysmal vertigo of childhood," consists of at least five episodes of severe vertigo lasting minutes to hours with normal audiogram and electroencephalogram, neurologic examination, and vestibular function between attacks. Vomiting and nystagmus may occur, as may headache. Antihistamines have been used to treat this condition (e.g., betahistine).

HEADACHE TREATMENT IN PREGNANCY AND LACTATION

As above, there is a paucity of good data, but recommendations exist for treatment of headache in pregnant women with migraine and during lactation (U.S. Headache Consortium).

Again, no drug has FDA approval. In pregnancy, all drugs should be avoided to the extent possible. Vomiting and dehydration may be injurious to the health of both the mother and the fetus. Non-pharmacologic measures are the treatment of choice. Fifty percent to 80% of women who have migraine without aura/menstrually associated migraine will have a significant reduction in headache attacks by the end of the first trimester (those who do not improve by then are unlikely to experience improvement as the pregnancy progresses). With any worsening of the headache pattern, the clinician should always consider the possibility that a secondary headache is declaring itself (e.g., pituitary tumor, stroke, venous sinus thrombosis, eclampsia).

Acute therapy of headache in pregnancy (Table 15–1) includes acetaminophen (suppositories may be preferable to the oral route if there is a lot of nausea/vomiting) and nonsteroidal anti-inflammatories (NSAIDs) (until week 32,

Table 15–1 Example of Treatment Options in Pregnancy

Treatment Option	Dose/Route	Comment
Acetaminophen	650 mg orally q4–6h prn	
Promethazine	25–50 mg orally q4–6h prn	
Meperidine	50–150 mg orally q4–6h prn	May be used IM as well
Prednisone	60 mg orally/daily for 3 days	Then taper over 4 days
Occipital nerve blocks	1 cc 1% lidocaine	May add steroid
Intravenous magnesium	1–2 g BID prn	Follow serum levels
Intravenous hydration	For dehydration	

after which they can cause premature closure of the ductus arteriosus). Opioids may be used within strict limits. Drug intake should be monitored to avoid analgesic rebound/medication overuse headache. Anti-emetics such as metoclopramide, prochlorperazine, and promethazine are quite useful. During a severe acute attack intravenous hydration and intravenous magnesium have been used and are safe. Judicious use of steroids may be considered. Occipital nerve blocks seem reasonable. Triptans do not have FDA approval in pregnancy, but the sumatriptan registry suggests no increased occurrence of birth defects, so mothers who inadvertently use sumatriptan prior to realizing they were pregnant may be reassured. Ergots must be strictly avoided as they are category X.

Preventive drug therapy during pregnancy is best avoided if possible. Recognition of medication overuse headache may allow a reduction in the amount of acute medication taken and allow for an improvement in the headache frequency. When necessary, several drugs are category C: propranolol, amitriptyline, topiramate, and verapamil (verapamil is tocolytic).

Regarding headache treatment during lactation, all drugs get into breast milk and therefore ideally should be avoided. While sumatriptan does not have an FDA indication for this use, the package insert suggests that infant exposure can be minimized by pumping/storing and then discarding breast milk for 8 to 12 hours after using sumatriptan.

HEADACHE IN THE ELDERLY

Primary headaches can continue into old age in patients or may begin de novo. Diagnoses to consider in this context include tension-type headache, migraine, cluster, chronic daily headache, SUNCT, medication overuse headache, and hypnic headache. Always consider the possibility of secondary headache, such as that due to mass lesion or giant cell arteritis (also known as temporal arteritis or Horton's disease). Trigeminal neuralgia (which may cause diagnostic uncertainty with or overlap with SUNCT) and post-herpetic neuralgia frequently affect the elderly. Headaches related to Parkinson's disease may respond to treatment of the parkinsonism itself. When choosing drug therapy in the elderly, remember the limitations of reduced hepatic and renal function and make appropriate dosage adjustments. Coronary artery disease becomes more likely with advancing age, and there are few safety data on using triptans in this age group.

Giant cell arteritis usually occurs in patients 50 years old and up, and they usually have an erythrocyte sedimentation rate (ESR) of at least 50 mm/hr. C-reactive protein may be useful to monitor disease activity. Giant cell arteritis can cause a headache that resembles any type of primary headache: constant or intermittent, localized or holocranial. There may be intermittent visual symptoms (e.g., amaurosis fugax), jaw claudication, tender scalp vessels, and polymyalgia rheumatica. This diagnosis must be considered in any individual 50 years old and up with a new or worsening headache. Headache is the most

common symptom, occurring in at least 90% of patients. Start steroids immediately (e.g., prednisone 60 to 80 mg/day) if you are entertaining this diagnosis
and arrange for a temporal artery biopsy relatively soon (ideally as soon as possible, within a week). Serial sections of the specimen are necessary due to the
presence of "skip lesions." If the first biopsy is negative, a biopsy of the contralateral side may prove rewarding. A positive biopsy is useful but not necessary to
fulfill ICHD-II criteria. If not treated successfully, 50% or more of patients with
giant cell arteritis may become blind; stroke may also occur, usually in the posterior circulation. The occipital artery may be tender and the patient may have
symptoms suggestive of "occipital neuralgia."

ICHD-II recognizes 10.6, "Cardiac cephalgia." These headaches may be
severe, with nausea, and aggravated by exertion, and are due to myocardial
ischemia. Chest pain may not be present. Treatment is directed toward the
underlying myocardial ischemia. Triptans and other vasoconstrictors obviously
should not be administered.

4.5, "Hypnic headache," is a dull headache that awakens the patient from
sleep (including from naps) and usually occurs more than 15 times per
month. It usually lasts more than 15 minutes and has an onset in patients
older than 50 years. Unlike trigeminal autonomic cephalgias, there are no
autonomic symptoms and no more than one of nausea, photophobia, or
phonophobia. Treatment options include caffeine, lithium, indomethacin,
and flunarizine.

Trigeminal neuralgia consists of attacks of lancinating pain lasting a fraction
of a second to a few minutes. The second and third divisions of cranial nerve V
are most frequently involved; the first division is involved less often. ICHD-II
describes the "classical" form (presumably due to compression of the nerve by
an aberrant vessel) and secondary forms (e.g., due to a mass lesion in the cerebellopontine angle). The classical form may have a refractory period after an
attack, while secondary forms may have associated sensory loss. Neuroimaging
is necessary (MRI/MRA with gadolinium). Treatment of the classical form
includes carbamazepine, baclofen, clonazepam, other anticonvulsants/mem-
brane stabilizers, and microvascular decompression. Trigeminal neuralgia may
cause diagnostic confusion or overlap with SUNCT.

HEADACHE IN RENAL DISEASE

Headache commonly occurs in patients with renal failure. Low magnesium levels have been implicated. Headache is the most common complaint in those
undergoing hemodialysis (up to 70% in some series). It is also seen in the disequilibrium syndrome, which includes headache, cerebral swelling, stupor, seizures, and coma. ICHD-II lists 10.2, "Dialysis headache." This consists of at
least three attacks in a dialysis patient of acute headache occurring in at least
half of sessions. The headache resolves within 72 hours after each session and
will cease after successful renal transplantation. The headache is usually bilateral,

may be dull or throbbing, and has a mean duration of 5 hours. Caffeine is highly dialyzable, so caffeine-withdrawal headache is in the differential. Risk factors for dialysis headache include hypertension, high BUN, low serum osmolality, and low serum magnesium.

Finally, gabapentin undergoes neither hepatic nor renal metabolism but it is renally excreted. Similar considerations apply to pregabalin.

SUMMARY

Treatment of patients in these special populations requires understanding the limitations imposed by their particular situations. For pregnant patients, concerns about safety and lack of information limit treatment options, and therefore non-pharmacologic options are important to remember. For children, while there are recommendations for treatment, there is limited evidence to guide therapeutic selection. Certain diagnoses come into consideration for the elderly, such as giant cell arteritis and other secondary headaches. Headache is a very common problem for patients with renal disease, and knowledge about this problem is of great practical value.

Review Questions

1. A 14-year-old girl comes to your office with a history of disabling migraine headaches associated with nausea and vomiting. She is missing 2 days of school per month and sometimes has difficulty when she is at school due to the headaches. Her positive family history of migraine, presence of triggers, and normal examination reassure you she has migraine. Which is the best choice for treating this patient?
   a. Aspirin in adequate doses both as an acute remedy and as prevention
   b. Adequate doses of ibuprofen and/or acetaminophen acutely
   c. Intranasal sumatriptan
   d. Prochlorperazine rectally
2. You base your choice mainly on:
   a. FDA recommendations for the drug
   b. AAN Practice Parameter
   c. Package inserts
   d. NIH research that guides practice
3. For a child with frequent migraine in need of prophylaxis, which choice is not thought to be effective?
   a. Propranolol
   b. Topiramate
   c. Cyproheptadine
   d. Fluoxetine

4. Headache may occur as part of the ICHD-II diagnostic criteria for:
   a. Cyclic vomiting
   b. Abdominal migraine
   c. Benign paroxysmal vertigo of childhood
   d. None of the above
5. For patients who are pregnant or lactating, which drug has FDA approval?
   a. Sumatriptan
   b. Topiramate, but only in patients who are lactating
   c. Dihydroergotamine nasal spray
   d. None
6. A 32-year-old pregnant woman has frequent severe attacks of migraine with intractable nausea and vomiting to the point of recurrent dehydration. You determine that the potential benefits of preventive therapy justify the risks of use. Which drug is absolutely contraindicated?
   a. Amitriptyline
   b. Methysergide
   c. Propranolol
   d. Topiramate
7. Which statement is true about giant cell arteritis?
   a. Headache is the most common symptom.
   b. Blindness occurs in more than 80% of untreated patients.
   c. ICHD-II criteria require a positive temporal artery biopsy.
   d. The presence of what seems to be "occipital neuralgia" suggests alternative diagnoses.
8. An 80-year-old man has headaches that awaken him from sleep. Which features are true of hypnic and cluster headaches that will enable you to differentiate them?
   a. Neither can have aura.
   b. Hypnic headache has no autonomic features, while cluster headache does.
   c. Cluster headache responds to lithium, while hypnic headache does not.
   d. Hypnic headache occurs only at night.
9. Trigeminal neuralgia:
   a. May have associated sensory loss if it is "secondary"
   b. Is likely to have associated sensory loss if it is "classical"
   c. Is easy to differentiate from SUNCT
   d. Responds to the same best therapy for idiopathic stabbing headache
10. You have a patient with multiple organ failure and on multiple drugs who needs headache prevention. You wish to use a drug that is neither hepatically nor renally metabolized. You select:
   a. Topiramate
   b. Valproate
   c. Gabapentin
   d. Tincture of opium

1. c
2. b
3. d
4. c
5. d
6. b
7. a
8. b
9. a
10. c

SUGGESTED READING

Antoniazzi, A.L., Bigal, M.E., Bordini, C.A., et al. Headache and hemodialysis: A prospective study. *Headache* 43 (2003): 99–102.

Antoniazzi, A.L., Bigal, M.E., Bordini, C.A., & Speciali, J.G. Headache associated with dialysis: The International Headache Society criteria revisited. *Cephalalgia* 23 (2003): 146–149.

Classification Committee of the International Headache Society. International Classification of Headache Disorders II. *Cephalalgia* 24, Suppl. 1 (2004): 1–160.

Gladstone, J., Eross, E., & Dodick, D.W. Migraine in special populations. Treatment strategies for children and adolescents, pregnant women, and the elderly. *Postgraduate Medicine* 115, no. 4 (2004): 39–50.

Göksan, B., Karaali-Savrun, F., Ertan, S., & Savrun, M. Haemodialysis-related headache. *Cephalagia* 24 (2004): 284–287.

Goksel, B.K., Torun, D., Karac, S., et al. Is low blood magnesium level associated with hemodialysis headache? *Headache* 46 (2006): 40–45.

Gutierrez-Morlote, J., & Pascual, J. Cardiac cephalgia is not necessarily an exertional headache: A case report. *Cephalalgia* 22 (2002): 765–766.

Jameson, M.D., & Weigmann, T.B. Principles, uses and complications of hemodialysis. *Medical Clinics of North America* 74 (1990): 845–960.

Lewis, D., Ashwal, S., Hershey, A., et al. Practice Parameter: Pharmacological treatment of migraine headache in children and adolescents. Report of the American Academy of Neurology Quality Standards Subcommittee and the Practice Committee of the Child Neurology Society. *Neurology* 63 (2004): 2215–2224.

Lipton, R.B., Lowenkopf, T., Bajwa, Z.H., et al. Cardiac cephalgia: A treatable form of exertional headache. *Neurology* 49, no. 3 (1997): 813–816.

Olesen, J., Goadsby, P.J., Ramadan, N.M., Tfelt-Hansen, P., Welch, K.M.A., eds. *The headaches*, 3rd ed. Philadelphia: Lippincott Williams & Wilkins, 2006.

Silberstein, S.D., Lipton, R.B., & Goadsby, P.J., eds. *Headache in clinical practice*, 2nd ed. Oxford: Isis Medical Media, Ltd., 2002.

U.S. Headache Consortium Guidelines. Available at: www.aan.com

Victor, S., & Ryan, S.W. Drugs for preventing migraine headaches in children. *Cochrane Database Systematic Reviews* 2003; (4): CD002761.

Ward, T.N. Headache disorders in the elderly. *Current Treatment Options in Neurology* 4, no. 5 (2002): 403–408.

Ward, T.N., & Levin, M. "Facial pain." In: *Principles and Practice of Pain Medicine*, 2nd ed., eds. Warfield, C., & Bajwa, Z. New York: McGraw-Hill, Inc. 2003, pp. 246–251.

Ward, T.N., & Levin, M. Headache in giant cell arteritis and other arteritides. *Neurologic Science* 26, suppl. 2 (2005): S134–S137.

Ward, T.N., Levin, M., & Wong, R.L. Headache caused by giant cell arteritis. *Current Treatment Options in Neurology* 6, no. 6 (2004): 499–505.

16

Inpatient Headache Treatment

Thomas N. Ward, MD

Headache patients are usually managed on an outpatient basis, but under certain circumstances inpatient treatment may be appropriate. There is limited literature about this, in part because few physicians and few facilities provide this option. If inpatient treatment is considered, then a clear plan for that admission with predetermined goals is necessary. Much can be accomplished in a short time with appropriate planning and patient selection.

REASONS FOR CHOOSING HOSPITAL ADMISSION

Patients who are doing poorly as outpatients may benefit from admission. Emergency situations due to psychiatric decompensation or refractoriness to adequate trials of outpatient therapy or if the patient and/or family and/or provider are at "wit's end" all are scenarios suggesting that inpatient therapy might be a reasonable option. Before considering an admission, various possible reasons for failure of outpatient therapy must be looked at. Medication overuse/analgesic rebound is often not recognized and renders patients refractory to preventive medications and worsens the overall headache pattern. Side effects of medications may be causing headache (e.g., proton pump inhibitors) or preventing compliance (e.g., gastrointestinal side effects from indomethacin). Confounding or comorbid medical conditions, such as the emergence of coronary artery disease in a patient who had responded well to triptans, may lead to therapeutic dilemmas. Occasionally medical mismanagement is the problem, including incorrect therapeutic selection leading to treatment failure (e.g., propranolol chosen to treat cluster headache). Beyond this, inadequate or improper medication trials and unreasonable expectations on the part of both patients and providers may lead to outcomes that are incorrectly perceived as "poor." Prior to admission for inpatient headache treatment, it is often advisable to obtain second opinions and consultations to ensure that outpatient therapy has been optimized.

GOALS OF INPATIENT ADMISSION

A therapeutic target for the admission needs to be identified. Some goals include controlling the anticipated withdrawal headache that occurs upon withdrawing medications perpetuating analgesic rebound, rehydrating a dehydrated patient with intractable headache and vomiting, obtaining multiple consultations rapidly (pain service, psychiatry, behavioral medicine), and obtaining further tests, such as thyroid-stimulating hormone levels, MRI, and lumbar puncture (including an opening pressure; look for increased intracranial pressure or low cerebrospinal fluid pressure).

Most patients who end up being admitted for "intractable headache" and then subsequently improve turn out to have analgesic rebound headache/medication overuse headache. The therapeutic goal is to remove the offending medications (and not to initiate other analgesic-rebound–inducing medications) and to control the ensuing withdrawal headache and associated symptoms until they subside. The duration of withdrawal symptoms due to triptan drugs is usually brief (1 to 2 days), while the period for analgesics, especially those containing butalbital, is longer (several days). Abruptly stopping butalbital, at higher doses, carries a risk of provoking delirium and/or seizures, so it can either be tapered or replaced with a bedtime dosage of phenobarbital, which has a much longer half-life (100 mg of butalbital is approximately equal to 30 mg of phenobarbital).

TREATMENT STRATEGIES IN THE INPATIENT SETTING

During inpatient treatment great attention must be paid to detail, as small errors in treatment protocols may result in treatment failure. Clonidine and especially neuroleptics can help suppress withdrawal symptoms, allowing for cessation of narcotics. Medications that can cause rebound must be avoided. Sedating medications can be especially useful during the withdrawal period. Strict bed rest may be necessary (e.g., intravenous chlorpromazine can cause impressive orthostatic hypotension), and if so, then measures must be instituted to lessen the risk of deep venous thrombosis (Table 16–1).

The pain service may be used to administer blocks (e.g., for neck pain, low back pain) if narcotics that were being used to treat pain from those chronic

Table 16–1 Examples of Inpatient Treatment Regimens

Protocol	Typical Doses
Modified "Raskin"	25 mg IV diphenhydramine/10 mg IV metoclopramide/0.5–1 mg DHE IV tid
Prochlorperazine	25 mg IV diphenhydramine/5–10 mg IV prochlorperazine/0.5–1 mg DHE IV tid
Chlorpromazine	25 mg IV diphenhydramine/10 mg IV chlorpromazine tid
Depacon	IV valproate 300–500 mg given over approximately 5–10 minutes
Magnesium	1–2 g IV magnesium over 10–20 minutes BID (follow serum levels)
Toradol	30 mg IV ketorolac q6h prn (limit 5 days)

conditions are being stopped. Occipital nerve blocks can be dramatically effective, particularly for unilateral headaches with neck pain.

The "Raskin" protocol uses repetitive intravenous metoclopramide 10 mg followed by the effective subnauseating dose of dihydroergotamine (DHE) (0.25 to 1 mg) tid. Akathisia or dystonic reactions can be ameliorated by intravenous diphenhydramine 25 mg or benztropine mesylate. The regimen is given tid, not q8h (to avoid awakening sleeping headache patients: you cannot have a headache when you are asleep!). Three days of therapy is typical, although some patients may benefit from longer stays. Most if not all analgesics must be stopped: a common error is to initiate or continue meperidine, which renders the protocol ineffective. Meperidine, by the way, is a potent serotonin uptake inhibitor, and data suggest it is potentially dangerous in our headache patients, who are often on multiple drugs that affect serotonin levels. Intravenous prochlorperazine 5 to 10 mg can be substituted for the metoclopramide, especially if sedation is desired. Dihydroergotamine must be avoided in pregnancy and should also be avoided in coronary artery disease.

Intravenous chlorpromazine (preceded by intravenous diphenhydramine or benztropine mesylate), titrated to a dose that renders the patient lightly asleep, is quite useful. A reasonable initial dose is 10 mg tid. If the patient becomes hypotensive during therapy, intravenous boluses of saline may be helpful; sometimes rather than advancing the doses of intravenous chlorpromazine, a dose of oral clonazepam (0.5 to 1 mg) may be added to tip the patient into unconsciousness.

Intravenous valproate has been advocated for acute headache therapy: 300 to 500 mg is run in rather rapidly over 5 to 10 minutes. This may be repeated. A serum pregnancy test prior to administration would be appropriate in females of childbearing potential (this would also apply prior to the initiation of DHE, which is pregnancy category X).

It makes good sense to use intravenous magnesium, although there is little evidence to support its use. It is certainly safe, and there are anecdotal reports of efficacy. In pregnant patients and in patients with hemiplegic migraine it can easily be justified as safe, and if it is ineffective it does not preclude trials of other measures. A dose of 1 g initially is given over 5 to 10 minutes. Some have used up to 2 g given intravenously bid (serum magnesium levels should be followed; although ionized magnesium levels would be more relevant, they are generally unavailable).

Intravenous ketorolac 30 mg given every 6 hours as needed for several days can be a helpful addition for breakthrough headaches during inpatient treatment. Sometimes steroids may provide benefit. When we are treating patients acutely we also typically begin prophylactic medication(s) so we know patients can tolerate them. We also educate patients about reasonable expectations of the therapy. Prior to discharge they are given an action plan for how to deal with acute headache attacks after discharge and a rescue plan to let them stop vomiting and achieve sleep when their usual acute therapy may fail. They are discharged with instructions to keep a headache calendar and to return for a headache clinic appointment 1 to 3 weeks after discharge.

With meticulous attention to detail, approximately 70% of such difficult patients are either headache-free or substantially improved upon discharge. Failure to improve portends a bad prognosis, but some of those patients do improve. Some require hospitalizations longer than the average 3-day stay of most of our patients. Failure to improve mandates a reassessment of the diagnosis, and some patients end up undergoing more invasive treatments such as occipital nerve stimulators or surgery for causes of headaches (e.g., upper cervical root entrapments).

SUMMARY

With appropriate planning and patient selection, most patients with intractable headaches benefit from inpatient treatment. Much can be accomplished in a relatively short time, such as 3 days. If reasonable expectations have been set, satisfaction for both the patient and practitioner can be achieved. During the admission, attention to detail is mandatory, and close follow-up after discharge can allow therapeutic gains to be maintained.

Review Questions

1. For inpatient headache admissions with suspected medication overuse headache, the goal is:
   a. To control the withdrawal headache and stop medications that can cause medication overuse headache
   b. To obtain video-EEG monitoring and other essential tests expeditiously
   c. To render the patient unconscious so he or she doesn't suffer
   d. To stop all medications to allow ascertainment of which medications are causing the refractory headache
2. A 42-year-old man who was taking 24 butalbital-containing pills per day is admitted to a community hospital, where his butalbital is stopped. Two days later he worsens dramatically. Which complication is least likely to be needed in the differential diagnosis?
   a. Increased intracranial pressure
   b. Increased headache
   c. Seizures
   d. Delirium
3. Which strategy is most likely to fail if you admit a patient on high doses of narcotics and you wish to avoid/suppress withdrawal symptoms?
   a. Give intravenous prochlorperazine.
   b. Use intravenous chlorpromazine.
   c. Use clonidine.
   d. Use ketorolac.

4. Which statement about the use of repetitive DHE therapy is untrue?
   a. The full 1-mg dose three times a day is optimal.
   b. Adding meperidine may be used to boost efficacy.
   c. It may be done for longer than 3 days.
   d. Prochlorperazine may be substituted for metoclopramide.
5. Which statement best describes intravenous magnesium therapy for migraine?
   a. It is safe.
   b. It has been proven effective.
   c. It can only be used safely during pregnancy.
   d. It cannot be used in conjunction with other drugs.
6. Your patient is 36 weeks pregnant and has intractable headache with vomiting. Which is the best treatment option?
   a. Intravenous ketorolac because it is now after week 32
   b. The repetitive DHE protocol (plus metoclopramide) because it is now the third trimester and major organ malformation and neural tube defects are no longer a limiting factor
   c. Intravenous magnesium and hydration
   d. Indomethacin suppositories
7. During an admission for intractable headache the most important thing is:
   a. To involve the chaplaincy service
   b. To stop all potentially offending medications and initiate as many medication trials as possible
   c. To get numerous consultations, especially with psychiatry and pain services
   d. To have a therapeutic goal communicated to the patient and a plan to implement it
8. In diagnosing a headache patient and using a lumbar puncture, which test should always be included?
   a. Closing pressure
   b. Opening pressure
   c. Opening and closing pressure
   d. Tumor necrosis factor-beta
9. You admit a 73-year-old man with daily headache that seems to be triggered by walking or running. He has no chest pain. Once admitted he develops his typical severe bilateral headache while walking on the unit. Which drug is most reasonable to give him initially while awaiting further (stat) workup?
   a. Dihydroergotamine 1 mg IV
   b. Sumatriptan 6 mg SC
   c. Zolmitriptan 5 mg intranasal
   d. Nitroglycerin 0.4 mg SL

10. In headache clinics the most common type of headache problem to improve with an admission is:
   a. Indomethacin-responsive headaches
   b. New daily persistent headache
   c. Medication overuse headache (analgesic rebound)
   d. Chronic cluster headache

10. c
9. d
8. b
7. d
6. c
5. a
4. b
3. d
2. a
1. a

SUGGESTED READING

Ashkenazi, A., Levin, M., & Ward, T.N. Treatment of chronic daily headache with intravenous chlorpromazine (abstract S135). Presented at the 44th Annual Scientific Meeting of the American Headache Society, Seattle, WA, June 2002.

Hand, P.J., & Stark, R.J. Intravenous lignocaine infusions for severe chronic daily headache. *Medical Journal of Australia* 172, no. 4 (2000): 157–159.

Katsarava, Z., Fritsche, G., Muessig, M., Diener, H.C., & Limmroth, V. Clinical features of withdrawal headache following overuse of triptans and other headache drugs. *Neurology* 57, no. 9 (2001): 1694–1698.

Krusz, J.C., Cagle, J., & Scott, V. Intravenous valproate for treatment of status migrainosus in the headache clinic: A retrospective look. *Headache and Pain* 17, no. 3 (2006): 121–123.

Krusz, J.C., Scott, V., & Belanger, J. Intravenous propofol: Unique effectiveness in treating intractable migraine. *Headache* 40, no. 3 (2000): 2224–2230.

Mathew, N.T., Kailsam, J., Meadors, L., Chernyschev, O., & Gentry, P. Intravenous valproate sodium (Depacon®) aborts migraine rapidly: A preliminary report. *Headache* 40, no. 9 (2000): 720–723.

Mathew, N.T., Kurman, R., & Perez, F. Drug-induced refractory headache—clinical features and management. *Headache* 30 (1990): 634–638.

Mathew, N.T., Reuveni, U., & Perez, F. Transformed or evolutive migraine. *Headache* 27, no. 2 (1987): 102–106.

Rapoport, A.M., & Sheftell, F.D. "Inpatient treatment of primary headache disorders." In *Headache disorders. A management guide for practitioners*, eds. Rapoport, A.M., & Sheftell, F.D. Philadelphia: WB Saunders, 1996: p. 148.

Rapoport, A.M., & Weeks, R.E. "Analgesic rebound headache." In *A clinician's guide to diagnosis, pathophysiology, and treatment strategies*, eds. Rapoport, A.M., & Sheftell, F.D. Costa Mesa, CA: PMA Publishing Corp., 1993: pp. 157–165.

Raskin, N.H. Repetitive intravenous dihydroergotamine as therapy for intractable migraine. *Neurology* 36 (1986): 995–997.

Silberstein, S.D., & Silberstein, J.R. Chronic daily headache: Prognosis following inpatient treatment with repetitive IV DHE. *Headache* 32 (1992): 439–445.

Smith, T.R. Low-dose tizanidine with non-steroidal anti-inflammatory for detoxification from analgesic rebound headache. *Headache* 42 (2002): 175–177.

Ward, T.N. Medication overuse headache. *Primary Care Clinician Office Practitioner* 31 (2004): 369–380.

17

Non-Pharmacologic Headache Treatment

Randall E. Weeks, PhD

Most clinicians agree that biobehavioral factors are important considerations in the assessment and treatment of headache patients. Psychological and behavioral issues become important treatment concerns if the frequency of a patient's headaches increases, there is increased disability secondary to headaches, and/ or there is inadequate response to usually effective pharmacotherapy. Patients with long histories of chronic headache are candidates for comprehensive treatment strategies that include both pharmacologic and non-pharmacologic treatment modalities. This chapter will offer an introduction to relevant behavioral variables that the physician should consider in the assessment and treatment of headache patients and an overview of non-pharmacologic treatment options for headache patients, including when available the evidence base for such treatments.

It should be emphasized that *non-pharmacologic treatments are not anti-pharmacologic*. The combination of both pharmacologic and non-pharmacologic treatments has been shown to be superior to each individually and appears to maximize long-term therapeutic benefit. In addition, effective non-pharmacologic strategies help to ensure pharmacologic treatment compliance, which has been shown to be a significant problem with headache patients.

In 2000, the U.S. Headache Consortium noted the following reasons that cause migraine patients to seek non-pharmacologic treatment for migraine headache:

1. Patient preference
2. Poor tolerance/poor response to preventive medications
3. Medical contraindications to medications
4. Pregnancy, planned pregnancy, or lactation
5. History of overuse of acute-care medications
6. Significant stress or deficient coping strategies

Goals of non-pharmacologic treatment included:

1. Reduced frequency/severity of headache
2. Reduced headache-related disability

3. Reduced reliance on poorly tolerated or unwanted pharmacotherapy
4. Enhanced personal control of pain
5. Reduced headache-related distress and psychological symptoms

Other authors have noted that non-pharmacologic treatment strategies should be considered for the following reasons:

- As viable treatment options to augment pharmacologic therapy
- As important treatment approaches for children and adolescents
- To maximize the long-term maintenance of pharmacologic treatment
- Most importantly, because they have been found to be effective

In sum, migraine and other types of headaches are highly prevalent and affect not only individual patients (and their families) but also society at large. Direct and indirect costs of disability have a negative impact on personal, social, and economic systems. Patients with complex headache histories (and those whose headaches have been refractory to usually effective pharmacotherapy) require careful assessment and comprehensive treatment, which frequently includes both pharmacologic and non-pharmacologic interventions.

BEHAVIORAL FACTORS TO CONSIDER IN HEADACHE TREATMENT PLANNING

No chapter on non-pharmacologic treatment of headache would be complete without a brief discussion of behavioral factors that should be considered in treatment planning and in setting goals for headache treatment. These factors have been shown to affect treatment efficacy whether the interventions are pharmacologic or non-pharmacologic. Effective treatment begins with an evaluation and understanding of the context in which a patient's head pain occurs. It is important to identify and treat the relevant environmental, behavioral, and psychological variables that may exist as triggers and/or may be maintenance factors in a patient's head pain.

A careful headache and medical history is essential to establish an ICHD-II diagnosis. Although there have been recent efforts to develop brief screening instruments to diagnose migraine headaches, most clinicians rely on structured, behavioral interviews to arrive at an initial diagnosis. These approaches are quite similar across settings, and they have been shown to be reliable and effective in diagnosing headache in both adults and children.

Headache data are gathered with respect to how many days out of the month that the patient is, in fact, dysfunctional. The impact that severe or incapacitating headache has on the patient's ability to function (e.g., decreasing pleasurable events, creating greater social isolation, causing enhanced feelings of guilt) should be recorded. Headache triggers and changes in the headache pattern based on alterations in stress levels, hormonal changes, dietary triggers, weather changes, and disturbance in behavioral routine (e.g., changes in sleep patterns, missing meals) are important to recognize and may require behavioral treatment.

Many headache patients present with a variety of concerns in addition to or secondary to their head pain. Patients may have optimistic or pessimistic feelings about treatment based on previous experiences. Effective diagnosis and treatment planning can occur only after an assessment of the specific needs of the individual patient. This is relevant, as studies have shown that differences can (and do) exist between patient and physician goals for treatment.

A significant problem in treating headache patients has been poor compliance with previous pharmacologic and non-pharmacologic interventions. There is a vast literature showing that headache and other medical patients fail to take abortive and preventive medications as prescribed. Treatment drop-out and inconsistency in keeping appointments are problems for the treating clinician. It is ironic that practitioners tend to change treatment strategies and medication regimens without doing a complete assessment as to whether the patient has been compliant with previous and/or present treatment. Adherence should be viewed as an ongoing treatment variable and should be addressed at the initial evaluation.

Recent research has identified "modifiable" risk factors for migraine and headache progression. These variables include attack frequency, obesity, medication overuse, stressful life events, caffeine overuse, and snoring/sleep apnea. Identification and aggressive treatment of such factors is critical. Non-pharmacologic treatment approaches (especially when implemented early in the patient's headache history) are indicated to address these risk factors.

Identification of subgroups of patients with medication overuse headache has been shown to predict treatment outcome. One approach divides these patients into two groups—those with type 1 or "simple" histories (relatively short-term drug overuse, relatively modest amounts of overused medications, minimal psychiatric contribution, and no history of relapse of after drug withdrawal) versus those with type 2 or "complex" histories (multiple psychiatric comorbidities and history of relapse). It is believed that the type 1 group should be treated aggressively to prevent them from evolving into type 2 patients. Non-pharmacologic treatments are strongly recommended in addition to appropriate pharmacotherapy. Type 2 patients must have both pharmacologic and non-pharmacologic treatments.

Obtaining an accurate, complete medication history is critical. It is important to assess not only what medication that the patient is taking (both prescription and over-the-counter preparations) but also at what point in the pain process that the patient medicates. Headache recurrence should be noted as well as the patient's feelings regarding the medication's efficacy. Previous medication overuse should be evaluated. Dose levels need to be assessed in terms of whether the patient had an adequate therapeutic trial and/or whether the medication (especially preventive agents) was taken in the presence of medication overuse headache. The patient's subjective sense of which medication has been the most effective in the past may also be revealing. In some cases, it may be necessary to establish "treatment boundaries" if there is more than one physician treating the patient for different medical conditions.

The patient's current and previous use of nicotine, caffeine, alcohol, and substances should be assessed. Sleep difficulties or disturbances should be evaluated. Consistency in eating habits, caffeine consumption, and sleep patterns should be assessed, as all can contribute to headache and may be markers of an underlying affective disturbance. Previous psychiatric history and symptoms should be noted.

There should be an assessment of the family's reaction to the patient's headaches, as well as any areas of family conflict. This is especially important in the evaluation of a child with headache. The impact of the patient's headaches on academic/vocational systems should be assessed. The number of absences and degree of disability should be noted. Variables such as job security in adults or the need for "homebound" tutoring with adolescents should be explored. Evidence of secondary gain from headache disability should be assessed.

In sum, effective treatment begins with building a positive, therapeutic relationship with patients during the initial consultation. Patients should be advised that they must be active participants in their headache care: there is a shared responsibility between the patient and clinician regarding headache improvement.

REVIEW OF NON-PHARMACOLOGIC TREATMENTS

The importance of non-pharmacologic treatments has been recognized by headache practitioners for many years. As with pharmacologic research, however, demonstration of the clinical effects of non-pharmacologic treatment has been limited by the lack of controlled studies to demonstrate efficacy, lack of diagnostic consistency between studies, lack of standardization between treatment and outcome measures, lack of control for medication overuse, and a myriad of other methodologic shortcomings. Despite these shortcomings, a summary of the clinical data will be offered.

In 2000, the U.S. Headache Consortium evidentiary panel conducted an evidence-based review and published their results regarding the behavioral treatment of migraine. The grading system used in determining the quality of evidence was as follows:

Grade A—Multiple well-designed randomized clinical trials, directly relevant to the recommendation, yielded a consistent pattern of findings.
Grade B—Some evidence from randomized clinical trials supported the recommendation, but the scientific support was not optimal.
Grade C—The consortium achieved consensus on the recommendation in the absence of relevant randomized controlled trials.

The consortium concluded the following with respect to behavioral treatments for migraine headache:

> *Grade A Evidence*—Relaxation training, thermal biofeedback combined with relaxation, electromyographic biofeedback, and cognitive-behavioral therapy may be considered as treatment options for the prevention of migraine.
>
> *Grade B Evidence*—Behavioral therapy may be combined with preventive drug therapy to achieve added clinical improvement for migraine.
>
> *Grade C Evidence*—Evidence-based treatment recommendations are not yet possible regarding the use of hypnosis, acupuncture, transcutaneous electrical nerve stimulation (TENS), cervical manipulation, occlusal adjustment, and hyperbaric oxygen as preventive or acute therapy for migraine.

A 2007 review by Andrasik (a "meta-analysis" of the meta-analyses of behavioral treatment) noted that early meta-analyses were overly inclusive. Such reviews compared studies that included limited sample sizes and were poorly designed with research that was well designed and adequately powered. Hence, it was difficult to interpret the results from each specific analysis of these early meta-analyses. A summary of references of meta-analyses of behavioral treatments for migraine and tension-type headaches is given in the Suggested Reading list at the end of the chapter.

With respect to the treatment of migraine headaches, analysis of the results of these studies suggested that behavioral treatments such as relaxation, temperature biofeedback, temperature biofeedback plus relaxation, electromyographic biofeedback, cognitive-behavioral therapy, and cognitive-behavioral therapy plus temperature biofeedback were superior to control conditions. There were no major differences between the behavioral treatments and medications in both direct and indirect comparisons.

In the analysis of meta-analyses evaluating behavioral treatment of tension-type headache, it was concluded that behavioral treatments such as relaxation, electromyographic biofeedback, electromyographic biofeedback plus relaxation, and cognitive-behavioral therapy were superior to control conditions. As with the migraine data, there was no significant difference between the behavioral treatments and medication.

Recent reviews have examined physical treatments for headaches. A 2004 Cochrane Review found evidence that cervical spinal manipulation may be an effective short-term treatment option, but evidence was weaker for a combination of TENS and electrical neurotransmitter modulation. Amitriptyline was found to be more effective than spinal manipulation in treating tension-type headaches, although the latter appeared to have longer-lasting benefit after treatment cessation. The relatively poor quality of research and lack of replication made such results difficult to interpret, however. Two later reviews failed to find consistent efficacy of spinal manipulation and other physiotherapy strategies in the treatment of migraine and tension-type headache. It was concluded that physical treatments should complement, not replace, better-validated forms of treatment; more methodologically rigorous studies are needed to strengthen the evidence base; and most physical treatments appeared not to be dangerous except "high-velocity" neck manipulation.

Recent reviews have also examined the efficacy of acupuncture in treating headaches since the preliminary findings of the Headache Consortium in 2000. Though recent independent studies have found acupuncture to be an effective headache treatment, three reviews failed to find consistent effects of acupuncture versus "sham" acupuncture in the treatment of either migraine or tension-type headaches. Larger-scale, better-controlled research is needed to evaluate more clearly the effects of acupuncture as a clinical treatment for headache.

SUMMARY

Clinicians who treat headache patients need to be aware of biobehavioral issues in both the assessment and treatment of such patients. A variety of non-pharmacologic strategies have been shown to be effective individually and to enhance the efficacy of pharmacologic treatment of headache. Non-pharmacologic treatments are *not* anti-pharmacologic: maintenance of headache reduction seems to improve with the combination of such treatments. Such comprehensive treatment is essential with patients with frequent headache and complex headache histories.

The evidence base includes grade A efficacy for relaxation training, thermal biofeedback combined with relaxation training, electromyographic biofeedback, and cognitive-behavioral therapy for the prevention of migraine. Relaxation training, electromyographic biofeedback, relaxation training combined with electromyographic biofeedback, and cognitive-behavioral therapy were found to be superior to control conditions in the treatment of tension-type headache.

With the identification of "risk factors" in headache progression, comprehensive treatment early in the patient's headache history is indicated using both pharmacologic and non-pharmacologic treatments. Identification of specific populations that are especially amenable to non-pharmacologic treatment heightens the need to consider such interventions. Finally, the therapeutic effects and sustained efficacy of pharmacologic treatments have consistently and dramatically been shown to improve when they are combined with non-pharmacologic treatments.

Review Questions

1. Which of the following was listed by the U.S. Headache Consortium as having Grade A evidence regarding treatment efficacy for migraine headache?
   a. Acupuncture
   b. Spinal manipulation
   c. Cognitive-behavioral therapy
   d. None of the above

2. Which of the following is *not* true?
   a. Non-pharmacologic treatment should be considered only if pharmacologic treatment fails.
   b. Non-pharmacologic treatment is not anti-pharmacologic.
   c. Non-pharmacologic treatment enhances pharmacologic treatment.
   d. All are true.

3. Which of the following has been shown to be a "modifiable" risk factor for the progression of migraine and is amenable to non-pharmacologic treatment?
   a. Obesity
   b. Medication overuse
   c. Stress and stressful life experiences
   d. All have been identified as risk factors that should be treated.

4. Which of the following was listed by the U.S. Headache Consortium as having Grade A evidence regarding treatment efficacy for migraine headache?
   a. Thermal biofeedback combined with relaxation training
   b. Imagery exercises
   c. Massage therapy
   d. None of the above

5. According to meta-analytic studies of behavioral treatment of tension-type headache:
   a. Relaxation training was superior to control conditions
   b. Thermal biofeedback was superior to control conditions
   c. Guided imagery was superior to control conditions
   d. All are true

6. According to meta-analytic studies of behavioral treatment of migraine headache:
   a. Relaxation training was superior to control conditions
   b. Temperature biofeedback was superior to control conditions
   c. Cognitive-behavioral therapy was superior to control conditions
   d. All are true

7. Which of the following was listed by the U.S. Headache Consortium as having Grade A evidence regarding treatment efficacy for migraine headache?
   a. Hypnosis
   b. Cervical manipulation
   c. Electomyographic biofeedback
   d. None of the above

8. With respect to the efficacy of acupuncture in the treatment of headache:
   a. Meta-analytic data are supportive of efficacy
   b. There have been some recent positive studies, but more are needed to demonstrate efficacy
   c. There are differences in outcomes based on the type of acupuncture used
   d. All are true

9. Adherence to pharmacologic and non-pharmacologic headache treatment:
   a. Should be considered to be an ongoing treatment variable
   b. Has been shown to be poor
   c. Frequently leads to unnecessary changes in treatment strategies
   d. All are true

10. Which of the following was noted by the U.S. Headache Consortium as being a reason why migraine patients seek non-pharmacologic treatment?
   a. Patient preference
   b. Medical contraindications to medications
   c. Pregnancy
   d. All were listed as reasons for seeking non-pharmacologic treatment

10. d
1. c
2. a
3. d
4. a
5. a
6. d
7. c
8. b
9. d

SUGGESTED READING

Andrasik, F. What does the evidence show? Efficacy of behavioural treatments for recurrent headaches in adults. *Neurologic Science* 28 (2007): S70–S77.

Andrasik, F., & Schwartz, M.S. Behavioral assessment and treatment of pediatric head-ache. *Behavior Modification* 30 (2006): 93–113.

Bigal, M.E., & Lipton, R.B. Modifiable risk factors for migraine progression. *Headache* 46 (2006): 1334–1343.

Biondi, D. Physical treatments for headaches: A structured review. *Headache* 45 (2005): 738–746.

Blanchard, E.B., & Andrasik, F. "Biofeedback treatment of vascular headache." In *Biofeedback: Studies in clinical efficacy*, Eds. Hatch, J.P., Fisher, J.G., & Rugh, J.D. New York: Plenum, 1987: pp. 1–79.

Blanchard, E.B., Andrasik, F., Ahles, T.A., et al. Migraine and tension headache: a meta-analytic review. *Behavioral Therapy* 14 (1980): 613–631.

Bogaards, M.C., & ter Kuile, M.M. Treatment of recurrent tension headache: A meta-analytic review. *Clinical Journal of Pain* 10 (1994): 174–190.

Bronfort, G., Nilsson, N., & Haas, M. Non-invasive physical treatments for chronic/recurrent headache. *Cochrane Database Systematic Review*, 2004.

Campbell, J.K., Penzien, D.B., & Wall, E.M. Evidence-based guidelines for migraine headaches: Behavioral and physical treatments (Consortium guidelines). Available at: http://www.aan.com/professionals/practice/pdfs/g10089.pdf

Goslin, R.E., Gray, R.N., McCrory, D.C., et al. *Behavioral and physical treatments for migraine headache* (Technical Review 2.2). 1999; Prepared for the Agency for Health Care Policy and Research under Contract No. 290–94–2025. (NTIS Accession No. 127946).

Grazzi, L., Andrasik, F., D'Amico, D., Leone, M., Usai, S., Kass, S., & Bussone, G. Behavioral and pharmacologic treatment of transformed migraine with analgesic overuse: Outcome at three years. *Headache* 42 (2002): 483–490.

Griggs, C., & Jensen, J. Effectiveness of acupuncture for migraine: A critical literature review. *Journal of Advanced Nursing* 54 (2006): 491–501.

Haddock, C.K., Rowan, A.B., Andrasik, F., et al. Home-based behavioral treatments for chronic benign headache: A meta-analysis of controlled trials. *Cephalalgia* 17 (1997): 113–118.

Headache Classification Subcommittee of the International Headache Society. The International Classification of Headache Disorders, 2nd ed. *Cephalalgia* 24, Suppl. 1 (2004): 1–160.

Holroyd, K.A., O'Donnell, F.J., Stensland, M., & Lipchik, G.L. Management of chronic tension-type headache with tricyclic antidepressant medication, stress-management therapy, and their combination: a randomized controlled trial. *JAMA* 285 (2001): 2208–2215.

Holroyd, K.A., & Penzien, D.B. Client variables and the behavioral treatment of recur-rent tension headache: A meta-analytic review. *Journal of Behavioral Medicine* 9 (1986): 515–536.

Hu, H.X., Markson, L.E., Lipton, R.B., Stewart, W.F., & Berger, M.L. Burden of migraine in the United States: Disability and economic costs. *Archives of Internal Medicine* 159 (1999): 813–818.

Lainez, M.J.A., Dominguez, M., Rejas, J., Palacios, G., Arriaza, E., Garcia-Garcia, M., & Madrigal, M. Development and validation of the Migraine Screen Questionnaire (MSQ). *Headache* 45 (2005): 1328–1338.

Lake, A.E. Medication overuse headache: Biobehavioral issues and solutions. *Headache* 46, Suppl. 3 (2006):S88–97.

Lake, A.E., Rains, J.C., Penzien, D.B., & Lipchik, G.L. Headache and psychiatric comorbidity: Historical context, clinical implications, and research relevance. *Headache* 45 (2005): 493–506.

Linde, K. Review of acupuncture as a headache treatment. *JAMA* 293 (2005): 2118–2125.

Lipton, R.B., Hamelsky, S.W., Kolodner, K.B., Steiner, T.J., & Stewart, W.F. Migraine, quality of life, and depression: A population-based case-controlled study. *Neurology* 55 (2000): 629–635.

Lipton, R.B., Hamelsky, S.W., & Stewart, W.F. "Epidemiology and impact of headache." In *Wolff's headaches and other head pain*, 7th ed., eds. Silberstein, S.D., Lipton, R.B., & Dalessio, D.J. Oxford: Oxford University Press, 2001, pp. 85–107.

Lipton, R.L., Bigal, M.E., Amatniek, J.C., & Stewart, W.F. Tools for diagnosing migraine and measuring its severity. *Headache* 44 (2004): 387–398.

London, L.H., Shulman, B., & Diamond, S. The role of psychometric testing and psychological treatment in tension-type headache. *Current Pain and Headache Reports* 5 (2001): 467–471.

McCrory, D.C., Penzien, D.B., Hasselblad, V., & Gray, R.N. *Evidence report: Behavioral and physical treatments for tension-type and cervicogenic headache* (Product No. 2085). Des Moines, IA: Foundation for Chiropractic Education and Research, 2001.

Nestoriuc, Y., & Martin, A. Efficacy of biofeedback for migraine: A meta-analysis. *Pain* 128 (2007): 111–127.

Packard, R.C. What does the headache patient want? *Headache* 19 (1979): 370.

Penzien, D.B., Holroyd, K.A., Holm, J.E., & Hursey, K.G. Behavioral management of migraine: Results from five dozen group outcome studies. *Headache* 25 (1985): 162.

Rains, J.C., Lipchik, G.L., & Penzien, D.B. Behavioral facilitation of medical treatment for headache—Part I: Review of headache treatment compliance. *Headache* 46 (2006): 1387–1394.

Rains, J.C., Penzien, D.B., & Lipchik, G.L. Behavioral facilitation of medical treatment for headache—Part II: Theoretical models and behavioral strategies for improving adherence. *Headache* 46 (2006): 1395–1403.

Sacks, O. *Migraine: Understanding a common disorder*. Los Angeles: University of California Press, 1985.

Silberstein, S.D., Lipton, R.B., & Goadsby, P.J. *Headache in clinical practice*, 2nd ed. London: Martin Dunitz Ltd., 2002.

Stewart, W.F., Lipton, R.B., Celentano, D.D., & Reed, M. Prevalence of migraine headache in the United States: Relation to age, income, race, and other sociodemographic factors. *JAMA* 267 (1992): 64–69.

VonKorff, M., Stewart, W.F., Simon, D.J., & Lipton, R.B. Migraine and reduced work performance: A population-based diary study. *Neurology* 50 (1998): 1741–1745.

Weeks, R. "Psychological assessment of the headache patient." In *Office practice of neurology*, eds. Samuels, M., & Feske, S. New York: Churchill Livingstone, 1996, pp. 1096–1101.

18

Procedures for Headache

Thomas N. Ward, MD

Various "procedures" can be employed to help alleviate headache. This section will focus on neurosurgical options and anesthetic blockade. These options vary from relatively noninvasive (e.g., neural blockade) to destructive and/or invasive to a significant degree. They rarely cure headache; medical management is usually still necessary. All carry some degree of risk, and therefore the age and general medical condition of the patient must be kept in mind.

CLUSTER HEADACHE

Cluster headache is said to be the most painful of all conditions. Most patients, fortunately, have the episodic form (with bouts and remissions). The unfortunate minority have chronic cluster, currently defined in ICHD-II as cluster headache occurring without significant remissions (for more than 1 year with either no remissions or with remissions lasting less than 1 month). Many such patients still achieve significant relief with vigorous medical therapy. For those who do not, surgical procedures become a consideration. As understanding of cluster pathogenesis has advanced, treatment options have expanded. Cluster also serves as a useful example of the various procedures that may be employed for head pain.

Anatomy and Neurophysiology

The trigeminal nerve is an important part of the cluster headache story. Cluster pain is usually most prominent in the first and less often the second division of cranial nerve V. Fibers pass via the Gasserian (trigeminal) ganglion in Meckel's cave to the brain stem and reach the trigeminal nucleus caudalis. Indirect (polysynaptic) connections involve the superior salivatory nucleus in the pontine tegmentum. This trigemino-autonomic reflex may help explain the cranial parasympathetic symptoms that occur during a cluster attack (e.g., lacrimation, rhinorrhea). The autonomic fibers travel in the nervus intermedius (sensory VII) and then with the greater petrosal nerve to the sphenopalatine ganglion. Postganglionic fibers then run to the various glands. Also of note, there are bilateral pathways descending from the hypothalamus to both the superior salivatory nucleus and the trigeminal nucleus caudalis. These bilateral projections may explain why cluster pain sometimes switches sides, especially after a procedure.

One of the most exciting findings now known about cluster pathophysiology is the abnormal activity (previously postulated) and anatomy shown by functional imaging and voxel-based MRI morphometry that occurs in the posterior hypothalamic gray matter.

Procedures for Cluster

Nervus intermedius section was pioneered by Ernest Sachs, Jr., MD, at Dartmouth. The procedure is invasive and involves a suboccipital craniectomy. This nerve usually runs between cranial nerves VII and VIII in the cerebellopontine angle; it is not always a separate bundle but may run admixed with the fibers of cranial nerve VIII. While Dr. Sachs reported generally good outcomes on a very small series of patients, other series have been less favorable. Adverse events include hearing loss, vertigo, loss of taste, and facial weakness.

Further along the autonomic pathway, the greater superficial petrosal nerve has been sectioned. Radiofrequency lesioning of the sphenopalatine ganglion has also been performed. While less invasive, results tend to be disappointing due to fairly frequent failures and recurrences.

The majority of procedures for alleviating cluster headache pain are directed against the sensory trigeminal nerve. Sometimes these are combined with procedures directed against the cranial parasympathetic pathways. Minimally invasive procedures on the supra- and/or infra-orbital nerves can be helpful. These nerves can be blocked temporarily with a local anesthetic such as lidocaine or bupivacaine. Longer benefit might be achieved using alcohol injection. Still longer-lasting results may be seen with neurectomy (avulsing the nerves). These procedures are minimally invasive and have fewer side effects, but recurrence rates are quite high. These options are most appropriate for older patients and others who are not suitable candidates for more invasive (but potentially more durable) procedures.

Procedures directed against the trigeminal ganglion are certainly much more invasive but may result in more durable outcomes. Injections of alcohol have given disappointing results. Glycerol may also be injected, with fairly high initial success rates but also fairly high recurrence rates. Perhaps 75% experience pain relief, but nearly half have recurrence, often with the year. It is fairly safe, so it can be done in elderly patients and does not require general anesthesia. It results in a mild sensory deficit, which patients tolerate. It can be repeated but may cause arachnoiditis, which then renders further such treatments ineffective.

The Gasserian ganglion may be "treated" with heat (radiofrequency). The device is inserted through the cheek and passed through the foramen ovale, and the lesioning is performed. The operator can control the amount of neural damage by assessing the amount of sensory deficit produced. Less deficit generally results in fewer side effects (which can be serious) but at the price of lower efficacy. About 50% of patients do very well, 20% less well, and about 30% fail to benefit. Side effects include corneal anesthesia (with the risk of corneal abrasions) and anesthesia dolorosa, which may become a more serious problem than the cluster pain was.

Sensory rhizotomy (section of the trigeminal root) involves sectioning the nerve at the root entry zone. Jarrar and colleagues at the Mayo Clinic reported their experience: 88% of patients had complete or near-complete symptom relief (mean follow-up was more than 6 years). Complete section gave better results than did partial sectioning. Adverse events included cerebrospinal fluid leak, weakness of masticatory muscles, and one case of (mild) anesthesia dolorosa. Some surgeons have added nervus intermedius sectioning to this procedure.

Gamma knife radiosurgery has also been directed against the trigeminal nerve and/or the nervus intermedius. Response may occur after days to weeks (or longer). There are few published reports, and long-term consequences are not known. Mistargeting has been reported when used for other indications and would therefore be possible in this situation.

Analogous to the Janetta procedure for trigeminal neuralgia, microvascular decompression has been applied to both the trigeminal nerve and nervus intermedius for cluster headache. Both arterial and venous compressive lesions have been reported. In Lovely's series, the initial success rate was about 75%, but recurrences lowered the longer-term success rate to slightly less than 50%. Repeat procedures were ineffective.

TRIGEMINAL NEURALGIA

Refractory trigeminal neuralgia has been treated with some of the same procedures as for cluster headache. These options can be directed against the peripheral nerve, the trigeminal ganglion, or the root entry zone. "Medullary tractotomy" has been abandoned. Most procedures are directed against the root entry zone or Gasserian ganglion. Trigeminal nerve cryosurgery, alcohol blockade, and neurectomy are less invasive but also less efficacious. The four major procedures are balloon compression of the ganglion in Meckel's cave, glycerol "gangliolysis" in the trigeminal cistern, radiofrequency lesioning of the fibers for the appropriate division of the fifth nerve ("retrogasserian"), and stereotactic radiosurgery directed at the root entry zone (this may require several months or longer to work, while the other methods have a much quicker onset of benefit). All these procedures tend to provide temporary relief, with recurrence in at least 50% of patients within 3 years Side effects include masseter weakness, corneal ulcerations, and anesthesia dolorosa.

The microvascular decompression procedure of Janetta has also been advocated. When performed, about 80% of patients are without symptoms at 1 year. The offending vessel is often found to be the superior cerebellar artery compressing the root entry zone of the fifth nerve. Adverse events include death, cerebrospinal fluid leak, eighth nerve damage, and stroke (cerebellar infarction).

INTRACRANIAL HYPERTENSION

Surgical procedures may be necessary for medically refractory intracranial hypertension. In idiopathic intracranial hypertension, surgery is considered when vision is deteriorating. Optic nerve sheath fenestration may not only preserve vision but sometimes ameliorates the head pain. It may be a preferable option to ventricular shunting. Shunts may be very efficacious but have numerous drawbacks, including the need for shunt revision/shunt failure, infection (which may be deadly), low-pressure headache, and acquired Chiari. Medical management may still be required.

NERVE BLOCKS AND NEUROSTIMULATION

Nerve blocks and neurostimulation have utility in treating some types of headache. There are not adequate controlled data supporting their use, but there is ongoing research. Occipital nerve blocks are easy to perform. Afridi and colleagues reported that 26 of 57 injections in 54 migraine patients resulted in either a complete or partial response, with a median duration of benefit of 21 days. A tender occipital nerve predicted response; the presence or absence of medication overuse did not. Obviously, the duration of response outlasts the presence of the local anesthetic. They postulated an alteration in central nervous system nociceptive pathways. These blocks also may lessen central sensitization/cutaneous allodynia. These blocks may work in hemicranial migraine/status migrainosus and in cluster as well as other headache types. They seem to be ineffective in tension-type headaches and paroxysmal hemicrania. It is uncertain whether they work in hemicrania continua. Sometimes supraorbital nerve blocks may be useful. Atlanto-axial joints may also be blocked. Deep CT-guided C2 and C3 root blocks may be diagnostic as well as (briefly) therapeutic.

"Neurostimulation" is an exciting development for treating some intractable headaches. Occipital nerve stimulation has been studied by numerous investigators, including Goadsby and Dodick. It may work in chronic/transformed migraine, posttraumatic headache, intractable cluster headache, new daily persistent headache and hemicrania continua. Prior response to occipital nerve blockade is not predictive of response to occipital nerve stimulation. A trial of a temporary stimulator is usually undertaken prior to placing a "permanent" device. Stimulation may be unilateral or bilateral. PET scan changes during stimulation are noted in the anterior cingulate cortex and dorsal pons. Complications include lead migration and infection.

Vagus nerve stimulation (VNS) has been reported, also anecdotally, to help some refractory headache patients. Transformed migraine and chronic cluster have been reported to sometimes respond. The total number of cases reported has been very small. VNS is known to have analgesic effects and has been used to treat seizures and depression (both known to be comorbid with migraine).

Finally, the most exciting reports of all have been on the use of deep brain stimulation for refractory cluster (see the reports by Leone and Schoenen) and also for SUNCT. Complications include infection, and there has been one death reported due to hemorrhage.

SUMMARY

Fortunately, only select populations of headache sufferers require the use of procedures to manage their pain. While some of these procedures are quite invasive and carry considerable risk, others, such as occipital nerve blocks, are easy to perform and may also offer considerable relief. Deciding when to consider offering these options to patients requires knowledge of the natural history of the headache type as well as the magnitude of the potential benefits and side effects of the various procedures.

Review Questions

1. The Gasserian ganglion is located in:
    a. Heschl's gyrus
    b. The ambient wing cistern
    c. Meckel's cave
    d. The sphenopalatine fossa
2. The superior salivatory nucleus resides in:
    a. Meckel's cave
    b. The midbrain
    c. The pons
    d. It does not exist in man; in animals it is found in the Gasserian ganglion.
3. Functional MRI shows abnormal activity in cluster patients in:
    a. The hypothalamus
    b. The cavernous sinus ipsilateral to the side of the headache
    c. Meckel's cave and the sphenopalatine ganglion
    d. The Edinger-Westphal nucleus
4. Your 34-year-old otherwise healthy patient with refractory chronic cluster headache has failed to respond to all medications. You feel he could benefit most durably from the most invasive of the following selections:
    a. Bilateral supraorbital nerve avulsions (to prevent side-switch)
    b. Trigeminal rhizotomy
    c. Radiofrequency lesioning of the Gasserian ganglion
    d. Occipital nerve stimulation

5. The least effective treatment but also the least invasive therapy for refractory chronic cluster might be chosen for a frail patient with a short life expectancy. You ask your favorite neurosurgeon to perform a:
    a. Trigeminal rhizotomy under local anesthesia
    b. Microvascular decompression
    c. Deep brain stimulation, intermittently
    d. Nerve avulsion

6. For tic doloureux (trigeminal neuralgia), which procedure has been largely abandoned?
    a. Medullary tractotomy
    b. Microvascular decompression
    c. Stereotactic radiosurgery
    d. Radiofrequency lesioning

7. You have a patient with medically refractory intracranial hypertension. Her vision is in jeopardy. Which statement about the following options is untrue?
    a. A shunt may preserve vision and treat the headache.
    b. A shunt may worsen or change the headache.
    c. Optic nerve sheath fenestration can prevent visual loss but cannot ameliorate the headache.
    d. Optic nerve sheath fenestration can relieve the headache but cannot preserve vision.

8. You decide to perform an occipital nerve block in a patient with otherwise refractory unilateral headache. Which statement about occipital nerve bocks is false?
    a. It is indicated, as response to occipital nerve blocks predicts response to occipital nerve stimulation.
    b. They can be done repetitively and are reasonably safe.
    c. They may act by decreasing central sensitization
    d. They do not work in medication overuse headache.

9. You have a 25-year-old patient with severe medically refractory headaches who also has epilepsy and depression. Which form of neurostimulation may help headaches and also treats her comorbidity?
    a. Electroconvulsive therapy
    b. Deep brain stimulation
    c. Vagal nerve stimulation
    d. Occipital nerve stimulation (done bilaterally)

10. Deep brain stimulation has been used successfully for:
    a. Refractory cluster headache and refractory migraine
    b. Refractory cluster headache and idiopathic stabbing headache
    c. Refractory cluster headache and new daily persistent headache
    d. Refractory cluster headache and SUNCT

10. d
9. c
8. a
7. c
6. a
5. d
4. b
3. a
2. c
1. c

SUGGESTED READING

Antonaci, F., Pareja, J.A., Caminero, A.B., & Sjaastad, O. Chronic paroxysmal hemicrania and hemicrania continua: Anesthetic blockades of pericranial nerve. *Functional Neurology* 12, no. 1 (1997): 11–15.

Ashkenazi, A., & Young, W.B. The effects of greater occipital nerve block and trigger point injection on brush allodynia and pain in migraine. *Headache* 45, no. 4 (2005): 350–355.

Barr, M.L., & Kiernan, J.A. *The human nervous system*, 4th ed. Philadelphia: Harper & Row, 1983.

Corbett, J.J., Nerad, J.A., Tse, D.T., & Anderson, R.L. Results of optic nerve sheath fenestration for pseudotumor cerebri: The lateral orbitotomy approach. *Archives of Ophthalmology* 106 (1988): 1391–1397.

Jarrar, R.G., Black, D.F., Dodick, D.W., & Davis, D.H. Outcome of trigeminal nerve section in the treatment of chronic cluster headache. *Neurology* 60 (2003): 1360–1362

Lovely, T.J., Kotsiakis, X., & Janetta, P.J. The surgical management of chronic cluster headache. *Headache* 38 (1998): 590–594.

Mauskop, A. Vagus nerve stimulation relieves chronic refractory migraine and cluster headaches. *Cephalalgia* 25 (2005): 82–86.

Nurmikko, T.J., & Jensen, T.S. "Trigeminal neuralgia and other facial neuralgias." In *The Headaches*, 3rd ed., eds. Olesen, J., Goadsby, P.J., Ramadan, N.M., Tfelt-

Hansen, P., & Welch, K.M.A. Philadelphia: Lippincott Williams & Wilkins, 2006.

Peres, M.F.P., Stiles, M.A., Siow, H.C., Rozen, T.D., Young, W.B., & Silberstein, S.D. Greater occipital nerve blockade for cluster headache. *Cephalalgia* 22 (2002): 520–522.

Pikus, H.J., & Phillips, J.M. Characteristics of patients successfully treated for cervicogenic headache by surgical decompression of the second cervical root. *Headache* 35, no. 10 (1996): 621–629.

Rozen, T.D. Interventional treatment for cluster headache: A review of the options. *Current Pain and Headache Reports* 6 (2002): 57–64.

Sachs, E. Jr. The role of nervus intermedius resection in facial neuralgia. Report of four cases with observations on the pathways for taste, lacrimation, and pain in the face. *Journal of Neurosurgery* 28 (1968): 54–60.

Schmidek, H.H., & Roberts, D.W., eds. *Schmidek & Sweet's operative neurosurgical techniques: Indications, methods, and results*, 5th ed. Philadelphia: Saunders Elsevier, 2006.

Schwendt, T.J., Dodick, D.W., Hentz, J., Trentman, T.L., & Zimmerman, R.S. Occipital nerve stimulation for chronic headache—long-term safety and efficacy. *Cephalalgia* 27 (2007): 153–157.

Sergott, R.C., Savino, P.J., & Bosley, T.M. Optic nerve sheath decompression: A clinical review and proposed pathophysiologic mechanism. *Australia & New Zealand Journal of Ophthalmology* 18 (1990): 365–373.

Sprenger T, Boecher H, Tolle TR, Bussone G, May A, Leone M. Specific hypothalamic activation during a spontaneous cluster headache attack. Neurology 62(3) (2004): 516-517

Weiner, R.L., & Reed, K.L. Peripheral neurostimulation for control of intractable occipital neuralgia. *Neuromodulation* 2, no. 3 (1999): 217–221.

Index

Note: Figures are indicated by *f* after the page number; tables are indicated by *t* after the page number.

Abdominal migraine, 68, 278
Acetaminophen, 211*t*, 212, 224, 277, 278
Acetazolamide, 150–51, 259, 260
Acupuncture, 267, 269, 297, 298
Allodynia, 30, 217, 306
Almotriptan (Axert), 212*t*, 218*t*, 219,
    220*t*–221*t*, 225
Amitriptyline
    chronic daily headaches, 267, 268, 269
    mechanism of action, 234
    migraine, 237*t*, 240, 241*t*, 248
    suppression of cortical spreading
        depression, 26
    tension-type headache, 248, 249, 297
AMPA (alpha-amino-3-hydroxy-5-methyl-
    4-isoxazolepropionic acid) receptors,
    15, 235
Anatomy of head pain
    dermatomes of the head and neck, 5*f*
    nociceptive anatomy of the face and head,
        12–13, 12*f*
    nociceptive innervation, 3–5, 4*t*
    pain-sensitive structures of the head,
        3–5, 4*t*
Aneurysms
    diagnosis, 130–31, 130*t*, 132*f*
    locations, 130, 131*f*
    saccular aneurysm, 128, 130*t*, 145
    symptoms and clinical features, 130
Angiitis, 138*t*, 139*t*, 144
Angiography headache, 141*t*
Angiopathy, benign (or reversible), 143*t*
Angiotensin-converting enzyme (ACE)
        inhibitors and angiotensin receptor
        blockers (ARBs), 235, 243–44, 258
    See also individual medications
Antiemetics
    children, 277
    cluster headache, 257
    migraine, 29, 216, 218, 223
    pregnancy, 279
Anti-epilepsy drugs (anticonvulsants)
    chronic daily headache, 267

hemicrania continua, 260
    migraine prevention, 235, 244–45, 244*t*
    new daily persistent headache, 260
    trigeminal neuralgia, 280
Anti-serotonin drugs, 235–36, 245–46
    See also individual medications
Arterial hypertension headaches, 181–83
Arteries
    anatomy and innervation, 4–5, 7*f*
    auriculotemporal artery, 5
    dural and cortical arteries, 4, 7*f*
    meningeal arteries, 5, 7*f*
    occipital artery, 5
    sensitivity of cerebral arteries, 4
    temporal artery, 5, 7*f*
    vertebral artery, 5
    See also carotid artery
Arteriovenous malformation (AVM), 130*t*,
    131, 134
Arteritis
    giant cell arteritis headache, diagnostic
        criteria, 134, 137*t*, 279
    giant cell arteritis headache, in the elderly,
        279–80
    giant cell arteritis headache, treatment,
        136, 280
    primary central nervous system angiitis
        headache, diagnostic criteria, 138*t*
    secondary central nervous system angiitis
        headache, diagnostic criteria, 139*t*
    treatment, 136, 280
Aseptic (non-infectious) meningitis, 155–56,
    156*t*, 157*f*, 164, 166
Aspirin
    migraine, 211*t*, 212, 246
    Reye syndrome in children,
        224, 277
    tension-type headache, 212
Ataxia, 25
Atenolol, 237*t*, 242, 242*t*, 260
Aura
    association with migraine, 21, 65
    definition, 64

Aura *(continued)*
    excitatory transmission and elevated
        extracellular potassium
        concentrations, 25
    hemiparesis, 21, 23
    heritability, 22
    symptoms and forms, 65–66
    See also migraine with aura (MA)

Bacterial meningitis, 165–66, 165*t*, 166*f*
Basilar-type migraine, 66, 67*t*
Benign (or reversible) angiopathy, 143*t*
Benign paroxysmal vertigo, 68, 278
Benzodiazepine, 266–67, 268
Benztropine mesylate, 287
Berkson's bias, 193–94
Beta-blockers
    chronic daily headache, 267
    cough, exertional, or sexual activity
        headache, 260
    hemicrania continua, 260
    mechanism of action, 234
    migraine, 242, 242*t*, 243*f*
    new daily persistent headache, 260
    See also individual medications
Botulinum toxin A, 267, 268, 269
Brain stem and mechanisms of migraine, 30–31
Bromocriptine, 144
Butalbital-containing medications, 211*t*,
        214–15, 266–67, 286
Butorphanol, 211*t*
Butterbur (*Petasites hybridius*, petasites), 236, 246

CADASIL. *See* cerebral autosomal dominant
        arteriopathy with subcortical infarcts
        and leukoencephalopathy (CADASIL)
Caffeine
    chronic daily headache risk, 50, 80
    combination analgesics, 213
    hypnic headache, 81
    spontaneous (idiopathic) low CSF pressure
        headache, 153–54
    tapering, 266–67
Calcitonin gene-related peptide (CGRP),
        27–29, 35, 178, 233
Calcium channel blockers, 234, 243, 258
    See also individual medications
Calcium channels, 15, 24–25, 232
Candesartan, 235, 244
Carcinomatous meningitis headache,
        160, 161*t*
Cardiac cephalalgia (cardiac cephalgia), 179,
        183, 280
Carotid artery
    anatomy, 5
    aneurysm, 132*f*
    in cluster headaches, 34, 94

pain sensitivity and referred pain, 5, 137
symptoms attributed to arterial dissection,
        137–38, 139*t*–140*t*, 140*f*
Cavernous angioma, 134, 135*f*, 135*t*, 136*f*
Celecoxib, 211*t*, 214, 259, 270
Cerebral autosomal dominant arteriopathy with
        subcortical infarcts and
        leukoencephalopathy (CADASIL), 25,
        142, 143*t*, 144, 145
Cerebral vasculitis, 4
Cerebral venous thrombosis, 82, 140–42,
        142*f*, 145
Cervical nerves, nociceptive innervation,
        4–5, 4*t*, 5*f*, 9
Cervical spine, anatomy, 10, 11*f*
Cervical vascular disorders and headaches,
        overview, 124, 125*f*–126*t*, 144–45
    See also specific types
Cervicogenic headache, 184, 184*t*
CGRP (calcitonin gene-related peptide)
        antagonists, 29, 223
Chiari malformation type 1
    cough headache, 101, 102, 102*t*, 162
    diagnostic criteria, 161–62, 163*f*, 164*t*
    low pressure from lumboperitoneal
        shunt, 151
    treatment, 162
Childhood headache
    abdominal migraine, 68, 278
    benign paroxysmal vertigo, 68, 278
    childhood migraine, diagnostic criteria, 68,
        68*t*, 277
    cluster headache, 92
    cyclical vomiting, 68, 265
    migraine, acute treatment, 224
    prevalence of headache in children, 42–43
    Reye syndrome and aspirin, 224, 277
    treatment, 277–78
Chlorpromazine, 286–87, 286*t*
Chromosomal loci associated with headache
    FHM1 mutations in the CACNA1A
        gene, 232
    FHM2 mutations in the ATP1A2 gene, 232
    FHM3 mutations in the SCN1A gene, 232
    migraines with or without aura, 22–23
    subcortical infarcts and leukoencephalopathy
        (CADASIL), 25–26, 143*t*, 145
Chronic, definition, 64, 73
Chronic daily headache
    bridge therapy strategies, 266–67
    classification and diagnosis, 66–68, 73
    epidemiology, 49–50, 73
    non-pharmacologic therapy, 268, 269
    pharmacologic prophylaxis, 266, 267–68
    primary chronic daily headache, 66–67
    primary forms of chronic headaches, 73, 74*t*
    risk factors, 50, 80

secondary forms of chronic headaches, 73
transformed migraine comorbidity with
psychiatric disorders, 199
transformed migraine epidemiology,
49–50, 73
treatment, overview, 265–66
Chronic migraine (transformed migraine)
diagnostic criteria, 67–68, 68t, 73–77,
75t, 76t
epidemiology, 49–50, 73
risk factors, 79–80, 80t, 295
Silberstein-Lipton (S-L) criteria, 67, 74,
75t, 265
transformed migraine comorbidity with
psychiatric disorders, 199
triptans, 75
Chronic post-bacterial meningitis headache,
165, 170, 172t
Civamide, 258
Classification of headache disorders
Ad Hoc Committee on Classification of
Headache of the National Institute of
Health, 60, 60t
history, 60–61
International Headache Society (IHS)
classification (ICHD-1), 60–61
overview, 59, 69
primary headaches, classification and
definition, 39, 60, 61
secondary headaches, classification and
definition, 39, 60, 61
See also diagnostic criteria for headaches;
International Classification of Headache
Disorders, 2nd ed. (ICHD-II)
Clomipramine, 237t, 248, 249
Clonazepam, 237t, 260, 280, 287
Clonidine, 237t, 267, 286
Cluster headache
acute (abortive) treatment, 256–57, 256t
anatomy and neurophysiology, 33–34, 303–4
autonomic manifestations, 33, 34, 35, 94
brain mechanisms, 33–35
chronic subtype, 33, 64, 92, 303
diagnostic criteria, 92, 93t
diencephalic structure, 33–34
epidemiology, 48–49, 92
episodic subtype, 92, 93t
genetics, 32–33, 48–49
orexin-2 receptor, 33, 34, 36
preventive treatment, 256t, 257–58
secondary mimics, 94
short-term preventive treatment, 256t
surgical treatment, 258–59, 304–5
symptoms and clinical features, 32–33,
92–94, 99t
therapy, overview, 255–56, 256t
Coenzyme Q10, 236, 246

Colloid cyst, 159f
Combination analgesics, 211t, 212–13
See also individual medications
Comorbidity of psychiatric disorders with
headache. See psychiatric comorbidity
with headache
Complications of migraine, 66, 67t
Concussion, 115–16, 117f
Cortical spreading depression (CSD), 26–27, 29,
30, 31, 231–33
Corticosteroids
acute migraine treatment, 222–23
carcinomatous meningitis, 158
cluster headache, 256t, 257
giant cell arteritis, 136, 280
inpatient treatment, 287
lymphocytic hypophysitis, 157
medication overuse headache, 222–23
in pregnancy, 223, 279, 287
side effects, 223
Tolosa-Hunt syndrome, 134, 189
withdrawal, 149, 150
COX-2 inhibitors, 211t, 214, 270
See also individual medications
Cranial bone disorders, 183
Cranial nerve V (trigeminal nerve)
anatomy and nociceptive sensation, 4–5,
4t, 8f, 9
causes of pain, 9
dermatomal distribution, 3, 5, 5f
mandibular branch, dermatomal
distribution, 4
maxillary branch, dermatomal distribution,
5, 5f, 9
ophthalmic branch, dermatomal
distribution, 4, 5, 5f, 9
spinal trigeminal nucleus (STN), 9, 13,
15, 16f
trigeminal ganglion (Gasserian or semilunar
ganglion), 8f, 9
Cranial nerve VII (facial nerve), 4t, 9, 13
Cranial nerve IX (glossopharyngeal nerve), 4,
4t, 9, 12, 13
Cranial nerve X (vagus nerve), 4t, 9, 13
Cranial nerves, anatomy and nociceptive
sensation, 4t, 9
Cranial neuralgias
glossopharyngeal neuralgia, 187–89, 188t
neck–tongue syndrome, 189
nervus intermedius neuralgia, 188t, 189
overview, 186–87
persistent idiopathic facial pain, 190
superior laryngeal neuralgia, 188t, 189
Tolosa-Hunt syndrome, 189–90
trigeminal neuralgia (TN), 186–87, 188t,
279, 280
Cranial parasympathetic fibers, 27, 29, 34–35, 304

Cranial vascular disorders and headaches,
   overview, 124, 125t–126t, 144–45
   See also specific types
Craniocervical dystonia, 184
Cryptococcal infection, 169, 170, 172f
CSF (cerebrospinal fluid) fistula headache,
   153, 154t
Cyclical vomiting, 68, 265
Cyproheptadine, 235–36, 245, 277–78

Deep brain stimulation, 33, 259, 307
Dental pain, 12
Dermatomes of the head and neck, 5f
Descending antinociceptive system,
   16–17, 16f
Dexamethasone, 218, 222, 225, 257, 269
DHE. *See* dihydroergotamine (DHE)
Diagnostic criteria for headaches
   alcohol-induced headache, 178
   aneurysms, 130–31, 130t, 132f
   angiitis headache, 138t, 139t
   angiography headache, 141t
   arterial dissection, 139t–140t
   arteriovenous malformation (AVM), 130t
   aseptic (non-infectious) meningitis,
      155–56, 156t, 157f
   bacterial meningitis, 165–66, 165t, 166f
   basilar-type migraine, 66, 67t
   benign (or reversible) angiopathy, 143t
   brain abscess, 168, 169f, 169t
   carcinomatous meningitis headache,
      160, 161t
   cardiac cephalalgia, 183
   cavernous angioma, 134, 135t
   cerebral autosomal dominant arteriopathy
      with subcortical infarcts and
      leukoencephalopathy (CADASIL),
      142, 143t
   cervicogenic headache, 184, 184t
   CGRP-induced headache, 178
   Chiari malformation type 1, 161–62,
      163f, 164t
   childhood migraine syndromes, 68,
      68t, 277
   chronic daily headache, 66–68, 73
   chronic migraine (transformed migraine),
      67–68, 68t, 73–77, 75t, 76t
   chronic post-bacterial meningitis headache,
      170, 172t
   cluster headache, 92, 93t
   complications of migraine, 66, 67t
   cranial or cervical vascular disorders,
      125t–126t
   CSF (cerebrospinal fluid) fistula
      headache, 154t
   dialysis headache, 181
   dural arteriovenous fistula, 134, 134t

   encephalitis, 166–67, 167f, 168t
   encephalotrigeminal or leptomeningeal
      angiomatosis (Sturge Weber
      syndrome), 136t
   giant cell arteritis headache, 134, 137t, 279
   headache attributed directly to neoplasm, 160t
   headache due to head and neck trauma,
      115–17, 116t
   headache induced by acute substance or
      exposure, 177–78
   hemicrania continua, 82, 82t, 107–8, 107t
   hemicrania epileptica, 161, 162t
   hemiplegic migraine, 66
   histamine-induced headache, 178
   hypertensive crisis (paroxysmal
      hypertension), 182
   hypnic headache, 81, 81t, 104–5, 105t, 280
   hypothalamic or pituitary hyper- or
      hyposecretion, 160, 161t
   idiopathic intracranial hypertension (IIH),
      149–50, 150t
   increased intracranial pressure or
      hydrocephalus caused by neoplasm,
      158, 159f, 160t
   intracranial hemorrhage, 128t, 129f, 129t
   intracranial hypertension secondary to
      metabolic, toxic or
      hormonal causes, 152t
   ischemic stroke (cerebral infarction)
      headache, 126, 126t
   lymphocytic hypophysitis, 156–57, 158t
   lymphocytic meningitis, 164, 166, 167f, 168t
   medication overuse headaches, 77–79, 78t,
      177, 178–79
   medication withdrawal, 179, 180t
   menstrually related migraine (MRM), 68
   migraine with aura (MA), 21, 65–66,
      65t, 66t
   migraine without aura (MO), 21,
      64–65, 65t
   migrainous infarction, 66, 126–27
   migrainous-triggered seizure, 66
   mitochondrial encephalopathy lactic acid
      and stroke (MELAS), 143t
   neurosarcoidosis, 154, 155t
   new daily persistent headache, 82–83, 83f,
      108–9, 109t
   nitric oxide (NO) donor–induced
      headache, 178
   ophthalmoplegic migraine, 66
   other non-infectious inflammatory
      diseases, 157t
   other nonvascular intracranial
      disorder, 165t
   paroxysmal hemicrania, 95–96, 95t
   PDE (phosphodiesterase) headache, 178
   persistent aura without infarction, 66

pituitary apoplexy, 144t
post-dural (post-lumbar) puncture
      headache, 151–52, 152t
post-endarterectomy headache, 141t
postictal headache, 161, 162t
post-traumatic headache, acute, 117–19,
      118t, 119f
post-traumatic headache, chronic, 119–20,
      119t, 120t
pre-eclampsia and eclampsia, 182
primary chronic daily headache, 66–67, 73
primary cough headache, 100–101, 102t
primary exertional headache, 101–2, 103t
primary headache associated with sexual
      activity, 102–4, 103t
primary stabbing headache, 80–81, 81t,
      100, 101t
primary thunderclap headache,
      105–6, 106t
psychotic disorder, headache
      attributed to, 201, 201t
pure menstrual migraine (PMM), 68
retinal migraine, 66
rhinosinusitis headache, 185–86, 186f
sleep apnea headache, 180
somatization disorder, 200–201, 200t
spontaneous (idiopathic) low CSF pressure
      headache, 153–54, 155f, 155t
status migrainosis, 68
subdural empyema, 168, 170t
SUNCT syndrome, 97t
systemic infection, 169, 170t
tension-type headache, 83–84, 84t, 85t
transient ischemic attack (TIA)
      headache, 128t
trigeminal neuralgia (TN), 187, 188t
whiplash, acute and chronic headaches,
      120–21, 120t, 121t
See also classification of headache disorders;
      International Classification of Headache
      Disorders, 2nd ed. (ICHD-II)
Dialysis headache, 181, 280–81
Diclofenac, 211t, 214
Diclofenac (diclofenac sodium), 211t, 214
Diencephalon, 33–34
Dihydroergotamine (DHE)
      cluster headache, 256, 256t, 257
      contraindications, 225, 287
      inpatient treatment, 217, 286t, 287
      migraine, 211t, 217–18, 224
      tapering process, 267
Diltiazem, 237t, 243
Diphenhydramine, 286t, 287
Dipyridamole, 178
Divalproex sodium, 26, 237t, 244
      See also valproate
Diving headache, 179

Dorsal horn region of cervical spinal cord,
      15, 16f
Doxepin, 237t, 240–41, 241t
Drug-induced aseptic meningitis (DIAM),
      155–56, 156t
Dural arteriovenous fistula, diagnostic criteria,
      134, 134t
Dural pain, 3

Eclampsia and pre-eclampsia, 182
Elderly patients, headache in, 279–80
Eletriptan (Relpax), 212t, 218t, 220t–221t,
      221, 225
Encephalitis, 166–68, 167f, 168t, 172f
Encephalotrigeminal angiomatosis, 136t
Epidemiology of headaches
      chronic daily headache, 49–50, 73
      chronic migraine (transformed migraine),
            49–50, 73
      cluster headache, 48–49, 92
      headache due to head and neck trauma,
            115, 117
      hypnic headache, 104, 280
      new daily persistent headache (NDPH), 109
      overview, 39, 40t
      paroxysmal hemicrania, 94
      prevalence of headache in children, 42–43
      prevalence of primary and secondary
            headaches, 40t
      primary stabbing headache, 81
      SUNCT syndrome, 97
      tension-type headache, 47–48, 49
      See also migraine, epidemiology
Epilepsy, 25, 160–61, 162t
Episodic, definition, 64
Ergot alkaloids, 27, 211t, 216–18, 245, 258, 267
      See also individual medications
Ergotamine and ergotamine tartrate, 211t,
      216–17, 225, 256t, 257
Eye disorder headaches, 185
Eyes, nociceptive innervation, 12

Facial nerve (cranial nerve VII), 4t, 9, 13
Familial hemiplegic migraine (FHM)
      channelopathies, 23–24, 234, 243
      elevated extracellular potassium, 24–25
      enhanced glutamatergic transmission, 24–25
      FHM1 mutation (CACNA1A gene), 23, 24f,
            25, 232, 234, 243
      FHM2 mutation (ATP1A2 gene), 23, 24f,
            25, 232
      FHM3 mutation (SCN1A gene), 23, 24f,
            25, 232
      glutamate transporter (GLAST/EAAT1),
            25, 232
      phenotype, 23–26, 24f
Fasting headache, 182–83

Flunarizine, 237t, 277
Fluoxetine, 237t, 241, 249
Flurbiprofen, 211t, 214
Frovatriptan (Frova), 212t, 218t, 219–22, 247

GABA (gamma-amino butyric acid),
        234, 235
Gabapentin
    chronic daily headache, 249, 267
    effectiveness in preventing migraine, 237t,
        243f, 244
    hemicrania continua, 270
    mechanism of action, 235
    primary stabbing headache, 81
    renal failure, 281
    SUNCT syndrome, 259
Gamma-amino butyric acid (GABA),
        234, 235
Gamma knife radiosurgery, 305
Gating mechanism of pain modulation,
        15, 15f
Giant cell arteritis, 134, 136, 137t, 279–80
Glossopharyngeal nerve (cranial nerve IX), 4,
        4t, 9, 12, 13
Glossopharyngeal neuralgia, 187–89, 188t
Glutamate receptors
    AMPA (alpha-amino-3-hydroxy-5-methyl-
        4-isoxazolepropionic acid) receptors,
        15, 235
    calcium channels, 15, 24–25, 232
    ionotropic, definition, 15
    kainate receptors, 15, 234, 235
    metabotropic, definition, 15
    NMDA (N-methyl-D-aspartate) receptors,
        15, 24
    sodium channels, 15, 24–25, 232–33
    stimulation of second-order nociceptive
        neurons, 14
Glutamate transporter (GLAST/EAAT1),
        25, 232

HaNDL syndrome, 156, 162–63, 164t
Headache due to head and neck trauma,
        overview, 115–17, 116t
    See also specific types
Hemicrania continua
    autonomic symptoms, 107–8
    chronic form, 108
    diagnostic criteria, 82, 82t, 107–8, 107t
    episodic form, 108
    misdiagnosis, 108
    secondary mimics, 108
    treatment, 82, 107, 108, 260, 269–70
Hemicrania epileptica, 161, 162t
Hemiparesis, 21, 23
Hemiplegic migraine, 21, 66
    See also familial hemiplegic migraine (FHM)

High-altitude headache, 179
HIV/AIDS headache, 170, 171f, 171t, 172f
Horner's syndrome, 33, 96, 137–38
Hospital admission, reasons and goals,
        285–86
Hydrocephalus, 150, 158, 159f, 160t
Hydrocortisone, 223
Hypertensive crisis (paroxysmal
        hypertension), 182
Hypertensive encephalopathy, 182
Hypnic headache
    diagnostic criteria, 81, 81t, 104–5, 105t, 280
    epidemiology, 104, 280
    secondary causes, 105
    treatment, 81, 260, 280
Hypothalamic or pituitary hyper- or
        hyposecretion, 159–60, 161t
Hypothyroidism, 183

Ibuprofen, 211t, 214, 237t, 249, 277
ICHD-II. See International Classification
        of Headache Disorders, 2nd ed.
        (ICHD-II)
Idiopathic intracranial hypertension (IIH),
        149–51, 150t, 151f
ID Migraine™ survey, 64
Imipramine, 237t, 241, 241t
Immunoglobulins, 155
Incidence, definition, 39
Indomethacin
    exertional and sexual activity
        headaches, 260
    hemicrania continua, 82, 107, 108, 260,
        269–70
    hypnic headache, 280
    migraine, 211t, 214, 237t
    paroxysmal hemicrania, 94, 96, 259
    primary cough headache, 101, 162, 260
    primary stabbing headache, 81, 100, 260
    side effects, 285
    thunderclap headache, 260
Infection
    bacterial meningitis headache, 165–66,
        165t, 166f
    brain abscess, 168, 169f, 169t
    cryptococcal infection, 169, 170, 172f
    encephalitis, 166–68, 167f, 168t, 172f
    HIV/AIDS, 170, 171f, 171t, 172f
    lymphocytic meningitis, 164, 166,
        167f, 168t
    subdural empyema, 168, 170t
    systemic infection, 169, 170t
Inpatient treatment, 285–88, 286t
International Classification of Headache
        Disorders, 2nd ed. (ICHD-II)
    appendix, 61–62, 62t
    decimal system for diagnosis categories, 63

nomenclature, 64
organization and format, 61–63, 62t
overview, 59
See also classification of headache disorders;
    diagnostic criteria for headaches
Intracranial hemorrhage
    diagnostic criteria, 128t, 129f, 129t
    intracerebral hemorrhage, 128t
    saccular aneurysms, 128, 130t
    subarachnoid hemorrhage, CT images,
        129f, 132f
    subarachnoid hemorrhage, symptoms, 3,
        106, 127–29, 130
Intracranial hypertension, 151, 152t, 306
Intracranial infection
    bacterial meningitis headache, 165–66,
        165t, 166f
    brain abscess, 168, 169f, 169t
    encephalitis, 166–68, 167f, 168t, 172f
    lymphocytic meningitis, 164, 166, 167f, 168t
    overview, 163–64
    subdural empyema, 168, 170t
Intracranial neoplasm
    carcinomatous meningitis headache, 160, 161t
    headache attributed directly to neoplasm, 160t
    hypothalamic or pituitary hyper- or
        hyposecretion, 159–60, 161t
    increased intracranial pressure or
        hydrocephalus caused by neoplasm,
        158, 159f, 160t
    mechanisms of headache in brain tumors,
        158–59, 158t
    pituitary tumors, 159–60, 161t
Ionotropic glutamate receptors, 15
Ischemic stroke (cerebral infarction) headache,
    126–27, 126t, 127f, 128t
Isometheptene combination analgesics, 213

Kainate receptors, 15, 234, 235
Ketoprofen, 237t, 246
Ketorolac, 214, 224, 225, 286t, 287

Lamotrigine, 237t, 245, 259, 270
Leptomeningeal angiomatosis, 136t
Lidocaine, 256t, 257, 259, 304
Lisinopril, 235, 244
Lithium, 81, 256t, 258, 260, 280
Locus ceruleus (LC), 28f, 31, 34, 233
Low CSF (cerebrospinal fluid) pressure
    headache, 153–54, 155f, 155t
Lumboperitoneal shunts, 151
Lymphocytic hypophysitis, 156–57, 158t
Lymphocytic meningitis, 164, 166, 167f, 168t

Magnesium
    acute headache treatment, 278t, 279, 286t, 287
    headache prevention, 236, 246

Matrix metalloproteinases (MMP), 232, 233
Medication overuse headaches
    bridge therapy strategies, 266–67
    chronic tension-type headache, 84
    combination analgesics, 213
    criticism and controversy over criteria, 77–79
    diagnostic criteria, 77–79, 78t, 177, 178–79
    overuse, criteria, 78, 179
    prevention, 224
    psychiatric disorders with medication
        overuse, 199–200
    "simple" and "complex" medical histories, 295
    treatment, 222–23, 266–67
MELAS (mitochondrial encephalopathy lactic
    acid and stroke), 26, 143t, 145, 161
Melatonin, 256t, 258, 259, 260
Meningitis
    aseptic (non-infectious) meningitis, 155–56,
        156t, 157f, 164, 166
    bacterial meningitis, 165–66, 165t, 166f
    carcinomatous meningitis headache,
        160, 161t
    chronic post-bacterial meningitis headache,
        165, 170, 172t
    cryptococcal meningitis, 166
    drug-induced aseptic meningitis (DIAM),
        155–56, 156t
    headache pain, 3
    lymphocytic meningitis, 164, 166, 167f, 168t
    Mollaret's meningitis, 166
Menstrually related migraine (MRM), 68,
    221, 247
Meperidine, 216, 287
Metabotropic glutamate receptors, 15
Methazolamide, 151
Methylergonovine, 235–36, 237t, 245–46
Methysergide
    5HT$_2$ receptor antagonist, 29
    cluster headache prevention, 256t, 258
    cough headache, 260
    mechanism of action, 235–36
    migraine prevention, 233, 235, 237t, 245
    suppression of cortical spreading
        depression, 26
Metoclopramide, 212, 286t, 287
Metoprolol, 237t, 242, 242t
Metronidazole, 258
Mianserin, 237t, 248
Microvascular decompression, 280, 305
Migraine, acute treatment
    basic principles of acute treatment, 210–11
    in children, 224
    in the emergency room, 223–24, 225
    intravenous medications, 225
    medications, overview, 211–12, 211t–212t
    pharmacologic treatment, overview,
        209–10

Migraine, acute treatment *(continued)*
  See also migraine, preventive treatment;
    specific medications
Migraine, epidemiology
  in adolescents, 43–44, 44*t*
  age of onset, 41, 41*f*
  burden to families, 46
  burden to individual, 45–46
  frequency patterns, 45–46
  incidence, by age and gender, 39–41, 40*f*
  incidence, cumulative, 41, 42*f*
  prevalence, overall, 42, 43*f*, 45
  by race and geographic region, 44
  societal impact, 46–47
  by socioeconomic status, 45
  transformed (chronic) migraine, 49–50
Migraine, genetics
  familial hemiplegic migraine (FHM)
    phenotype, 23–26, 24*f*
  FHM1 gene mutation, 23, 24*f*, 25, 232, 234, 243
  FHM2 gene mutation, 23, 24*f*, 25, 232
  FHM3 gene mutation, 23, 24*f*, 25, 232
  migraines with or without aura, 22–23
  mitochondrial encephalopathy lactic acid
    and stroke (MELAS), 26, 145
  subcortical infarcts and leukoencephalopathy
    (CADASIL), 25–26, 143*t*, 145
  twin studies, 22
Migraine, pathophysiology
  central sensitization, 15, 30, 233, 306
  cortical spreading depression (CSD),
    26–27, 29, 30, 31, 231–33
  denervation hypersensitivity, 15
  migraine with aura (MA), 21
  migraine without aura (MO), 21
  overview, 21–22, 31–32, 32*f*
  symptoms, 21–22
  trigeminovascular system (TGVS) changes,
    27–29, 28*f*, 30, 32*f*, 233
  vascular hypothesis, 27
Migraine, preventive treatment
  goals and guidelines, 236, 238–40, 266
  mechanisms of preventive medications, 233–36
  overview, 231
  pathophysiology of preventive medications,
    231–33
  review of non-pharmacologic
    treatments, 297
  short-term prevention, 246–47, 247*t*
  See also migraine, acute treatment; *individual*
    medications
Migraine with aura (MA)
  diagnostic criteria, 21, 65–66, 65*t*, 66*t*
  pain mechanisms, 231, 233
  See also aura
Migraine without aura (MO)
  diagnostic criteria, 21, 64–65, 65*t*

ID Migraine™ survey, 64
  pain mechanisms, 231, 233
Migrainous infarction, 66, 126–27
Migrainous-triggered seizure, 66
Migralepsy, 160
Mirtazepine, 249
Mitochondrial encephalopathy lactic
    acid and stroke (MELAS), 26, 143*t*,
    145, 161
Modulation of pain, 15, 15*f*, 16–17, 16*f*, 17
Monoamine oxidase inhibitors (MAOIs),
    213, 242
Monoclonal antibodies, 155
Muscles of the head and face, 3, 6*f*

Nadolol, 237*t*, 242, 242*t*
Naproxen, 211*t*, 214, 237*t*, 246
Naratriptan (Amerge), 212*t*, 218*t*, 219–22,
    225, 247
Neck–tongue syndrome, 189
Neck trauma, 115
  See also headache due to head and neck
    trauma
Nerve blocks, 257, 269, 279, 286–87, 306
Nerves of the head and face, 3–5, 4*t*, 5*f*, 10*f*
  See also individual nerves
Nervus intermedius neuralgia, 188*t*, 189
Nervus intermedius section, 304
Neurokinin A, 27
Neuropathic pain, 13
Neurosarcoidosis, 154, 155*t*
Neurostimulation, 306–7
New daily persistent headache (NDPH)
  diagnostic criteria, 82–83, 83*f*, 108–9, 109*t*
  epidemiology, 109
  possible infectious etiology, 109
  secondary mimics, 82, 109–10
  treatment, 260, 270
Nifedipine, 237*t*, 258
Nimodipine, 106, 128, 237*t*, 258, 260
Nitroglycerine, 29
NMDA (*N*-methyl-D-aspartate) receptors,
    15, 24
Nociceptive pain, definition, 13
Non-pharmacologic treatments
  chronic daily headache, 268, 269
  migraine, 297
  reasons for, 293–94
  review of, 296–98
  tension-type headache, 269, 297
Nonsteroidal anti-inflammatory drugs
    (NSAIDs)
  COX-2 inhibitors, 211*t*
  drug-induced aseptic meningitis
    (DIAM), 155
  migraine, 211*t*, 214
  retropharyngeal tendinitis, 184

subdural hematoma, 153*f*
See also individual medications
Nortriptyline, 237*t*, 240, 241*t*
Nucleus raphe magnus (RM), 16, 16*f*, 31, 231

Obesity
    link to increased migraine frequency, 50
Obesity and headache risk, 50, 80
Occipital nerve vulnerability to trauma, 9
Octreotide, 257
Ondansetron, 29, 217, 223
Ophthalmoplegic migraine, 66
Opiate analgesics, 211*t*, 213, 215–16, 267
Opioid antagonists, 16, 17
Opioids, 16, 215, 279
Optic nerve sheath fenestration, 151, 306
Orexin-2 receptor mutations, 33, 34, 36
Orgasmic headache, 103–4, 103*t*
Overview, 186–87
Oxygen therapy, 256–57, 256*t*

Pain phase of migraine, 27–29
Pain-sensitive structures of the head, 4*t*
Paroxetine, 237*t*, 248, 268
Paroxysmal hemicrania
    chronic form, 95*t*, 96, 99*t*
    diagnostic criteria, 95–96, 95*t*
    epidemiology, 94
    episodic form, 95*t*, 96, 99*t*
    secondary mimics, 96
    symptoms and clinical features, 95–96, 99*t*
    treatment, 94, 96, 259
Paroxysmal hypertension, 182
Patent foramen ovale, 31, 268
Periaqueductal gray region (PAG), 16, 28*f*,
    31, 231
Periostea, 3
Persistent aura without infarction, 66
Persistent idiopathic facial pain, 190
Petasites, 236, 246
Pharmacologic treatment of headache,
    overview, 209–10
Phenelzine, 237*t*, 242
Phenobarbital, 267, 286
Pheochromocytomas, 181–82
Phosphodiesterase (PDE) headache, 178
Physiology of head pain
    descending antinociceptive system, 16–17, 16*f*
    gating mechanism of pain modulation, 15, 15*f*
    lateral/discriminative pain pathway,
        13–14, 14*t*
    medial/affective pain pathway, 13–14, 14*t*
    modulation of pain, 15, 15*f*, 16–17, 16*f*, 17
    nociceptive anatomy of the face and head,
        12–13, 12*f*
    three-neuron pathway, 13
See also migraine, pathophysiology

Piroxicam, 211*t*, 270
Pituitary apoplexy, 144*t*
Pituitary tumors, 159–60, 161*t*
Pizotifen, 235–36, 237*t*, 245, 278
Post-dural (post-lumbar) puncture headache,
    151–52, 152*t*, 153*f*
Post-endarterectomy headache, 141*t*
Posteromedial inferior diencephalon, 33–34
Post–head trauma syndrome, 115, 119,
    120, 121
Postictal headache, 161, 162*t*
Post-traumatic headache, acute, 117–19, 118,
    118*t*, 119*f*
Post-traumatic headache, chronic, 119–20,
    119*t*, 120*t*
Prednisone, 136, 256*t*, 257, 259
Pre-eclampsia and eclampsia, 182
Pregnancy and lactation
    ergotamine and DHE risks, 217, 287
    headache treatment, 223, 278–79,
        278*t*, 287
    pre-eclampsia and eclampsia, 182
    valproate risks, 287
Premonitory symptoms, definition, 64
Preorgasmic headache, 103, 103*t*
Prevalence, definition, 39
Primary cough headache, 100–101, 102*t*, 260
Primary exertional headache, 101–2,
    103*t*, 260
Primary headache associated with sexual
    activity, 102–4, 103*t*, 260
Primary headaches
    classification and definition, 39, 60, 61
    epidemiology, 40*t*
    primary forms of chronic headaches,
        73, 74*t*
    treatment, 81
    See also specific types
Primary stabbing headache
    diagnostic criteria, 80–81, 81*t*, 100, 101*t*
    epidemiology, 81
    secondary causes, 100
    treatment, 100, 260
Primary thunderclap headache
    diagnostic criteria, 105–6, 106*t*
    in the emergency room, 223
    secondary causes, 106
    subarachnoid hemorrhage, 3, 106, 127–29,
        129*t*, 130
    treatment, 106, 128, 223, 260
Probable, definition, 64
Propranolol
    in children, 277–78
    cough, exertional, and sexual activity
        headaches, 260
    effectiveness in preventing migraine, 231,
        237*t*, 242, 242*t*

Propranolol *(continued)*
  suppression of cortical spreading
    depression, 26
Proton pump inhibitors, 214, 269, 285
Protriptyline, 237*t*, 240, 241*t*
Pseudomigraine with pleocytosis syndrome. *See*
    transient headache and neurological
    deficits with cerebrospinal fluid
    lymphocytosis (HaNDL) syndrome
Psychiatric comorbidity with headache
  anxiety disorders and migraine, 195,
    197–98, 198*t*
  bipolar spectrum disorders and migraine,
    197, 197*t*
  chronic daily headache, 199–200, 269
  depression and migraine, 194–97, 195*t*, 198
  mechanisms of comorbidity, 194
  medication overuse with psychiatric
    disorders, 199–200
  mood disorders and migraine, 194–97
  obsessive–compulsive disorder and
    migraine, 198
  overview and definitions, 193–94
  panic disorder and migraine, 197–98
  selection bias in comorbidity studies,
    193–94
  stress and migraine, 193
  suicide attempts and migraine, 196
  transformed migraine comorbidity with
    psychiatric disorders, 199
  See also psychiatric disorder, headache
    attributed to
Psychiatric disorder, headache attributed to,
    200–201, 200*t*, 201*t*
  See also psychiatric comorbidity with
    headache
Psychological factors and headache
  behavioral factors to consider in treatment
    planning, 294–96
  effect on pain, 17
  psychological interactions with headache,
    193, 293
  reasons for non-pharmacologic treatments,
    293–94
  review of non-pharmacologic treatments,
    296–98
  "simple" and "complex" medical histories,
    295–96
  See also psychiatric comorbidity with
    headache
Pure menstrual migraine (PMM), 68

Radiofrequency lesioning, 304, 305
Raskin protcol, 286*t*, 287
RCT (randomized controlled trials), 231
Rebound headache. *See* medication overuse
    headaches

Referred pain, 12, 14, 137, 173
Renal disease, headache in, 181, 280–81
Retinal migraine, 66
Retropharyngeal tendinitis, 184
Rhinosinusitis headache, 185–86, 186*f*
Riboflavin (vitamin B$_2$), 236, 237*t*, 246
Rizatriptan (Maxalt), 212*t*, 218*t*, 219–21, 225
Rofecoxib, 211*t*, 214, 270
Rostral ventromedial medulla (RVM),
    16, 31

Secondary headaches
  classification and definition, 39, 60, 61
  prevalence of, 40*t*
  secondary forms of chronic headaches,
    73, 74*t*
Sella turcica, empty, 150, 151*f*
Sensitization of pain
  allodynia, 30, 217, 306
  central sensitization, 15, 30, 233, 306
  denervation hypersensitivity, 15
  NMDA receptors, 15
  peripheral sensitization, 30, 233
Sensory rhizotomy, 305
Serotonin, role in migraine, 29
Serotonin norepinephrine reuptake inhibitors
    (SNRIs), 241
Serotonin receptors, 27, 29, 30
Serotonin reuptake inhibitors (SSRIs), 222, 225,
    241, 248–49
Short-lasting unilateral neuralgiform headaches
    with conjunctival injection and tearing
    (SUNCT syndrome)
  deep brain stimulation, 259, 307
  diagnostic criteria, 97*t*
  epidemiology, 97
  secondary causes, 98
  symptoms and clinical features, 97–98, 99*t*
  treatment, 259
  triggers, 98
Sildenafil, 178
Sinuses and headache, 4*t*, 5, 9–10, 185–86, 186*f*
Sleep apnea headache, 179
Sodium channels, 15, 24–25, 232–33
Somatization disorder, 200–201, 200*t*
Sphenopalatine (pterygopalatine)
    ganglion, 8*f*
Spinal trigeminal nucleus (STN), 9, 13,
    15, 16*f*
Spontaneous (idiopathic) low CSF pressure
    headache, 153–54, 155*f*, 155*t*
SSRIs (serotonin reuptake inhibitors), 222, 225,
    241, 248–49
Status migrainosis, 68
Sterile inflammation, 27, 29
Steroids. *See* corticosteroids
Sturge Weber syndrome, 136*t*